CLASSIC PAPERS IN
ASTHMA

VOLUME TWO

CLASSIC PAPERS IN
ASTHMA
VOLUME TWO
Treatment

EDITOR:
R A L BREWIS
Consultant Physician
The Royal Victoria Infirmary
Newcastle upon Tyne, UK

ALLEN & HANBURYS
Limited

This publication was supported by an educational grant from Allen & Hanburys

science press

British Library Cataloguing in Publication Data
Classic Papers in Asthma
Vol 2
1. Man. Bronchi. Asthma
I. Brewis, R.A.L. (Robert Alistair Livingston).
616.2'38

ISBN 1-870026-21-7

Designed by Robin Dodd FCSD
Printed and bound in the United Kingdom by Bell & Bain Limited, Glasgow

INTRODUCTION

I n the last 20–30 years the treatment of asthma has become markedly more effective, so that most people with asthma are now able to lead a full and active life. This improvement in outlook is largely attributable to the proper application of a relatively small number of effective medicines belonging to one of the following five groups: *atropine derivatives*, *xanthines*, *sympathomimetics*, *corticosteroids* and *cromones*. Few of the preparations in common use today were available 40 years ago and some were not available 20 years ago or even more recently. With the exception of corticosteroids, however, drugs in the other four major groups derived from plants have a long history stretching back, in some cases, many centuries.

Most of the papers reproduced in this volume record individual steps in the evolution of modern drug treatment. Some of the papers announced the discovery of a new finding, others provide confirmation of earlier findings and have been included either because they were important and influential papers in their day, or because they offer an interesting summary of the treatment practices prevailing at the time. The concentration here on the drugs used in asthma reflects their importance, but does not deny the place of non-medicinal elements in treatment, some of which have interesting histories of their own. Some classic writings have had an important effect on the way in which drugs are used, even though the development of drug treatment has not been their main subject. This is reflected in the inclusion of papers dealing with death from asthma and the measurement of airflow obstruction.

This collection of papers reflecting the development of treatments for asthma is necessarily a personal and arbitrary selection from the enormous range of publications available. There are notable omissions, most particularly the omission of publications in other languages. Pharmacological chemistry was extremely strong in Germany in the late 19th and early 20th centuries and the more recent development of ipratropium was first reported in German publications.

ANCIENT TREATMENT

The treatment of asthma is as old as medicine itself. In ancient times it seems likely that remedies followed the prevailing beliefs about causation. In ancient China medical practice was guided by respect for certain cosmic principles such as the celestial Yan (embodied in light, heat and life) and Yin (darkness, cold and death). Many diseases were perceived to be due to an imbalance between Yan and Yin and also to inappropriate distribution of male and female principles in different parts of the body. These concepts, and acupuncture, which developed in parallel, are of great antiquity. The ancient Chinese also developed the use of herbal and other natural products which included a traditional remedy known as Ma Huang. This is an extract of the plant *Ephedra sinica* containing ephedrine, which is believed to have been in use in China from before 3000 BC.

INTRODUCTION

In India, as early as 4000 BC, inhalation had developed as a treatment for respiratory ailments and amongst the remedies in use was *Nardostachys jatamansi* (*Datura*) which, when heated, evolved an anticholinergic alkaloid[1]. Sanskrit accounts of Ayurvedic medicine, which evolved from 700 BC onwards, record adverse effects of overindulgence in medicines which clearly had atropine-like effects. It is not known how the plant was originally used, but in a 17th century account of Indian medicine it is recorded that the root of a plant of the *Datura* species was ground with ginger, peppers and arsenic and the powder made into a paste with the addition of ghee (butter) and then smoked in a pipe. This practice may have continued essentially unchanged for over a thousand years. It is of interest that the same remedy was prescribed as a treatment for epilepsy and mania, which is in keeping with the essentially neural concept of asthma which prevailed through many centuries in different cultures (see Volume one). *Datura* in the form of *Datura metel* has continued to be smoked as an antiasthmatic remedy in India until modern times[2].

The ancient Egyptians are also recorded as using an atropine-like drug for breathing disorders in the form of henbane (*Hyoscyamus muticus*), which yielded hyoscine (1-scopolamine) and hyoscyamine. A method of administration was by inhalation of the vapour given off by heating the plant on hot bricks.

The ancient Greeks evolved concepts of disease based on the influence of the four elements: fire, air, earth and water. These had four qualities: heat, dryness, coldness and moisture; they were expressed in the body as the humours: blood, phlegm, yellow bile and black bile. Imbalance of the essential humours was thought to be responsible for disease and treatment was generally designed to encourage nature, with rest and diet being prominent features. Drugs were in use, but it is not clear whether any specific remedies were directed to the treatment of asthma. Roman medicine was heavily influenced by Greek tradition; indeed many Roman physicians were Greeks. Early in the Christian era physical means of treating asthma were in vogue. It is recorded that Celsus recommended bleeding, purgatives, hot and cold compresses, diuretics and so forth[3] for asthma, and probably for other forms of dyspnoea. These physical remedies were essentially the same as those used in Europe in the 17th century, some of which continued into the 19th century. Celsus also followed the principle of similitude: treating like with like.

Galen, practising in the second century AD, had a profound influence on therapeutics throughout medicine. Sometimes regarded as the father of experimental physiology, he elaborated the existing system of Greek medicine based on the influence of the four elements and humours, combining it with some basic precepts of his own into an all-embracing philosophy of polypharmacy which was to persist as the main guide to physicians in Europe for the following 14 centuries. He used numerous simple vegetable remedies which continued to be referred to as 'galenicals' until the 19th century. Some of the remedies were bizarre; his advice on asthma included the drinking of owl's blood in wine.

Aetius of Amida, a Greek physician writing in the sixth century, recommended inhalations and fumigations of pine resins, gums, turpentine (a distillate of pine resin), mastic and arsenic salts. Ammoniacal salts and vinegar were also used together with external applications in the form of poultices or plasters. It is of some interest that altitude is mentioned as bringing about the cure for asthma in these early writings, although no suggestion seems to emerge that the effect might be due to removal from the influence of an external agent.

In the seventh century Severus is known to have recommended the use of an acrid therapeutic enema for the treatment of asthma. This form of treatment was still in use in Europe a thousand years later. Also writing in the seventh century, Paulus Aegineta recommended treatment which was clearly aimed at dissolving the impacted secretions of asthma.

'. . . The affection arises from thick and viscid humours becoming infarcted in the bronchial cells of the lungs. Dyspnoea is a common symptom which accompanies these and many other complaints. The indication of cure in asthmatic complaints is to consume the viscid and thick humour by attenuant and detergent medicines. Wherefore the Vinegar of Squills will answer well with them and oxymel prepared from it . . .'[4]

Oxymel of squills* was yet another treatment still being recommended a thousand years later.

Arabic medicine flourished from about the eighth century and produced some outstanding physicians. One of the greatest, Abur Bakr Muhammad ibn Zakariy'ya (AD 860–932), known as Rhazes, documented the views of others extensively in his writings but was of independent mind. On asthma he writes:

'Ben Mesue said "Let persons troubled with asthma take two drachms of dried and powdered fox lung in their drink.' Galen said that many cure asthma with owl's blood given in wine. I say that owl's blood is not to be given, for I have seen it administered, and it was useless.'

Dried fox lung had been used by Celsus in Rome and was thus at least 700 years old as a remedy when Rhazes wrote this. Rhazes favoured a simple remedy comprising juice from soaked wheat bran to which sugar and ground almonds were added before being thickened by warming and evaporation.

The Arabian period saw the beginnings of modern pharmacy and the systematic observation of the physical actions of particular medicines, together with the development of basic chemical processes which were applied to the modification of remedies. Camphor, musk and laudanum were promoted as treatments by Arab physicians during the early middle ages and these were to find application in the field of respiratory medicine for many centuries. Later, in the 12th century, a major monograph on asthma was produced by Rabbi Moses ben Maimon, known as Moses Maimonides, primarily to advise the Sultan Saladin on the proper management of his asthmatic son. As well as presenting an outstanding account of the clinical features, his *Treatise on Asthma* also laid out a detailed prescription for treatment which centred on diet, personal conduct, cleanliness (including clean air), and the regulation of the emotions, sleep, coitus, exercise, respiration and bowel habit[5,6]. Medicinal treatment played a relatively minor part. Features of his writing which were to reappear for many centuries afterwards included the avoidance of bulky and gas-producing vegetable foods, and the use of chicken soup. Chicken soup in one form or another appears repeatedly in the treatment of asthma and other chest conditions from the time of the Ancient Greeks, but the origin of the association is obscure. Maimonides was well aware of the potentially harmful effects of treatment in asthma, specifically warning against the dangers of opiates and excessive purging, and advising all physicians to follow the teaching of Hippocrates: *primum non nocere* (above all, do no harm).

TREATMENT IN THE 16TH AND 17TH CENTURIES

One of the most celebrated cases of asthma was successfully treated in 1552 by Girolamo Cardano, a physician and renowned polymath from Milan. Such was his reputation that he was summoned to Scotland by John Hamilton, Archbishop of St Andrews who, as primate of Scotland and brother of the Regent, was a powerful and important figure. In a prolonged

---

*The term 'oxymel' referred to a mixture of vinegar and honey. Simple oxymel was taken without any additions but it was common for other remedies to be added to the basic mixture. 'Squill' was derived from the bulb of a plant of the lily family related to the Scilla and in Europe was derived from the sea onion (*Urginea maritima*). Squill contained glycosides resembling digitalis and was widely used as an emetic and expectorant.

consideration of the case lasting some months, Cardano made a recommendation that the Archbishop should forgo his feather bedding. This was followed by a miraculous remission of his intractable asthma[7]. It seems quite likely that allergy to either feathers or house dust mite might have been responsible for the Archbishop's asthma and it is pleasing to regard this as the first instance of specific allergen avoidance, although it is far from certain that Cardano regarded the bedding as a source of noxious inhalations.

A century later, Jean van Helmont was certainly aware of the propensity of certain foods to precipitate asthma in predisposed individuals. He described a monk who had alarmingly severe acute asthma after consuming fish fried in oil; in circumstances like this, avoidance was presumably practised.

The teachings of Galen received a vigorous overhaul in the early 16th century by Paracelsus, who publicly burned his published works. Paracelsus's own ideas were, however, far-fetched and based on ludicrously simple chemical theory which was unfounded on observation. Despite numerous attempts to replace Galen's concept of the humours by other philosophical systems, the Galenic approach continued to survive into the 17th century as the basis for interpreting disease and determining its treatment. The concept of the original Greek and Roman elements and humours were by now extended to explain temperaments – sanguine, phlegmatic, melancholy and choleric – terms which have persisted to the present day.

At the beginning of the 17th century an enormous range of sometimes bizzare remedies was available. The first edition of *The London Pharmacopoeia*, published in 1618, contains nearly 2000 entries and includes reference to a linctus containing an extract of fox lungs for the treatment of asthma. Astrology, the workings of the devil and superstitions of one sort or another were still powerful influences. Physicians were often also astrologers so that the timing of, say, purging might be critically determined by the position of the planets. Observation and experiment gained ground only slowly over the received truths of centuries as the basis for medical practice. The 16th century saw the introduction of tobacco smoking in Europe. It is of interest that initially it was smoked for therapeutic reasons.

In the mid-17th century Thomas Willis, famous for his analysis of the cerebral circulation, was regularly in demand for his expertise in the understanding and treatment of asthma. He had largely broken away from the Galenic method. Willis distinguished between treatment aimed at terminating the asthmatic attack and treatment designed to prevent recurrence. A preliminary to treatment was to loosen constricting clothing and to reduce abdominal encroachment on breathing by the use of enemas. Willis used opiates when all else failed but not without great circumspection because:

'...*whereas more or less they hinder breathing (which already is difficult and too much hindred) they frequently bring the patient into danger of life.*'

He prescribed medicines which were considered to be antispasmodic or anticonvulsive. This treatment was used for other convulsive conditions such as epilepsy and was thus in keeping with Willis's view of asthma as essentially a nervous disorder. Part of his therapeutic approach was to 'direct the pneumonic spirits from their convulsions by molesting them in other places'. Some idea of the trials endured by the asthmatic patient can be obtained from his account of the treatment offered to a nobleman with 'dreadful asthma'.

'*Take of spirit of gum Ammoniacum distilled with salt of Tartar three drams, take from 15 to 20 drops in a spoonful of the following Julep, drinking after it five spoonfuls, repeat it every sixth hour.*

Take elder flower, camomile, and penny-royal water of each four ounces, snail-water two ounces, one ounce, mingle them, between whiles he took a dose of the following powder with the same Julep or pectoral decoction.

Take powder of Crabs eyes two drams, sal prunella a dram and a half, slat of Amber half a dram, mix them, divide into eight doses.

Large vesicatories were applied on the inside of his arms near the armpits, Clysters daily administered and frequent frictions. By the use of these he received sudden and unexpected help and within a few days became wholly free from the fit.*'

The Nobleman apparently took further doses from time to time thereafter whenever he felt the onset of symptoms and remained tolerably well and *'void of any outrageous invasion from his habitual asthma.'*

Amongst other remedies mentioned by Willis is a special form of chicken soup. He directed that orris, *Enula campane*, dill, scraped liquorice and stoned raisins should be sewed into the belly of an old cock and boiled, and that doses of the decoction should be taken regularly.

Thomas Sydenham (1624–1689), a major figure in British medical history, reviver of Hippocratic methods of observation and masterly describer of disease, had little to say on asthma. In his *Complete method of curing almost all diseases* he dealt with the treatment of asthma in less than a page. Of 'an obstinate asthma in sanguine constitutions' he distinguished three kinds: dyspnoea, asthma and orthopnoea. It is not certain that he was clearly distinguishing between bronchial asthma and other forms of acute respiratory distress. The treatment he advised[9], apart from the almost routine blood letting and purging, was simple and vegetable in nature.

'Take away ten ounces of blood from the right arm and next day give the common purging potion, which must be repeated twice more, once every third day. On the intermediate days of purging let the following medicines be used.

Take of the seeds of anise, finely powder'd, two drams; Locatellus's balsam, enough to bring it into a mass for pills, and make six pills of a dram, three of which are to be taken every morning, and at five in the afternoon, drinking four ounces of the bitter decoction without purgatives, warm after them.

If the disorder do not go off, let the whole process be repeated.'

Sir John Floyer (1649–1734), a renowned physician of Lichfield and a sufferer from asthma himself, was generally despairing in his description of the available regimens. He had tried a number of medicines popular in his day including Gill and Hysig, Syrup of Sulphur and Spirit of Hartshorn (ammonia) as well as bleeding and purgining-all to no avail. In his book *A Treatise of the Asthma*[10] he distinguishes between measures which aim to prevent asthma and those intended to ameliorate the attack. Of the treatments reviewed, he favours the old

---

*Gum ammoniacum was probably derived from shavings of deers' antlers, the early source of ammonia. Salt of tartar or tartar emetic was very popular for a variety of ailments. Emetics were thought to be helpful to expectoration in respiratory disease. A julep was a syrup. A 'pectoral' was a medicine directed to chest complaints and a decoction was any juice derived by boiling. The reference to crabs' eyes is less exotic than might be imagined and denotes chalk. The term originated from the white nodules found in the stomach of large crustaceans which were at one time believed to be the eyes of devoured sea creatures. Analysis showed them to be made from calcium carbonate and for many years calcium carbonate was commercially known as 'crabs' eyes'. The term 'vesicatory' sometimes indicated a corrosive skin irritant used to produce vesicles and excoriation but here 'large vesicatories' may refer to the use of cupping, an ancient practice in which a heated receptacle is applied to the skin. On cooling, suction raised a swelling and, if the skin had been incised earlier, bleeding and oozing of serum would result (wet cupping). Cupping as a treatment for respiratory ailments was still being practised in some parts of Europe in the 20th century. 'Clysters' were enemas.

galenicals to the 'new chymical ones'. Amongst the general measures recommended are early rising, the avoidance of irritating fumes (precisely the advice given by Moses Maimonides) and fasting during an attack. He considers that bleeding should be used only in extremis and then only in small amounts and notes that treatment may include cupping of limbs and shoulders, but indicates that he is not really in favour of this. He declares that clysters are useful-once weekly-but that violent purging is to be avoided. He encourages vomiting, noting that emetics promote expectoration of sputum, and suggests that a feather in throat may sometimes be used. His favourite medicine is squills, either the oxymel or the vinegar preparation. Opiates may be used in small doses to assist sleep. The recommended diet includes flesh meat once daily with good bread, *'well fermented and well baked and the Bran not too well dressed out'*. Floyer's suggestions contain clearly recognizable elements present in the recommendations of Severus and Moses Maimonides, respectively about 1000 years and 500 years before him. Coffee is mentioned once in passing but is given no special praise.

'All hot Liquors, as Coffees, Teas of Cephalic Herbs, as Sage etc. or Stomachic; as Buckbean, which is a Centaury*, I have tried, but find none so good as Toast and Water.'

Coffee receives firmer recommendations in Floyer's other work *Medicina Gericomica or, The Galenic Art of Preserving Old Men's Healths*[11] but this extends only to its use as an aid to the digestion.

John Millar (1733–1805) contributed a later but impressive monograph *Observations on the asthma and on the hooping cough*[12], drawing, like Floyer, on his personal experiences as a sufferer from asthma. He too distinguished between 'tempering the violence' of an attack and measures designed to prevent further attacks. In addition, he dealt separately with the question of ameliorating chronic asthma. He accepted a small amount of blood letting and the use of musk, but later abandoned it. He favoured the use of spiritus mendereri or simple oxymel or the use of squills to promote a discharge of phlegm.

'To prevent a return of the paroxysm a blister was put between the shoulders; emollient fomentations were directed for the stomach and belly; anodyne liniments were rubbed on these parts, and applied externally to the fauces and throat, antispasmodic clysters were injected; and a caution was given that the air the child breathed should not be infected with smoke or sulphureous steams and that it should, as much as possible, be constantly preserved in a moderate temperature.'

He goes on to recommend that the bowel should be strengthened and the cause of the distension be removed by gentle laxatives, aromatic carminitive and astringent medicines including magnesia, rhubarb, species aromatica and sal martis.

He used an oriental aromatic substance known as 'Gum assafoetida' with some enthusiasm, and also recommended 'the Peruvian bark'. The bark was brought to Europe in 1632. It had been used by Countess de Chincon, Vicereine of Peru, and may have been known to Peruvian Indians for some time. Chincona bark was widely used at the time for a variety of conditions and had an important influence on therapeutics generally, because it was recognized that it had an effect on fevers which was clearly not related to emesis or purgation. This led to a pharmacological understanding of drug action.

In the case of chronic asthma Miller urged a light animal diet in order to avoid producing air and regular mild emetics. The cure was to be encouraged by taking regular cold baths *'to restore tone to the lax fibres of the air passages'*. Millar believed that the way to avoid the gradual development of progressive disabling disease was by opposing the acute phases as vigorously as possible, a proposition of some interest even today and still to be properly examined.

---

*Centaury: pink single-stemmed annual wild flower *Centaureum umbellatum* (Gentianaciae).

In the later 18th century the idea of harnessing the healing power of nature came to dominate therapeutics. Bathing in hot and cold water and drinking cold water became central activities in the treatment of a wide variety of diseases. A change in climate was regularly advised in cases of asthma. Bizarre treatments were gradually less in evidence and some of today's drugs began to emerge, for example the use of *Atropa belladonna*. By the 19th century stramonium and lobelia were being particularly recommended from a large range of available treatments[13]. Lobelia was obtained from the dried leaves of *Lobelia inflata* (Campanulaceae) in North America and was smoked by native Indians. The alkaloid lobeline is the main active constituent with pharmacological properties resembling those of nicotine. It was used in America as an emetic, expectorant and antiasthmatic[14]. Sedatives such as chloral hydrate and injections of morphine were commonly used in severe episodes. Potassium iodide and ipecacuanha became widely used in chronic disease.

ANTICHOLINERGICS

Anticholinergic treatments have a long history. The inhalation of *Datura*, yielding atropine, in ancient India and of *Hyoscyamus*, a species yielding hyoscine (1-scopolamine) and hyoscyamine, in ancient Indian and Egyptian cultures, has already been referred to. A variety of henbane (*Hyoscyamus niger*) which was widely available in the countryside of England is known to have been in use in the 17th century and probably earlier. It was withdrawn from the London Pharmacopoeia in 1746 and 1788 but restored in 1809. In 1802 a Dr Anderson of Madras, who had found smoking of *Datura* an effective treatment for his own asthma, gave some of the plant to General Gent to bring back to Britain. Very soon the plant was in great demand and acquired a reputation as an infallible remedy. The introduction and reception of *Datura* is reported in correspondence relayed in the *Edinburgh Medical and Surgical Journal* of 1812[15], which is reprinted here (page 1). The species introduced by General Gent was *Datura ferox* but it was soon realized that the closely related and widely available Thorn apple *Datura stramonium* yielded equally effective relief. William English, an asthmatic surgeon, reported his satisfaction with smoking this form in 1811[16]. Many early accounts are unclear about which part of the plant was used and which was the most effective. Good effects were reported from smoking the leaf and stalks but Salter (*see below*) stressed that the seeds were the most concentrated source of the effective agent. By the middle of the 19th century lobelia, belladonna leaves, stramonium and hyoscyamus (from henbane) were in common use as treatments for asthma. A variety of forms of inhalation were devised, including cigarettes or cheroots in which tobacco was mixed with other substances including stramonium, hyoscyamus, opium, and cannabis. Atropine was isolated as the effective agent from belladonna by Geiger and Fesse in 1833[17] and in 1867 it was shown that it blocked the effect of vagal nerve stimulation on the heart. Demonstration that it exerted a similar blocking effect on the vagus in respect of bronchial constriction seems to have been long delayed.

The most renowned authority on the treatment of asthma in Britain in the second half of the 19th century was Henry Hyde Salter, who perceived the effectiveness of representatives of anticholinergic, xanthine and adrenergic substances. He was a physician to Charing Cross Hospital and later Kings College Hospital, London, and suffered from asthma himself. In his masterly monograph *On Asthma: Its Pathology and Treatment* published in 1860[18], the section on treatment covers seven chapters and 100 pages and makes interesting reading. Three chapters are reproduced here (page 5) because of the light they cast on several other treatments besides stramonium which were employed at the time. His consideration of tobacco smoking is interesting. He distinguishes between sedative and depressant effects and considers that the latter may be helpful in the asthmatic paroxysm. The depressant effects he refers to are those produced by large doses of tobacco smoke inhalation in those who are unaccustomed to it. Almost as interesting is his passing reference to the belief of many of his asthmatic patients that regular cigarette smoking has some protective effect against asthma. In recent years there has been renewed interest in the effect of smoking on asthma and other allergic lung disease. There is evidence that in some circumstances these processes may be suppressed by regular cigarette smoking.

By 1869 Salter had paid greater attention to the use of atropine in the form of tincture of belladonna. He reported his observations and opinions in the *Lancet* (page 49)[19]. The summary of his impressions is extraordinarily advanced:

> '*If I were to express what appears to me to be the peculiar excellence of belladonna as a sedative in asthma, I should say it consisted in its power of diminishing reflex irritability...*'

The observation would not have been out of place in a review a hundred years later.

The use of smoking powders or cigarettes remained popular throughout the remainder of the 19th century. A variety of commercial cigarettes was available which usually contained stramonium, lobelia and sodium or potassium nitrate, sometimes together with aresenic (*Cigarettes de Joy*), henbane and opium (*Espics*) and sometimes accompanied by tobacco or cannabis[1]. The importance of treatments containing atropine diminished in the early 20th century with the development of adrenergic and methyl xanthine treatments. However, Dautrebande in France and later Herxheimer in Britain[20] were sufficiently interested to confirm that spirometric improvement followed use of atropine. Herxheimer's paper indicates that in 1959 stramonium cigarettes were still in use, although by then they were becoming something of a curiosity. He found that atropine methonitrate cigarettes were effective and superior to both wet nebulization of atropine methonitrate and stramonium cigarettes. Atropine methonitrate received more attention from Altounyan (who was later to develop sodium cromoglycate) in a paper published in 1964 and reproduced here (page 51)[21]. He investigated a wide range of atropine-like substances in a large number of asthmatic subjects, including himself. It was found that compounds with a longer *N*-alkyl chain than the methyl derivative had reduced bronchodilatory properties and that quaternary substances had prolonged action. Atropine methonitrate was the most effective available and was singled out for further investigation. In addition to showing that the effect of atropine methonitrate was slower and more persistent than that of the beta agonist isoprenaline, Altounyan revealed that individuals responded differently to the two substances. Patients with inadequately treated asthma showed a prominent response to isoprenaline and little further response to atropine, whereas those with non-asthmatic airways obstruction or treated asthma showed a small response to isoprenaline and a relatively greater response to atropine. Atropine methonitrate and isoprenaline were for some years given in combination by inhalation is a favoured asthma remedy. The rationale of this combination had been demonstrated clearly by Chamberlain and colleagues, who showed that speed of action was combined with duration of action[22].

Another quaternary atropine derivative, ipratropium bromide, was later developed which combined effectiveness by inhalation with lack of important atropine-like side effects[23,24]. The first published clinical assessment of ipratropium, which is frequently quoted as a reference (and probably little read), is a study by Poppius and his colleagues[25], reproduced on page 61. Ipratropium has established a place for itself in the treatment of airways obstruction and is now regularly used by some clinicians in the treatment of bronchial asthma, most of whom are probably unaware that the inhalation of atropine-like agents has a history which extends back about 6000 years.

METHYL XANTHINES

The use of infusions of tea leaf (*Camellia sinensis*) to produce stimulation began in India and China and, although the origins are obscure, the practice is undoubtedly of great antiquity. Tea owes its stimulatory effects to the alkaloids theophylline and caffeine. The Greeks were familiar with the properties of tea, which they referred to as *the divine leaf*. The origins of coffee drinking are as unclear as those of tea. Coffee grows naturally in the Ethiopian highlands and parts of the Middle East as a berried shrub. It is said to have been used in Christian monasteries in the middle ages as a stimulant to assist the monks in night prayers, a device suggested by the observant prior of a Middle-Eastern convent who noted that if lambs ate coffee berries they gambolled about all night instead of sleeping. Drinking coffee as a social stimulant became very popular in Great Britain to such an extent that the coffee houses of London and other large cities became in effect the centres of commerce. Despite this widespread and sometimes intensive use, coffee received only subdued medical recommendation. It was not until Henry Hyde Salter wrote his important paper first mentioned in the Edinburgh Medical Journal in 1859[26] that its true importance was declared. Salter clearly regarded the benefits of coffee as part of the common experience of many asthmatic patients. He describes at some length the effect of sleep on asthma and the then known stimulatory effects of coffee which oppose sleep. He concluded that the effects of coffee must be connected with the central nervous stimulant actions. The relationship was consistent with his firm view of asthma as a disorder of the nervous system. He also drew an analogy between the effects of coffee and the short-term improvement in asthma which may be caused by sudden alarm. Here, of course, he had actually made an acute observation on the effect of sympathetic stimulation. Salter's perceptiveness is astonishing. In his writings around 1860 his own observations seem to be sufficient to alert him to the effects of substances representing three of the five major groups of antiasthmatic medicines. Reference has already been made to his monograph '*On Asthma: Its Pathology and Treatment*'[18], an excerpt from which is reproduced here (page 5). Coffee was also recommended by Foucart in 1860[27], who noted that, as well as Floyer (but see above), Withering, Musgrave, Bree, Laennec and Trousseau had all described benefit from coffee. Salter does not refer to any previous authority on the subject of coffee even though in general he freely refers to earlier authors wherever his extensive reading revealed something worthwhile. The active component of coffee, caffeine (trimethyl xanthine) was synthesized quite soon afterwards by von Strecker in 1861[28] but the direct effect of caffeine on the airways rather than by a central effect was not demonstrated until the experiments of Trendelenberg[29] and Pal[30] in 1912. In 1888 the active agent in tea leaves was isolated by Kossel, who was also responsible for its name, theophylline. In 1895 he isolated dimethyl xanthine from cocoa. A soluble theophylline derivative, aminophylline, was produced in 1908 by Dessauer[31], and found some clinical use primarily as a diuretic.

The first use of theophylline in asthma may have been that recorded by Hirsch in 1922[32]. He examined the bronchodilatory effect of xanthine derivatives in three asthmatic subjects using a suppository consisting of two-thirds theophylline and one-third theobromine, and found the treatment successful. Hirsch also examined the effect *in vitro* of the same theophylline/theobromine mixture he had used in patients by means of an isolated preparation of bovine bronchus.

The use of theophyllines was given a new boost by a paper from Hermann and Aynesworth in 1937[33]. They had conducted earlier systematic work on the treatment of cardiac failure. In the report reproduced here (page 70), they describe the effect of aminophylline in a mixed group of patients with respiratory distress in whom acute severe bronchial asthma was the prevailing disorder. This paper was very influential in its day. In the same year Greene *et al.*[34] (page 84) also reported the successful use of intravenous aminophylline in bronchial asthma. Like Hermann and Aynesworth they had been primarily interested in the treatment of cardiac failure. The principal thrust of their paper concerns intrathecal and venous pressure changes during treatment. Almost as an afterthought, they report on the experience of 15 patients with bronchial asthma, five of whom were studied during an acute attack. They found symptomatic improvement in all 15 patients and an increase in vital capacity was observed in eight of the 10 subjects in whom it was measured.

The paper by Hermann and Aynesworth stresses the effectiveness of aminophylline in 'adrenalin-fast status asthmaticus' and is interesting for its description of what was the customary treatment at the time. Intravenous adrenaline in a dose of 0.1–0.2 ml of 1/1000 solution was often used, as was the injection of calcium chloride or calcium gluconate and of hypertonic solutions of glucose. It is a little surprising that such interest was inspired by aminophylline in 1937, since it had been produced nearly 20 years earlier and was known to be active. It seems likely that the obvious effectiveness of adrenaline in a majority of cases may have distracted attention from other medicines. By the late 1930s aminophylline had very largely replaced adrenaline in the emergency treatment of severe asthma. Since then, intravenous aminophylline has remained a standard treatment for acute severe asthma, giving way in more tractable cases in recent years to the inhaled selective β_2-sympathomimetic drugs such as salbutamol and terbutaline. By the early 1940s oral preparations of aminophylline were in increasing use, often combined with ephedrine. Choline theophyllinate became available in 1954. Oral theophylline preparations declined slightly in use over the next decade, but then increased in popularity with the development of slow-release preparations. Theophyllines have an established place in the treatment of chronic disease. There are marked differences in prescribing behaviour on both sides of the Atlantic. In Great Britain, theophyllines tend to be reserved for the more intractable cases of chronic asthma in whom regular inhaled treatment with corticosteroid aerosols or cromoglycate together with a β-agonist does not produce adequate control. In the United States, oral theophylline treatment is commonly employed as the principal regular treatment. There is still uncertainty about quite how theophyllines exert their effects in asthma. The simple view of a decade ago, in which the drugs were seen as bronchial smooth muscle relaxants acting by means of inhibition of intracellular phosphodiesterase and resultant increase in intracellular levels of cyclic monophosphate, is no longer tenable.

ADRENERGIC DRUGS

The earliest adrenergic drug was ephedrine, known to the ancient Chinese as Ma Huang, which is included in many compound Chinese traditional remedies and which seems to have been in use for at least 5000 years[35]. Ma Huang was derived from the plant *Ephedra sinica*, a low shrub found at altitudes of around 1500 m (5000 feet) in Northern China. Related species of Ephedracieae are found elsewhere in Asia and Europe. The plant is an evergreen Gymnosperm (i.e. related to conifers) and has slim jointed branches and twigs without actual leaves. Ephedrine and pseudoephedrine can be obtained from the green twigs[36]. In one form the drug is taken by chewing short dried sticks. The properties of Ma Huang were investigated in the late 19th century and the alkaloid ephedrine was isolated and named by Nagai in 1887. Experiments by Nagai and others around this time demonstrated that the drug had what would now be called adrenergic effects on the pupil, intestinal muscle and circulation. The work on ephedrine seems to have stimulated little interest in English medical literature until Chen and Schmidt[35] published a new investigation of the properties of Ma Huang in 1924 (reproduced here on page 87). By this time adrenaline was established as an important treatment for asthma. Although Chen and Schmidt broke little truly new ground and provided almost no information on the bronchodilatory properties of ephedrine, their paper and others by Miller[37] and Leopold[38] helped to revive interest in ephedrine as an orally active substitute for adrenaline with a more sustained action, which led to its wider use as a decongestant and bronchodilator.

The demonstration in 1895 by Oliver and Sharpey-Schäfer[39] that injection of an extract of the adrenal gland had a striking effect on blood pressure opened a new chapter in the pharmacology of bronchial asthma. These workers, however, made no observations on the effect of adrenal extracts on the bronchi and confined their respiratory observations to the effect on regulation of breathing. The active substance, adrenaline (epinephrine), was isolated by Abel of Johns Hopkins Hospital just 3 years later. Pure crystalline adrenaline hormone was extracted by Takamine[40] and also by Aldrich[41] in 1901. Adrenaline was introduced as a treatment by injection in 1900 and later by inhalation.

Solis-Cohen, Professor of Medicine in Philadelphia at the turn of the century, was one of the first to report the use of adrenal substances in the treatment of asthma and hay fever[42]. He gave adrenal extract orally under the impression that patients with asthma suffered from 'vasomotor ataxia of the relaxing variety'. The first successful use of injected adrenaline in severe asthma was reported by Bullowa and Kaplan in 1903[43] (page 106). Over the next decade it found increasing use by intravenous injection in severe exacerbations of asthma. The direct bronchodilator effect of adrenaline was demonstrated by Kahn in 1907, who showed relaxation of isolated trachea by adrenaline[44].

By the 1920s enthusiasm for adrenaline as a treatment was probably at its height. Sir Arthur Hurst, an eminent physician of his day who suffered from asthma himself, gives some insight into how asthma and its treatment was regarded in his review of 1921[45] (page 110). Although Hurst did not contribute experimental work in the field of asthma, he was undoubtedly influential and there are still physicians who remember relying on 1/1000 adrenaline injected at 'a minim a minute', which he promoted as the mainstay of treatment in severe asthma. It is of interest that Hurst, like other physicians of his day, advocated subcutaneous injection by the patients themselves, a practice which has reappeared in recent years in patients prone to abrupt severe asthma, usually employing salbutamol or terbutaline in place of adrenaline. Hurst warns against the inhalation of fumes from burning materials, presumably disapproving of such things as stramonium cigarettes. He favoured the use of atropine inhaled from an atomizer. Hurst makes interesting reference in his autobiography[46] to a visit to Le Mont Doré in France where fresh air inhalation and hydrotherapy (still practised) were extremely popular. He noted that scars from cupping for asthma were commonly seen on the torsos of French patients.

Dr P.W.L. Camps, a general practitioner in Teddington, is generally credited with the introduction of inhaled adrenergic treatment for asthma to Britain through his delightfully frank report of 1929[47] reproduced here (page 115). Treatment administered by nebulization using oxygen had been developed earlier in Germany, where various compact forms of atomizer had also been developed. Inhalation of adrenaline as a 1/100 solution received closer scrutiny from Graeser and Rowe in 1935[48], by which time it had already become an accepted treatment. They clarified the topical nature of its action (the inhaled route having, until then, been seen merely as a convenient alternative to injection of a substance which was inactive given orally).

Adrenaline gradually displaced atropine-like agents but some mixtures of adrenaline with other agents such as atropine and papaveretum ('Brovon') were very popular, as were the very efficient hand-held nebulizers with which they were used. Isoprenaline became available during the 1940s and was found to produce fewer cardiovascular side effects than adrenaline and ephedrine. Both chronotropic and inotropic effects, however, were still quite pronounced soon after inhalation and the overall beneficial effect was still short-lived. Isoprenaline was nevertheless important. It became the principal inhaled treatment for asthma for about 20 years and allowed Ahlquist[49] to distinguish α and β receptors in 1948 on the basis of the difference between bronchial response to noradrenaline and to isoprenaline. In 1967 Lands and colleagues[50], using the same technique as Ahlquist, showed that β receptors could be subdivided further into β_1 and β_2 types and that cardiac effects could be largely separated from bronchodilator effects (this paper is reproduced in Volume 1). Strategic substitution at two different sites in the adrenaline molecule led to the development of agents with greater bronchial selectivity and much longer duration of action. The first selective β_2-bronchodilator was isoetharine, the synthesis of which made it possible to confirm Lands's theory that two types of β receptor existed in man[51]. Isoetharine, although selective, had the same brief duration of effect as isoprenaline. Duration of action was improved by substitution at a different site in the molecule. Probably the most successful of the bronchodilators showing both selectivity and longer duration of action has been salbutamol, which was first described[52,53] in 1968 (pages 118 and 119). Numerous studies later confirmed its clinical effectiveness, amongst the first being that by Choo-Kang, Simpson and Grant[54] reproduced on page 121.

The problem of administering a measured dose of inhaled agent in a convenient manner was solved by an American engineer, Philip Maschberg, who devised a special valve for use with an inhaler in which the drug was discharged with an inert volatile propellant[55]. By the 1960s pressurized metered-dose inhalers were used by millions of patients with asthma for the inhalation of bronchodilator treatments. In the 1970s other drugs besides bronchodilators began to be delivered by this means. Pressurized aerosols have remained important because of their convenience. Nevertheless, some patients experience difficulty in using pressurized aerosols and there is increasing concern about the effect of some volatile propellants on the earth's atmosphere. It remains to be seen whether the development of increasingly effective and convenient dry-powder inhalers will result in the early replacement of pressurized metered-dose inhalers.

CORTICOSTEROIDS

The first written investigation reporting the use of adrenal hormone in asthma, however, dates back to 1933, when Fineman[56] described the results of administering extracts of adrenal gland to five patients. Fineman tried adrenal extract because he observed that patients with severe and prolonged asthma often had exteme weakness, loss of appetite, weight loss and exhaustion, features which he thought might be due to underlying adrenal insufficiency. For the wrong reasons he had stumbled upon the most important form of treatment yet discovered for bronchial asthma. His paper makes interesting reading (page 124) but reaches no certain conclusions, with one of his four patients experiencing marked improvement, one moderate improvement, one slight improvement and one no improvement. Nevertheless, he clearly suspected some activity and encouraged further trials. Cold water was poured on the idea by a subsequent report by Cohen and Rudolph[57], in which negative results were obtained in four patients (the first treated as early as 1930), all with chronic severe disease. The adrenal cortical extract was of uncertain potency since the only means of standardizing activity at the time was comparison of the life-prolonging potential of similarly prepared extracts with recorded survival of untreated patients with Addison's disease (a form of calibration which involved reference to Addison's original data!).

The first administration of synthesized cortisone took place in 1948 when Hench and colleagues treated a woman with rheumatoid arthritis using a series of intramuscular injections with impressive resolution of her symptoms. The report of the treatment included results from 13 other patients, two of whom had also received ACTH (adrenocorticotrophic hormone). The effect of the report was sensational. Within a year the authors had become Nobel laureates and cortisone or ACTH had been applied to a variety of other inflammatory diseases. Within 6 months of the publication of Hench's paper Bordley and colleagues[58] had tried the effect of ACTH in five patients with asthma and had submitted an account of their exciting observations. This classic short paper is reproduced on page 133. Ten months later the same group had carried out a more detailed assessment of ACTH and cortisone in 23 patients with chronic asthma (page 136)[59]. Although the assessments were only partly controlled and objective measurements were sparse, by the standards of the day the work was carefully carried out and it offered substantial support to the earlier dramatic announcement as well as exploring such things as the effects of repeated courses of treatment and the effect upon skin tests). By this time other workers had begun to explore the clinical effects of ACTH[60] and intramuscular injections of cortisone[61,62] in asthma. Early in 1951 Schwartz published an account of three cases of intractable asthma successfully treated with oral cortisone (page 164)[63], supporting this later in the same year with a series of 22 similarly treated patients[64].

Over the next few years cortisone became generally available and was used with enthusiasm in a variety of inflammatory conditions with impressive results. Because of the inherently variable nature of asthma and the uncontrolled character of the initial reports on cortisone treatment there was a degree of scepticism in Britain about the value of the treatment, together with concern about the widespread use of a potentially harmful drug. Two multicentre controlled trials were established by a subcommittee of the Medical Research Council and resulted in the publication in 1956 of two papers[65,66] dealing with chronic and acute severe asthma. These papers are classics of their type and illustrate the difficulty that scientifically proper studies may have in discerning important clinical effects. They are reproduced here (pages 167 and 173). In chronic asthma corticosteroid treatment narrowly escaped being declared inert since only slight benefit was noted in the patients receiving cortisone and this had disappeared after 8 weeks of treatment. This surprising result may be a consequence of the modest dose of cortisone used and the lack of objective measurements except the recording of vital capacity at the beginning and end of 24 weeks of treatment in some patients. The study of 'status asthmaticus' showed a detectable benefit in patients receiving cortisone and certainly contributed to establishing corticosteroids as part of the treatment of this condition. It is interesting to note that more than 20 years later the importance of corticosteroid treatment in the management of chronic asthma was established beyond question but there was, for a time, argument about its place in the treatment of acute severe asthma[67–69]. With the availability of prednisone and prednisolone oral corticosteroid treatment eventually became of prime importance in the long-term management of severe chronic asthma and in the short-term management of acute exacerbations of asthma.

In the early days of corticosteroid treatment little attention was given to dosage. It soon became apparent that a heavy price was being paid in the form of severe hypercorticoid side effects which were noted in a high proportion of patients treated. This unfortunate experience resulted in extreme reluctance on the part of many doctors to prescribe steroids for asthma, an understandable over-reaction which undoubtedly denied many patients effective treatment of their asthma in the years which followed and which still influences prescribing today.

The idea of treating asthma by inhalation of cortisone first seems to have been taken up by Reeder and Mackay, who in 1950 treated a patient apparently suffering from pneumonia. Even in the first years of cortisone availability the motive for topical treatment was to avoid steroid side effects. An interesting account of treating asthma by repeated bronchoscopic instillation of cortisone appeared in 1951, in which the authors seriously proposed the outpatient treatment of chronic asthma by repeated tracheal cannulation[70]. In the same year, however, Gelfand[71] reported the treatment of five patients with long-standing asthma using a nebulized solution of cortisone. Ten-hourly inhalations were given every day for 2 weeks. Four of the five patients appeared to derive benefit and no side effects were noted on a daily inhaled dose of about 50 mg. It was realized, however, that cortisone was relatively inactive locally. Hydrocortisone became available in 1952 and reached Britain in 1954. Its effect on severer skin diseases was soon shown to be dramatically better than that of cortisone. Hydrocortisone in powder form was used as inhaled treatment for asthma by Foulds in 1955 in an open uncontrolled study in which good results were obtained in doses of 7.5 or 15 mg daily. Brockbank was initially sceptical[72], as he found no response in a double-blind controlled trial. Later, however, he repeated the study using powdered hydrocortisone and confirmed Foulds's results[73] using very small doses of hydrocortisone, so that there was no longer any doubt that the principal effect must be a local one. Over the next 10 years chemists worked persistently to try to produce topically active steroid molecules. The work was guided by McKenzie and Stoughton's discovery that topical activity appeared to be closely related to the ability of the agent to cause blanching when applied to the skin surface. Hydrocortisone in this test showed poor blanching, but the most effective molecules to emerge were betamethasone-17-valerate and beclomethasone dipropionate. These were the focus of subsequent development. Clinical reports on the effectiveness of both drugs in asthma were initially subdued until the publication of a study by Brown and colleagues in 1972[74]. This offered a straightforward demonstration that patients who had previously required regular systemic steroid treatment could have their asthma satisfactorily controlled by aerosol steroid while the oral treatment was reduced or withdrawn. In many instances better control was achieved by the steroid aerosol. Despite the fact that this was not a controlled study and was accordingly subjected to a certain amount of criticism, it was an extremely influential report quoted in hundreds of subsequent publications. Its conclusions were amply borne out by other controlled work and eventually by everyday clinical experience in the management of asthma. This classic paper is reproduced on page 177. Subsequent investigators confirmed in controlled work that the treatment was effective[75] and showed that there was usually good recovery of the pituitary-adrenal axis on conversion to regular aerosol treatment with beclomethasone dipropionate[76,77] or betamethasone valerate[78], suggesting that the systemic effects of the inhaled steroid were unimportant. In fact some patients suffered significant hypoadrenal symptoms when converted from regular oral treatment to aerosol steroids, with good control of their asthma, and the nature of the new non-respiratory complaints was not always recognized. Subsequently, budesonide was developed and shown to be effective in clinical terms[79] and to have favourable features for a topical steroid similar to those of beclomethasone dipropionate and betamethasone valerate.

In the early days of topical steroid treatment there was widespread confusion over the nature of selective topical activity. Although betamethasone valerate and beclomethasone dipropionate were originally selected because of their effect in the skin blanching test, the property which was to be just as important as local penetrance and inherent activity was that of susceptibility to first-pass degradation in the liver. Without active liver metabolism a potent absorbable steroid drug would tend to cause systemic effects when given by aerosol because of the relatively high proportion of the delivered dose swallowed. The fact that the compounds which caused blanching possessed this characteristic is fortunate and largely fortuitous.

Later developments in the clinical use of inhaled corticosteroids in asthma have centred firstly on improved means of dispersing the substance and secondly on exploration of the effect of higher doses in the more resistant cases of asthma. Improved efficiency of inhalation has been achieved with dry-powder inhalers, which many patients find easier to use, and also with spacer devices into which pressurized inhalers are discharged. These devices have been shown to give a more favourable distribution of particle size and to reduce the proportion of the inhaled dose which impacts in the mouth and pharynx. Steroid aerosol treatment has probably been the single most important development to bring benefit to the average patient with troublesome asthma. It has gradually come to be accepted that chronic asthma or recurrent asthma which is more than truly trivial can be best managed by early introduction of regular aerosol steroid treatment with suppression of the underlying inflammatory process rather than by repeated partial reversal of the element of smooth muscle constriction using bronchodilators alone.

CROMOGLYCATE

Khellin is a substance (aglycone) derived from the seeds of the plant *Ammi visnaga* of the family Apiaciae. It is known in Egypt, and perhaps more widely in the eastern Mediterranean, as kella. It was used for centuries as a traditional treatment for chest disorders and in the 20th century had found some use in the treatment of angina pectoris[80]. It was known to have some bronchodilator effect but development had not been pursued because of its tendency to cause nausea and difficulties arising from its low solubility.

In an attempt to improve the bronchodilator effects and diminish the nauseating effects of khellin, a research group from Fisons Pharmaceuticals produced and tested a variety of related synthetic cromone derivatives in the early 1960s. In the absence of a satisfactory animal model the testing and refinement of substances was carried out on an asthmatic volunteer and the effect of new preparations on asthma induced by either antigen inhalation of non-specific stimuli such as inhalation of histamine or a cholinergic agent was noted. It was found that compounds with di-carboxychromone structure, although lacking a bronchodilator effect, had a remarkable ability to prevent the development of antigen provoked asthma in the volunteer. The discovery of this effect and its later refinement is attributable to Dr Roger Altounyan, who was himself both the experimenter and the asthmatic volunteer. Over a period of 9 years Altounyan underwent hundreds of challenges in the course of testing compounds at varying doses taken at different times before or after several forms of inhalation challenge. It is notable that the dose of inhaled allergen was adjusted so that in control experiments the one-second forced expiratory volume fell by 45%, more than twice as severe as the conventional level of challenge used in laboratory assessments of bronchial responsiveness. Altounyan's experiments were sufficient to lead to the development of disodium cromoglycate, a completely new type of drug in the treatment of asthma. The substance was inert when taken orally and difficult to dissolve; novel means were therefore devised for its delivery by inhalation as a fine dry powder through a breath-actuated turbine device, the Spinhaler–also the product of Altounyan's inventiveness. The classic paper recording the crucial initial testing of cromoglycate is an unassuming but much-quoted abstract occupying less than a page (page 183)[81], which appeared in 1967 at about the same time as the first report on clinical testing of the compound in asthmatic patients[82] (page 184). The official announcement of the structure and characteristics of cromoglycate was published a few months later (page 188)[83]. Cromoglycate became available on the British market in the same year and within a few years had become generally accepted as a valuable anti-asthma medicine permitting good control in a useful proportion of patients with asthma, many of whom might otherwise have required continuous oral corticosteroid treatment. It found particular favour in the treatment of childhood asthma. Since the development of cromoglycate a great deal of energy has been directed towards the synthesis of more potent compounds with similar effects[84]. One such product, nedocromil, has become established as having useful activity by inhalation but, so far, no effective oral agent with cromoglycate-like properties has been developed.

IMMUNOTHERAPY

The idea of a treatment which could produce a lasting alteration of the predisposition to asthma has always had a compelling attraction. Apart from allergen avoidance as a strategy, the only measure which has seemed to offer a lasting change in asthma severity has been immunotherapy or desensitization to specific external antigens to which the asthmatic subject has become hypersensitive. The principle of inducing a state of resistance or tolerance through repeated injections of the external 'toxin' (in this case grass pollen) was first outlined by Charles Noon in a paper in the *Lancet* in 1911[85]. This paper and its sequel by Freeman[86] were to have great influence on the management of asthma over the next few decades, which is why they are reproduced here (pages 190 and 192). In the United States the practice of allergology developed and flourished to the point where it dominated the management of asthma. The paper's influence was perhaps less marked in Britain where, in general, specialization was slower to develop. Despite the intense interest in desensitization as a form of treatment its value never ceased to be a matter of controversy, partly because of the great scarcity of high quality controlled work on the subject[87]. Hay fever was the most popular target for desensitization and studies of hay fever yielded the best evidence for an effect. In time other treatments for hay fever and asthma were developed which were both more effective and more convenient than immunotherapy. Concern about the danger of severe hypersensitivity reactions associated with immunotherapy eventually led to its virtual abandonment in Britain as a treatment for asthma.

MEASUREMENT

The inclusion of a paper describing a measuring instrument in a collection of classic papers on asthma treatment may seem strange, but it is a reflection of the fact that the use of peak flow measurement has become an integral part of the management of asthma in Britain. Its use seems set to develop further with the recent introduction of the facility to prescribe a meter as easily as a drug. Before the development of peak flow measurement the idea of making frequent repeated measurements in individual patients was not really practical. In 1959 Wright and McKerrow[83] announced (page 196) a new index of pulmonary function, peak expiratory flow rate (PEFR, later shortened to PEF), which was related to the maximum instantaneous rate of expiratory airflow at the mouth. This was in turn shown to be closely related to other indices of maximum airflow such as the forced expiratory volume in one second (FEV_1). The index was in practice defined by the characteristics of the original instrument itself. The new instrument was portable and robust and yielded reasonably reliable results. It enabled doctors to measure the severity of airways obstruction in their surgeries and in patients' homes, but it was a relatively expensive piece of precision engineering. The later development of cheap plastic meters which patients could use themselves to make repeated measurements of PEF in their own homes was almost as significant a development as the original invention. The most successful of these was another instrument designed by Wright, the Wright Mini-Peak Flow Meter, introduced in 1978 (page 203). The ability of the patient to make regular measurements allows progressive refinement of treatment by doctor and patient in partnership on the basis of the results achieved. Patients can be trained to make sensible alterations to their own treatment (or seek help) if there are notable changes in PEF. The regular measurement and charting of peak flow has become pivotal to the assessment of progress and regulation of treatment in patients admitted to hospital with acute severe asthma. The peak flow meter has also played an important part in the development and testing of new anti-asthma preparations.

DEATH IN ASTHMA

Mortality from asthma has not decreased over the last 100 years and may well be increasing. As it is generally accepted that a substantial proportion of the deaths are probably preventable by appropriate treatment, understanding of the treatment received by patients in the period leading up to death from asthma should have a direct influence on management. Amongst the most important publications on death from asthma, but by no means the earliest, were a pair of papers published in 1968 by Speizer, Doll, Heaf and Strang[90,91], reproduced on pages 205 and 210. It was realized during the 1960s that deaths from asthma had increased sharply in England and Wales. Initially it was widely believed that the deaths might be in some way related to the excessive use of steroid treatment about which there was already much concern. The first paper examined the evidence and concluded that there was a real rise in death rate, which was most striking in the young. The second paper examined the use of drugs before death. One of the most important findings is represented in Table IV which shows that, far from receiving excessive doses of corticosteroids, the patients dying from asthma had received rather light steroid treatment. Only 23 of the 173 patients dying from asthma were receiving high-dose treatment before death; 81 had received no steroid at all in the last illness and the remainder had received moderate, decreasing or low doses of steroid. It is noted that deaths were frequently sudden and unexpected, occurring outside hospital. The paper indicates a possible link with the increased use of pressurized aerosols, which at the time usually contained isoprenaline. Some possible mechanisms are advanced, including direct cardiotoxicity and relief of bronchoconstriction without relief of hypoxia. The causes of the 'epidemic' of asthma deaths in the 1960s are still debated today but the prevalent view is that the excess of deaths was probably not attributable to simple isoprenaline cardiotoxicity. It is more probable that the important factors were, firstly, undertreatment with steroid drugs so that the underlying asthmatic inflammatory process was far advanced and, secondly, the effect of the potent bronchodilator, which may have trapped patients into tolerating dangerously severe airways obstruction in the belief that relief might still be obtained from the inhaler. Several well conducted studies have now examined the circumstances of death from asthma and a number of common findings have emerged. It is notable that recent studies point to the continuing importance of undertreatment with corticosteroid drugs and underrecognition of the severity of the asthma, features described over 20 years ago by Speizer and colleagues.

CONCLUSION

The present collection of papers was assembled with the idea of allowing the clinician interested in the treatment of asthma convenient access to some papers which were influential in their day, are still sometimes referred to today, and make interesting reading in their own right. Those who read the papers in sequence are unlikely to draw any general conclusions from an irregular selection of publications but one or two themes may emerge.

Classic papers evidently have no particular characteristics. It certainly seems to be true that there is no relationship between the length or prominence of a publication and the degree of novelty of its contents. Some of the shortest papers here had the most profound implications. Some very influential papers, moreover, report uncontrolled work or have other shortcomings which might well prevent their publication today. The collection is, of course, limited to papers which were actually published. It may occur to the reader that some of the most important and innovative reports may still be housed in the files of pharmaceutical companies. This tendency may become more pronounced as the financial pressures surrounding drug development increase so that a degree of secrecy is inevitable in the early stages of a drug's development. In some cases the papers reproduced here necessarily represent the first (usually influential) announcement of successful clinical trials with patients rather than the pioneering laboratory work on molecules, animals and volunteers.

One cannot fail to be impressed by the fact that the ancients recognized the effectiveness of botanical precursors of all of today's important drugs, with the exception of the corticosteroids, when they had such rudimentary concepts of disease. The theme has its modern counterpart since, in general, drugs have been shown to be effective and brought into widespread use long before the emergence of any clear understanding of their mode of action. To date new drugs seem to have played a larger part in developing understanding of the underlying mechanisms in asthma than *vice versa*. The papers also reflect some other general rules which seem to apply in medicine: progress in one field often occurs as a result of a development in another, and progress is occasionally the consequence of good fortune combined with acute observation rather than long-term strategic planning.

Alistair Brewis
Newcastle upon Tyne, 1991

REFERENCES

1. Gandevia B. Historical review of the use of parasympatholytic agents in the treatment of respiratory disorders. *Postgraduate Medical Journal* 1975; **51** (suppl 7): 13.

2. Lewis WH, Memory PFE. *Medical Botany: Plants Affecting Man's Health.* New York, John Wiley 1977.

3. Celsus. *De Medicina Vol 1* translated by Spencer WG. London, Heinemann (Loeb Classical Library) 1935: 385

4. Capel LH. A history of the pulmonary catarrhs and airways obstruction. *British Journal of Diseases of the Chest* 1966; **60**: 113.

5. Muntner S. *The Medical Writings of Moses Maimonides. Treatise on Asthma.* Philadelphia, Lippincott 1963.

6. Rosner F. Moses Maimonides' treatise on asthma. *Thorax* 1981; **36**: 245.

7. Dana CL. The story of a great consultation. *Annals of Medical History* 1921; **13**: 122.

8. Willis T. *Pharmaceutice Rationalis.* London, Thomas Dring 1679.

9. Sydenham T. *The complete method of curing almost all diseases. To which is added an exact description of their several symptoms. Written in Latin by Thomas Sydenham and now faithfully Englished.* London, Randall Taylor 1694.

10. Floyer J. *A Treatise of the Asthma.* London, R. Wilkin 1698.

11. Floyer J. *Medicina Gericomica or, The Galenic Art of Preserving Old Men's Healths.* London, J. Isted 1725.

12. Millar J. *Observations on the Asthma and on the Hooping Cough.* London, T. Cadell 1769.

13. Lefevre A. Recherches médicales sur la nature et le traitement de la maladie connue sous le nom d'asthme. *Journal Hebdomadaire* 1835; **97**: 193.

14. Volle RL, Koelle GB. Ganglion stimulating and blocking agents. In *The Pharmacological Basis of Therapeutics*, 3rd edn, edited by Goodman LS, Gilman A. New York, Macmillan 1965.

15. Sims J. Communications relative to the Datura stramonium, or thorn apple: as a cure or relief of asthma. *Edinburgh Medical and Surgical Journal* 1812; **8**: 364.

16. English W. Case of asthma cured by smoking the *Datura stramonium. Edinburgh Medical Journal* 1811; **7**: 153.

17. Geiger PL, Fesse H. Darstellung des Atropins. *Annalen der Chemie* 1833; **5**:43.

18. Salter HH. *On Asthma: Its Pathology and Treatment.* London, J. Churchill 1860.

19. Salter HH. On the treatment of asthma by belladonna. *Lancet* 1869; 152.

20. Herxheimer H. Atropine cigarettes in asthma and emphysema. *British Medical Journal* 1959; **2**: 167.

21. Altounyan REC. Variation of drug action on airway obstruction in man. *Thorax* 1964; **19**: 406.

22. Chamberlain DA, Muir DCF, Kennedy KP. Atropine methonitrate and isoprenaline in bronchial asthma. *Lancet* 1962, **ii**: 1019.

23. Deckers W. The chemistry of new derivatives of tropane alkaloid and the pharmacokinetics of a new quaternary compound. *Postgraduate Medical Journal* 1975; **51** (suppl 7): 76.

24. Engelhardt A, Klupp H. The pharmacology of a new tropane alkaloid derivative. *Postgraduate Medical Journal* 1975; **51** (suppl 7): 82.

25. Poppius H, Salorinne Y, Niljanen AA. Inhalation of a new anticholinergic drug, Sch 1000, in asthma and chronic bronchitis: effect on airway resistance, thoracic gas volume, blood gases and exercise-induced asthma. *Bulletin de Physio-pathologie Respiratoire de Nancy* 1972; **8**: 643.

26. Salter H. On some points in the treatment and clinical history of asthma. *Edinburgh Medical Journal* 1859; **4**: 1109.

27. Foucart A. Du café dans le traitement de l'asthme nerveux ou essentiel. *La France Médicale et Pharmaceutique* 1860; 300.

28. Strecker AFL. Untersuchungen über die chemischen Beziehungen zwischen Guanin, Xanthin, Theobromin, Caffein und Kreatinin. *Liebeg's Annalen der Chemie und Pharmacie* 1861, **118**: 151.

29. Trendelenburg P. Physiologische und pharmakologische Untersuchungen an der isolierten Bronkialmuskulatur. *Archiv für Experimentale Pathologie und Pharmakologie* 1912; **69**: 79.

30. Pal J. Ueber die Wirkung des Kaffeins auf die Bronkien und die Atmung. *Deutsche Medizinische Wochenschrift* 1912; **38**: 1774.

31. Dessauer P. Euphyllin, ein neues Diuretikum. *Therapeutische Monatschrifte* 1908; **22**: 401.

32. Hirsch S. Klinischer und experimenteller Beitrag zur krampflösenden Wirkung der Purin Derivative. *Klinische Wochenschrift* 1922; **1**: 615.

33. Hermann GR, Aynesworth MB, Martin J. Successful treatment of persistent extreme dyspnea, 'Status asthmaticus' – use of theophylline ethylene diamine (aminophylline, U.S.P.) intravenously. *Journal of Laboratory and Clinical Medicine* 1937; **23**: 135.

34. Greene JA, Paul WD, Faller AE. The action of theophylline with ethylenediamine on intrathecal and in venous pressures in cardiac failure and on bronchial obstruction in cardiac failure and in bronchial asthma. *Journal of the American Medical Association* 1937; **109**: 1712.

35. Chen KK, Schmidt CF. The action of ephedrine: the active principle of Chinese drug Ma Huang. *Journal of the American Medical Association* 1937; **109**: 1712.

36. Morton JF. *Major Medicinal Plants: Botany, Culture and Uses*. Springfield, Illinois, Charles C. Thomas 1977.

37. Miller T, Grier A. A consideration of the clinical value of ephedrin. *Amercian Journal of Medical Science* 1925; **170**: 157.

38. Leopold SS. The use of ephedrine in bronchial asthma and hay fever. *Journal of the American Medical Association* 1927; **88**: 1782.

39. Oliver G, Sharpey-Schäfer EA. The physiological action of extract of the suprarenal capsules. *Journal of Physiology* 1895; **18**: 230.

40. Takamine J. The blood-pressure raising principle of the supra-renal glands. *Therapeutic Gazette* 1901; **17**: 221.

41. Aldrich TB. A preliminary report on the active principle of the suprarenal gland. *American Journal of Physiology* 1901; **5**: 457.

42. Solis-Cohen S. The use of adrenal substances in the treatment of asthma. *Journal of the American Medical Association* 1900, **34**: 1164.

43. Bullowa JJM, Kaplan DM. On the hypodermic use of adrenalin chloride in the treatment of asthmatic attacks. *Medical News (N.Y.)* 1903, **83**: 787.

44. Kahn RH. Zur Physiologie der Trachea. *Archiv für Physiologie* 1907, 398.

45. Hurst AF. An address on asthma. *Lancet* 1921, **i**: 1113.

46. Hurst A. *A Twentieth Century Physician*. London, Edward Arnold 1949.

47. Camps PWL. A note on the inhalation treatment of asthma. *Guy's Hospital Reports* 1929, **79**: 496.

48. Graeser JB, Rowe AH. Inhalation of epinephrine for the relief of asthmatic symptoms. *Journal of Allergy* 1935, **6**: 415.

49. Ahlquist RP. A study of the adrenotropic receptors. *American Journal of Physiology* 1948, **153**: 586.

50. Lands AM, Arnold A, McAuliff JP, Luduena FP, Brown TG Jr. Differentiation of receptor systems activated by sympathetic amines. *Nature* 1967, **214**: 597.

51. Collier JG, Dornhorst AC. Evidence for two different types of β-receptor in man. *Nature* 1969, **223**: 1283.

52. Hartley D, Jack D, Lunts LHC, Ritchie AC. New class of selective stimulants of β-adrenergic receptors. *Nature* 1968; **249**: 861.

53. Brittain RT, Farmer JB, Jack D, Martin LE, Simpson WT. α-[(t-Butylamino)methyl]-4-hydroxy-*m*-xylene-α¹,α³-diol (AH.3365): a selective β-adrenergic stimulant. *Nature* 1968, **219**: 862.

54. Choo-Kang YFJ, Simpson WT, Grant IWB. Controlled comparison of the bronchodilator effects of three β-adrenergic stimulant drugs administered by inhalation to patients with asthma. *British Medical Journal* 1969, **2**: 287.

55. Ganderton D, Jones TM. *Drug Delivery to the Respiratory Tract*. Chichester, Ellis Horwood 1987.

56. Fineman EH. The use of suprarenal cortex extract in the treatment of bronchial asthma. *Journal of Allergy* 1933; **4**: 182.

57. Cohen MB, Rudolph JA. Studies on the relation of the adrenal glands to allergic phenomena. 3. On the specific therapeutic effects of cortical adrenal extract in asthma. *Journal of Allergy* 1934; **5**: 279.

58. Bordley JE, Carey RA, Harvey AM, *et al*. Preliminary observations on the effect of adrenocorticotropic hormone (ACTH) in allergic diseases. *Bulletin of the Johns Hopkins Hospital* 1949; **85**: 396.

59. Carey RA, Harvey AM, Howard JE, Winkenwerder WL. The effect of adrenocorticotropic hormone (ACTH) and cortisone on the course of chronic bronchial asthma. *Bulletin of the Johns Hopkins Hospital* 1950, **87**:387.

60. Rose B, Paré JAP, Pump K, Stafford RL. Preliminary report on adrenocorticotrophic hormone (ACTH) in asthma. *Canadian Medical Association Journal* 1950; **62**: 6.

61. Carryer Koelsche GA, Prickman LE, Maytum CK, Lake CF, Williams HL. Effects of cortisone on bronchial asthma and hay fever occurring in subjects sensitive to ragweed pollen. *Journal of Allergy* 1950; **21**: 282.

62. Randolph TG, Rollins JP. Effect of cortisone in bronchial asthma. *Journal of Allergy* 1950; **21**: 288.

63. Schwartz E. Oral cortisone in intractable bronchial asthma. *Journal of Allergy* 1951; **22**: 1.

64. Schwartz E. Oral cortisone therapy in intractible bronchial asthma. *Journal of the American Medical Association* 1951; **147**: 1734.

65. Medical Research Council. Controlled trial of effects of cortisone acetate in chronic asthma. Report to the Medical Research Council by the Subcommittee on Clinical Trials in Asthma. *Lancet* 1956; **ii**: 798.

66. Medical Research Council. Controlled trial of effects of cortisone acetate in status asthmaticus. Report to the Medical Research Council by the Subcommittee on Clinical Trials in Asthma. *Lancet* 1956; **ii**: 803.

67. McFadden ER, Kiser R, de Groot WJ, Holmes B, Kiker R, Viser G. A controlled study of the effects of single doses of hydrocortisone on the resolution of acute attacks of asthma. *American Journal of Medicine* 1976; **60**:52.

68. Luksza AR. Acute severe asthma treated without steroids. *British Journal of Diseases of the Chest* 1982; **76**: 15.

69. Fanta CH, Rossing TH, McFadden ER. Glucocorticoids in acute asthma: a critical controlled trial. *American Review of Respiratory Diseases* 1982; **125**: 94.

70. London McK, Alexander FW. Topical application of cortisone in intractable bronchial asthma. *Journal of Allergy* 1951; **21**: 518.

71. Gelfand ML. Administration of cortisone by the aerosol method in the treatment of bronchial asthma. *New England Journal of Medicine* 1951; **21**: 518.

72. Brockbank W, Brebner H, Pengelly CDR. Chronic asthma treated with aerosol hydrocortisone. *Lancet* 1956; **ii**: 807.

73. Brockbank W, Pengally CDR. Chronic asthma treated with powder inhalations of hydrocortisone and prednisolone. *Lancet* 1958; **i**: 187.

74. Brown HM, Storey G, George WHS. Beclomethasone dipropionate: a new steroid aerosol for the treatment of allergic asthma. *British Medical Journal* 1972; **1**: 585.

75. Gaddie J, Petrie GR, Reid IW, Sinclair DJM, Skinner C, Palmer KNV. Aerosol beclomethasone dipropionate in chronic bronchial asthma. *Lancet* 1973; **i**: 691.

76. Clark TJH. Effect of beclomethasone dipropionate delivered by aerosol in patients with asthma. *Lancet* 1972, **i**: 1361.

77. Lal S, Harris DM, Bhalla KK, Singhal SN, Butler AG. Comparison of beclomethasone dipropionate aerosol and prednisolone in reversible airways obstruction. *British Medical Journal* 1972; **3**:314.

78. Roscoe P, Choo-Kang YFJ, Horne NW. Betamethasone valerate in corticosteroid-dependent asthmatics. *British Journal of Diseases of the Chest* 1975; **69**: 240.

79. Ellul-Micaleff R, Handson E, Johansson SA. Budesonide: a new corticosteroid in bronchial asthma. *European Journal of Respiratory Diseases* 1980; **61**: 167.

80. Anrep GV, Barsoum GS, Kenawy MR, Misrahy G. Therapeutic uses of khellin; method of standardization. *Lancet* 1947; **i**: 557.

81. Altounyan REC. Inhibition of experimental asthma by a new compound – disodium cromoglycate 'Intal'. *Acta Allergologica* 1967; **22**: 487.

82. Howell JBL, Altounyan REC. A double-blind trial of disodium cromoglycate in the treatment of allergic bronchial asthma. *Lancet* 1967; **ii**: 539.

83. Cox JSG. Disodium cromoglycate (FPL 670) ('Intal'): a specific inhibitor of reaginic antibody-antigen mechanisms. *Nature* 1967; **216**: 1328.

84. Buckle DR. Disodium cromoglycate and compounds with similar activities. In *Development of Antiasthma Drugs* edited by Buckle DR, Smith H. London, Butterworths 1984: 297.

85. Noon L. Prophylactic inoculation against hay fever. *Lancet* 1911; **i**: 1572.

86. Freeman J. Further observations on the treatment of hay fever by hypodermic inoculations of pollen vaccine. *Lancet* 1911; **ii**: 814.

87. Lichtenstein IM. An evaluation of the role of immunotherapy in asthma. *American Review of Respiratory Diseases* 1978, **117**: 191.

88. Wright BM, McKerrow CB. Maximum forced expiratory flow rate as a measure of ventilatory capacity with a description of a new portable instrument for measuring it. *British Medical Journal* 1959; **2**: 1041.

89. Wright BM. A miniature Wright peak-flow meter. *British Medical Journal* 1978; **2**: 1627.

90. Speizer RE, Doll R, Heaf P. Observations on recent increase in mortality from asthma. *British Medical Journal* 1968; **1**: 335.

91. Speizer RE, Doll R, Heaf P, Strang LB. Investigation into the use of drugs preceding death from asthma. *British Medical Journal* 1968; **1**: 339.

CONTENTS

CONTENTS

CONTENTS

CONTENTS

ACKNOWLEDGEMENTS

The publishers would like to acknowledge the help given to them by the Library of the Royal Society of Medicine.

The papers below are reproduced by permission of the respective copyright holders.

Thorax
Papers 4, 31

Bulletin de Physio-pathologie Respiratoire de Nancy
Paper 5

Nature
Papers 12, 13, 24

British Medical Journal
Papers 14, 21, 27, 28, 29, 30

The Johns Hopkins University Press
Papers 16, 17

Journal of Allergy and Clinical Immunology
with permission from the CV Mosby Company
Papers 15, 18

Medical Research Council
Papers 19, 20

JBL Howell
Paper 23

Munksgaard International Publishers Ltd
Paper 22

IX.

Communications relative to the Datura Stramonium, or Thorn-apple : as a Cure or relief of Asthma : addressed to the Editor of the Monthly Magazine ; several of them never before published. Lond. 1811. pp. 90.

IT is a trite observation, that on the introduction of new, or revival of neglected remedies, two opposite faults are frequently committed. By some they are extolled for powers which they do not possess, while others deny them all virtues ; and it is seldom, until after repeated fluctuations, that their real value is at last ascertained and generally admitted.

The subject of this treatise furnishes a striking example of the truth of these remarks. Stramonium was for a short time extolled

1   as

Datura stramonium or thorn apple as a cure or relief for asthma. *Sims J*

as an almost infallible remedy in the cure of mania and melancholia, and then fell into total neglect. Once more it has become fashionable, for the cure of a totally different disease, and its newly ascribed powers are still a matter of keen controversy.

The first public notice of these was in a letter to the Editor of the Monthly Magazine, signed *Verax*, but now acknowledged by Mr Sills, a respectable merchant in London, who had derived great benefit from its use. The history, however, of its introduction, is very concisely detailed in the following letter, from Dr Sims of Guildford Street.

" Some time in the year 1802, I received from General Gent a remedy that he had not long before brought from Madras, which, the General informed me, was used there as a specific for relieving the paroxysm of asthma, and that it was prepared from the roots of the wild purple-flowered thorn-apple (Datura *ferox*). The roots had been cut into slips as soon as gathered, dried in the shade, and then beat into fibres resembling coarse hemp. The mode of using it was by smoking it in a pipe at the time of the paroxysm, either by itself or mixed with tobacco, according as the patients were previously addicted to smoking or not. General Gent procured this remedy from Dr Anderson, physician-general at Madras, who both recommended it, and, I believe, used it himself.

" I happened at this time to be attending the daughter of an eminent physician, labouring under phthisis pulmonalis, combined with asthma, as appeared to me from the frequent paroxysms of difficulty of breathing, not usual in pure phthisis, at least in so early a stage of the disorder. With a view of alleviating these distressing paroxysms, I recommended a trial of this remedy, which to me was at that time perfectly new. The relief obtained was far beyond expectation, and, although gradually sinking under an incurable disease, this amiable lady continued to experience great satisfaction in its use, almost to the fatal termination.

" Soon after this, meeting with Mr Toulmin, surgeon of Hackney, at a time when he was much harassed by frequent paroxysms of asthma, under which he had been suffering for several years, I recommended the same remedy to him. He received so much benefit from its use, that I gladly transferred all of the remedy that I had left to him. But the quantity not being sufficient to last long, he was obliged to have recourse to our common thorn-apple (Datura Stramonium), of which I had advised him to try the stalks, as the roots of this species are small and fibrous. Mr Toulmin experienced nearly the same relief from this as from the East India plant : he likewise tried the leaves, but could hardly distinguish these from tobacco, either in taste or effects. From Mr Toulmin, the knowledge of this remedy was communicated, among others, to your correspondent (Mr Sills).

" I have two purposes to answer by the above communication. In the first place, it will serve to point out the history of the introduction of a remedy which promises to become an important addition to the Materia Medica ; not that I can claim any merit from the share that I have accidentally had in it ; but the principal intention I have had in view, was

Datura stramonium or thorn apple as a cure or relief for asthma. *Sims J*

was to show that the original remedy, as used in the East Indies, is not exactly the same as what is used here. It is indeed highly probable that both species have nearly similar virtues, but the one may perhaps be more efficacious than the other. It is to be hoped that prepared roots will be imported from Madras, in order that such patients as may not have experienced the promised relief from smoking the stalks of Datura Stramonium, may have an opportunity of trying whether the roots of Datura Ferox may be efficacious.

More care ought to be taken in the preparation of the stramonium than is usually done. The stalks ought to be cut into slender slips while recent, and dried quickly. In our climate the general direction of drying in the shade is injurious to most herbs; the quicker they are dried the more they contain of the taste and colour, and consequently of the virtues of the fresh plants. I observe, that, of late, the whole plant is sold in the physic herb-shops, as a remedy for the asthma. Now it ought to be generally known that the leaves, and more especially the unripe capsule and seeds of the thorn-apple, are a very powerful, nay even a deleterious narcotic, if taken internally, and probably cannot, in all cases, be even smoked with impunity. Yet the leaves, according to the experience of Mr Toulmin himself, are not possessed of the same powers, in allaying the asthmatic paroxysms, as the comparatively mild and innocent stalks and roots.

We shall now make a few quotations from the cases contained in these letters. Mr Sills first describes the symptoms of his asthma, and the effect of the stramonium upon him, and his manner of using it.

The asthmatic paroxysm usually came on about two o'clock in the morning, when I was suddenly surprised from sleep with violent convulsive heavings of the chest; and I was scarcely allowed time to place myself upright in a chair, where I sat resting myself upon my elbows, and with my feet upon the ground (for I could not bear them in an horizontal posture,) before I underwent a sense, as it were, of immediate suffocation. The fits generally continued, with short intermissions, from thirty-six hours to three days and nights successively; during which time I have often, in the seeming agonies of death, given myself over, and even wished for that termination of my miseries.

An amiable friend and most respectable surgeon at Hackney (Mr Toulmin), first persuaded me to smoke the divine Stramonium, to which I owe altogether my present freedom from pain and renewed capacity of enjoyment.

It is the root only, and lower part of the stem of this plant, which seem to possess its anti-asthmatic virtue: these should be cut into small pieces, and put into a common tobacco-pipe, and the smoke must be swallowed, together with the saliva produced by the smoke; after which the sufferer will, in a few minutes, be relieved from all the convulsive heavings, and probably drop into a comfortable sleep, from which he will awake refreshed, and, in general, perfectly recovered: at least, this is the invariable effect produced upon myself. He should, by all means, avoid drinking with the pipe, a too ordinary accompaniment of smoking.

I

Datura stramonium or thorn apple as a cure or relief for asthma. *Sims J*

I once took some brandy and water with the pipe, but it proved a very improper combination : a dish of coffee, however, I often take after it, and find it highly refreshing. I should mention that strong coffee has frequently been recommended to me, but never produced any beneficial effect as a cure for asthma.

This plant is delightfully fragrant : and although it has been regarded hitherto as of a poisonous nature when taken inwardly, yet I have smoked a dozen pipes at a time, without experiencing from them any other inconvenience than a slight excoriation, or soreness of the tongue.

Dr Reid says, that, in several other instances of similar disease, the success has been equally remarkable and complete. Mr Willis of Bristol states its success in his own case ; likewise Mr Young of Aberdeen. Mr Woodrow of Norwich states, that he has smoked the stramonium since last September, and almost invariably experienced great relief in respiration ; but he did not find that it diminished the daily accumulations of phlegm. Mr Radborn of Alveston in Derbyshire, a sepuagintarian, was also greatly benefited by it ; but it must be remarked that he used the stalks and seeds-vessels. The last testimony in favour of the stramonium which we shall notice, is in the following letter from Mr Sills.

" You are at perfect liberty to make every use of my name respecting the stramonium you think proper, and may add, that I continue to derive increased good effects from the use of it. In truth, the asthma is destroyed! I drink beer, eat of every thing ; and if my mind was as free from perplexity as my body is from asthma, I should again enjoy my existence. I never experienced torpor or any ill effect whatever ; and I would rather be without life than without stramonium.

This evidence, though far from decisive, is sufficient to entitle the stramonium to a fair and varied trial, under the superintendence of attentive practitioners. Of the activity of many parts of the stramonium, there are unfortunately too many proofs on record, and we fear that its indiscriminate use as a popular remedy may be attended with danger, especially as we well know that the leaves and seed-vessels, and even the poisonous seeds, are often used instead of the principal stalk, which is the part specially recommended, and is *said* to be comparatively mild and innocent. We should also think that the direction given to swallow the saliva excited by inhaling its smoke, ought to be followed with great caution. From the analogy of tobacco, we should fear that it would be extremely apt to derange the stomach, for we know that experienced smokers carefully avoid swallowing the saliva impregnated with the condensed fumes of the smoke. Besides, we consider the novelty and advantage of the practice of *smoking* stramonium, to consist in applying the remedy directly to the seat of the disease. The coloured engraving, said to represent the *Datura Stramonium* in flower, is execrable, and gives no idea of the plant. It is easily cultivated, like any other hardy annual.

X.

Datura stramonium or thorn apple as a cure or relief for asthma. *Sims J*

161

CHAPTER VIII.

TREATMENT OF THE ASTHMATIC PAROXYSM.— TREATMENT BY DEPRESSANTS.

Preliminary measures.—Ipecacuanha. Tobacco. Tartar-emetic. — Their *modus operandi*.—Their relative value and methods of administration. —Cases.—Value of tobacco in hay-asthma.—Cases.—Caution with regard to tobacco.—Importance of early administration of these remedies.—Practical observations.

THE treatment of asthma, like that of all paroxysmal diseases, naturally divides itself into the treatment of the paroxysm and the treatment in the intervals of the paroxysms, and although the last is the real treatment of the disease, while the treatment of the paroxysm is merely the treatment of a symptom, yet the paroxysm being in asthma, potentially though not essentially, the disease, (for it is its sole manifestation, the only source of suffering, and the cause of those organic changes in the heart and lungs by which alone asthma threatens life,) its treatment holds the first place in the therapeutics of the affection. If the paroxysms are mitigated the disease is rendered proportionally trifling—if they are prevented the disease is extinguished. The persistence of the asthmatic tendency is of not the slightest consequence as long as the fits are warded off, or indefinitely postponed; and thus the mere negative treatment of abstention from the exciting cause of the paroxysm may amount to a virtual and final cure.

The first thing to be done on being called to a patient in a paroxysm of asthma, is to ascertain if there is any exciting

M

162   TREATMENT OF ASTHMATIC PAROXYSM.

cause actually present and in operation, and if so to remove it. An undigested meal or a full rectum may, as peripheral irritants, produce bronchial spasm ; the one I think through the pneumogastric nerve, the other through the sympathetic, and thus an emetic which relieves the one, and an enema, (or any other means,) which evacuates the other, may put a stop to the attack. I have previously mentioned a case in which the occurrence of an attack was entirely determined by the loaded or empty condition of the rectum : if the patient retired to bed without the bowels being relieved, he was sure to be awoke in the night with asthma ; if they were moved before going to bed, he awoke at the usual time in the morning well. The relief obtained by an emetic is well known.

At once ascertain then the condition of the patient in these respects, inquire what he last ate and when he ate it, and if his bowels are loaded ; and if there is any source of offence in either situation—stomach or lower bowel—secure its immediate evacuation. Ascertain, too, the state of the air he is breathing, if there is in it any known or unknown irritant, any of those subtle emanations of which asthmatics are so sensible, if there is a hay-field near, or ipecacuanha powder in the room, or dust, or smoke, and if so, let the removal from these influences be the first step taken. Inquire, too, if the patient has ever been seized with an attack in the same place before, if he has had any reason to imagine that that particular air did not agree with him, or if in any local peculiarities it resembles places that he has previously found offend his asthma. If so, get him away at once, never mind how difficult it is to move him, transport him to some place or some *kind* of situation known to agree with him ; very likely before he has gone a mile or two he will be quite well; whereas, all treatment will be powerless as long as he is under the influence of the injurious air.

Let it be your first care, too, to place your patient in a

favourable position ;—get him out of bed and bolster him up in an arm-chair, and place before him a table of convenient height, with a pillow on it, on which he may rest his elbows and throw himself forward. It is quite surprising, almost incredible, how much comfort this will give, and not only so, but how it will actually relieve the breathing and dispose the spasm to yield. Sometimes the patient's breath is so bad that he cannot sit ; the same arrangements must then be made for him in a standing posture.

But if, as will probably be the case, the spasm persists in spite of these preliminary measures, and if no exciting cause can be discovered by whose removal the paroxysm may be at once arrested, our next step is to cast about for some remedy by which we may hope to cut it short. In our choice of this we shall be very much influenced by our patient's former experience. Few asthmatics suffer long from their disease without having discovered what particular remedy is most efficacious in their case, and in this respect different cases of asthma vary so much, and display such a caprice, that I really know of no other guide except the patient's experience.

Of all the different kinds of evidence on which we build our theories of the pathology of diseases, there is none more convincing, or that tells a plainer tale, than that which is derived from therapeutics. The success of a remedy given on certain principles proves the correctness of the principles on which it was given, and the known action of a medicine directly implies the nature of the pathological state that it relieves, as it shows that in any case of its successful administration the pathological state must have been such as that known action would antagonize or correct. This reflected evidence has all the force of the fulfilment of a prediction, like the re-appearance of Halley's comet at the exact time that its discoverer foretold.

M 2

164   TREATMENT BY DEPRESSANTS.

My purpose in this chapter is to direct attention to the great efficacy and value, in the treatment of asthma, of certain drugs belonging to a class whose therapeutical action is very strongly marked, and about whose *modus operandi* there is no doubt, and which throw, therefore, a very clear light on the nature of the pathological condition that they relieve—the class of direct *depressants* or *contra-stimulants*. It is a class of remedies that exercises the most singular and powerful influence over the asthmatic condition, greater and more immediate than any other that I know, except, perhaps, mental emotion. As soon as their characteristic effect is established, the dyspnœa ceases—completely ceases from that moment; no matter how intense the spasm may have been, the moment the sensations characteristic of collapse are felt it yields, the respiration is free, and the patient passes from agony to ease. It is one of the most striking things to witness, in the way of the effect of a remedy, that can be imagined.

The three drugs of this class with whose use in asthma I am most familiar are, ipecacuan, tartar-emetic, and tobacco. No doubt they all act in the same way—by lowering innervation, depressing nervous vitality or irritability, or whatever we may call it, and enfeebling the contraction of the bronchial muscle, just as they weaken the heart's action, or relax the grasp wherewith a strangulated hernia is constricted, or relieve urethral stricture, or the spasm of colic.

With regard to their *modus operandi* in asthma I think a good deal of misconception very generally prevails; they are thought by some to act as emetics, by some as so-called expectorants. I believe they act neither as one nor the other, but as direct depressants, relaxing the spasm of the bronchial tubes in the way I have mentioned. In illustration of this I will just relate a case in which I had ample opportunity for some years of watching the effect of ipecacuanha.

IPECACUANHA. 165

The patient was a youth who had been asthmatic from his infancy. His attacks had increased in frequency till, at the time to which I refer, they occurred with tolerable regularity once a week. His asthma generally awoke him about four or five o'clock in the morning, and soon compelled him to sit up and wheeze in bed, or get out of bed and stand against some piece of furniture for support. In two or three hours he would be able to dress himself, and perhaps in the forenoon the severity of the dyspnœa would a little abate; but towards the afternoon and evening it would deepen, and towards bed-time get so intense that without an emetic there was no chance of sleep. The emetic would be taken, and in half an hour he would be perfectly easy, without the slightest trace of asthma. He would then take a light supper, go to bed, sleep like an infant, and have no more asthma till that day week. In this way he would have fifty attacks, or thereabouts, in a year; and cut them short at night with fifty emetics. If he did not take the emetic he passed a miserable, sleepless night, and was still bad the next day; indeed there was no definite end to the attack without it. I think *now*, that if he had taken it earlier in the day, or even in the morning on first waking up asthmatic, he would have cut short the attack equally well, and have saved himself a great deal of suffering. I never knew it fail. The dose taken was always twenty grains of the ipecacuanha powder; and, although he repeated it so frequently, it neither lost its efficacy nor did him any harm. It was clearly not as an emetic that it acted, but as a depressant, for the relief took place before the vomiting. About ten minutes or a quarter of an hour after swallowing the draught a sense of nausea would be felt, accompanied with a slight faintness, and dampness on the skin, and a profuse secretion of saliva which came from his mouth in a little clear stream. It was then that the spasm gave way, before a single act of retching had occurred; and his attendants would immediately know when the first sense of nausea was felt by the relief of the breathing that invariably accompanied it. Besides, the stomach was always perfectly empty; there was nothing of which it could be relieved.

The effect of *tobacco* is exactly the same, only the depression that it produces is more profound and amounts to actual collapse, and the relief, therefore, more speedy and complete. In those who have not established a tolerance of tobacco, its use is soon followed by a well-known condition of collapse, much resembling sea-sickness—vertigo, loss of power in the limbs, a sense of deadly faintness, cold sweat, inability to speak or think, nausea, vomiting. The moment this condition can be induced the asthma ceases, as if stopped by a charm. In one case in particular I have frequently watched its effects. In the case that I refer to the asthmatic fortunately never established a tolerance of the drug, and thirty whiffs of a pipe or half a cigar would at any time induce a condition of collapse. I have known him begin to smoke when his breathing has been so difficult that he could hardly draw his pipe; he would draw a feeble whiff or two and then stop to recover his breath, and then another whiff, and so on. By and by he would lay down his pipe with a look of intelligence at his attendant, as much as to say, "it's all right now;" his face would become pallid and damp with perspiration, his limbs relaxed, his breathing long and sighing,—but his asthma was gone. His object was to smoke just so much as to produce this condition, and no more, so that the moment he felt the sensation coming on he stopped. After this qualmy condition had continued for twenty minutes or half an hour, it would go off and leave him well—the attack cured. Sometimes, however, he would take a little too much, and then the operation of the drug would go on to vomiting, and sometimes he would overdo it altogether, and produce a deadly and protracted collapse, from which it seemed as if he would never recover. I have known his pulse hardly perceptible for nearly two hours, in spite of ammonia and brandy freely administered. It is this circumstance—the fear of this horrible and unmanageable collapse —that makes one so unwilling to employ tobacco; it is indeed a dreadful remedy, almost as bad as the disease ; but the asthmatic is willing to undergo anything to get quit of his sufferings.

The following account, illustrative of the effect of tobacco, I have received from an intelligent patient long subject to severe asthma :—

" I have always found perfect relief from smoking tobacco in the attacks of spasmodic asthma to which I have been liable. In describing my own experience, I should say that no relief is felt till the poison gives evidence of having taken effect by its disagreeable consequences; and just in proportion to the sickness and faintness and other miserable sensations, is the relief of the difficult breathing. I never knew this remedy fail. As the use of tobacco was new to me it affected me very powerfully, and produced the most miserable prostration and faintness. The cure of the asthmatic spasm was very speedy, and frequently it was forgotten altogether in the horrors of a sensation known to all novices in smoking, so that I was often unconscious of its disappearance, or of the mode or time of its departure; the asthma seemed supplanted by another condition, and cold perspiration and fear of collapse closed the scene. I am not aware whether this was followed by expectoration, and the presence of mucus in the throat removed by the usual process—the common action of ' clearing the throat,' as it is called— which invariably appears when an attack of asthma spontaneously subsides, and which always accompanies the slower cure resulting from the mild use of ipecacuanha, which of late years I have preferred to tobacco, as my asthma is not of sufficient intensity to require so violent and distressing a remedy. I imagine these more natural and ordinary symptoms of recovery would always accompany the use of ipecacuanha, and that an increased dose would only accelerate the process of recovery up to the interruption by vomiting. The difference between the characteristics of these two modes of cure appears to me to be strongly marked and very important. I conceive this to arise from the intensity of the depression caused by the poison of tobacco, which cannot be the case in the use of ipecacuanha, as it is a simple emetic, and I doubt if the same kind of sensations and depression could be produced by ipecacuanha, even if its effect could be carried on and the medicine were not rejected by the stomach, which is invariably the case when the effect is increased to a certain point. I have not gone beyond the stage of perspiration and a feeling of sickness, and I have always found the cure to resemble the natural process of mucous discharge and clearing of the air-passages, only more promptly induced and more rapidly performed. I have frequently had short spasms of asthma produced by laughing, lighting a lucifer-match, or some other special irritant, from which I have recovered as rapidly as when under the influence of ipecacuanha, going through the stages of silent asthma, audible asthma, and the expectoration mentioned above, in about the space of ten minutes or a quarter of an hour. The distinction between these two modes of cure or relief is worthy the attention of medical men and their patients, as much distress and perhaps injurious results might be avoided if the ipecacuanha is found to be as efficacious as tobacco. My only doubt is whether tobacco might not be preferable in desperate and suffocating spasms on account of its speedy and violent action.''

No doubt there is such a difference as that indicated

above in the action of tobacco and ipecacuan. Ipecacuan, I think, could never produce such collapse as that caused by tobacco; but that it does not always act as an expectorant or emetic, but as a direct depressant, is shown by the case that I related just now. The fact is, ipecacuan acts very differently on different individuals: in some, producing vomiting with little more irritation than sulphate of zinc; in some, producing collapse to a considerable degree. Moreover, by relaxing the bronchial spasm, it renders free cough and expectoration possible, which were previously impossible from inability to get sufficient air into the lungs to effect them; so that the expectoration is the consequence of the relief, and not the relief of the expectoration.

In that mild but annoying form of asthma that accompanies the other symptoms of hay-fever, and is known as hay-asthma, tobacco pushed *ad nauseam* gives more relief than any other remedy. In a relative of mine who is very much afflicted with this troublesome complaint, tobacco-smoking is the only thing that gives any relief. During the hay season and all the early hot summer weather, he suffers (besides the sneezing and running at the eyes, and tumid burning of the nose and throat, characteristic of hay-fever) from paroxysms of a wheezing dyspnœa of the true asthmatic type, coming on exclusively at night, so as almost to deprive him of sleep. During the rest of the year he never smokes, as it is disagreeable to him, and in other respects prejudicial; but during this season he is quite dependent on his cigar for any degree of comfort or alleviation of his symptoms. The following graphic account of the relief he finds from tobacco I cannot do better than give in his own words:—

" There is no remedy during a paroxysm of hay-asthma that has anything like the effect of smoking tobacco; and though this is especially the case in the latter stage of the

170   TREATMENT BY DEPRESSANTS.

attack, when the asthmatic element of the phenomena is most developed, still in the earlier stage, when the lachrymation, sneezing, and faucial irritation are most distressing, tobacco-smoke has, in my case, a very marked influence in soothing and diminishing these symptoms.

" No doubt any of those medicines which Dr. Pereira has called ' *cardiaco-vascular depressants*' would produce a somewhat similar result; but none is of so easy application, or can be used so readily or pleasantly as tobacco. During the hay-asthma season—that is, in my case, from about the 15th of May to the 10th or 12th of July—I regularly smoke a cigar the last thing before going to bed, or perhaps more frequently after I am in bed. The effect is, that (excepting during the last fortnight in June, when I never get a night's rest) the sedative influence of the tobacco prevents the occurrence of any asthmatic spasm. If during this period I omit my cigar, I seldom sleep beyond four o'clock; usually three o'clock finds me awake, hopelessly, though generally only slightly, asthmatic for the rest of the night; till, indeed, about nine o'clock, when almost always the asthma completely leaves me. This night-cigar is taken as a preventive. But tobacco will cure the asthmatic spasm when it is fairly on; only it requires a larger dose of the poison and in a stronger form. The sedative influence of the cigar will usually ensure me a fair night's rest; but the powerful depression of strong shag-tobacco is necessary to cut short the spasm when it is established. Even when I do smoke my night-cigar I not unfrequently have to get up about three or four o'clock in the morning and smoke; and during the last fortnight in June this happens almost nightly.

" Distressing as are the sensations of collapse from tobacco-poisoning, they are an unspeakable relief when contrasted with the impending suffocation of asthma. I shall never

TOBACCO. 171

forget an attack which I once had, and the joy with which I hailed the approach of collapse from tobacco-poisoning. It was late in July, many years ago. I had gone into Dorsetshire to stay with a relative in a country house. Immediately surrounding the house were grazing fields—not hay-fields—and they had not been mown. In these fields was a grass—*Nardus stricta*, I think—still blooming luxuriantly; for it is a grass which cattle will not eat; and thus, though past the usual time for hay-asthma, I was accidentally surrounded by its most potent cause—grass in flower. The night came, and I had not been an hour in bed when I was attacked with the most violent asthma I ever experienced. There were no cigars in the house; but one of the servants had some rank shag-tobacco. I smoked one pipe, then another; and as my face blanched, and my pulse failed, and the cold sweat stood on my forehead, miserable as were the sensations of collapse, they were Paradise to the agonies of suffocation. I shall never forget those moments of relief.

" The story of this attack of asthma, by the way, is a very instructive one; and I may just add it here, in brief:—I left my friend's house the day after this paroxysm, and went to the sea-side, where I was as usual perfectly well. Two days after, I received a letter from him asking me to return, as he had had the grass, in flower about his house, cut down. I did so, and remained with him a fortnight, sleeping every night as placidly as an infant. The *Nardus stricta* had given me the asthma: the scythe had cured it.

" To return to the tobacco. A hay asthmatic should never smoke tobacco but for his malady. Smoking should never be to him a habit or a meal, for it then ceases to be a medicine. Indeed to him it should be as a deadly drug, for it is by poisoning that it cures."

Not long ago I was conversing on the subject of his ma-

172   TREATMENT BY DEPRESSANTS.

lady with a surgeon of some distinction in this city who is grievously victimized with hay-asthma, and on asking him what he found do him any good, he replied, "Tobacco; tobacco is the only thing; nothing does me any good but smoking;" and he went on to tell me, that whenever he finds his asthma very bad, and that he shall get no sleep without it, he immediately resorts to a cigar. But the smoking does him no good unless it produces a condition of collapse; the mere sedative effect of it is of no use to him whatever; and having lost, from the habit of smoking, an easy susceptibility to tobacco influence, he adopts the following device to secure its more potent effect: he fills his mouth with tobacco-smoke, and then, instead of breathing it out again at once, as is usual in smoking, retains it in his mouth for several seconds, perhaps a quarter of a minute, then takes another mouthful, and so on. In this way, he finds that the tobacco is more rapidly absorbed by the mucus membrane of the oral cavity, and that a state of collapse is speedily induced. The moment the faintness and sickness come over him the asthma ceases, he turns into bed, and has a good night.

The effect of antimony nearly resembles that of tobacco, and it acts in the same way, but the nausea and collapse it produces are long and tedious.

Of the three drugs, I should say ipecacuanha is the most manageable, and entails the least suffering; tobacco the most speedy and effectual.

There are one or two practical points on which I would add a few words.

Remedies of this kind, given with the view of cutting short the paroxysm, should be given as early as possible; and for two reasons. First, because it is much easier to break through the asthmatic condition when it is but just established, while the longer it is allowed to go on, the more in-

IMPORTANCE OF EARLY ADMINISTRATION.   173

veterate and uncontrollable it becomes, and the more difficult
it is to arrest it; indeed its giving way at all may depend
on the earliness with which the remedy is applied.   I have
known treatment powerless after the dyspnœa has continued
for some hours, which never failed if administered as soon
as it declared itself.   Just at starting, in the earliest stages
of the paroxysm, a very slight thing will determine its advance or retreat, and in proportion as it advances and deepens,
in just such proportion do remedies become inoperative.   The
other reason is, that if the spasm *does* yield in spite of
having been some time established, the recovery is not so
complete as if the remedy had been applied immediately on
its appearance.   The longer the bronchial stricture lasts, the
greater is the arrears of breathing and the resulting pulmonary congestion; and if this goes on unchecked and increasing for many hours the disturbance of the vascular balance
becomes so great, the capillaries of the lungs so loaded, that
it is a long time, many hours, or perhaps even days, before
that balance is restored, and the vessels recover their normal
condition : and although the bronchial spasm may completely
give way, there remains a certain amount of shortness of
breath and an incapacity for exertion, and it is not until an
abundant expectoration of mucus has taken place, by the
pouring out of which the loaded vessels have relieved themselves, that the chest becomes clear and the breathing free.
In asthma at once cut short there is no such accumulated
congestion—no mucous exudation, and when the bronchial
spasm ceases all dyspnœa vanishes.   If on first awaking with
the sensations of asthma the asthmatic nauseates himself
with tobacco, or smokes his nitre-paper, or keeps himself in
a standing posture, or in any other way cuts short the
paroxysm, he will be throughout the succeeding day exactly
the same, with the exception of the sleep he has lost, as if
nothing had occurred; but if he suffers the fight between

174   TREATMENT BY DEPRESSANTS.

asthma and sleep to go on long, and then on the first remission of the dyspnœa lies back and goes to sleep, he will pro-
tract the asthmatic state, deepen the consequent pulmonary
arrears, and not only postpone his recovery for many hours,
but make it then slow and imperfect.   I know an asthmatic
who now never loses a day by his disease, in consequence of
the promptitude with which he meets its first appearance in
the early morning, but who formerly, from continuing to lie
in bed and try to get sleep after the asthma had begun,
protracted his sufferings through the day.   He is attacked
as often as ever, and at the same time—about three or four
o'clock in the morning—but the moment he finds his asthma
on him he takes measures to keep himself wide awake,
stands leaning against a piece of furniture, and, if necessary,
induces tobacco collapse, so that instead of a day's asthma
he has half an hour's, and, as far as all the engagements of
life go, has ceased to be an asthmatic.

It is a difficult thing for the asthmatic, I know, over-
whelmed with sleep as he is, and generally with a peculiarly
heavy drowsiness upon him, to leave his bed or light and
smoke his pipe; but he *must* do it; he must rouse himself
fairly up and adopt at once those remedies that in his particular case are most efficacious.   In fact, the treatment of the
asthmatic paroxysm should be so prompt as to be almost
rather preventive than curative: in the treatment of no
disease is the injunction "*obsta principiis*" of more vital
importance.

One is sometimes asked—Which is the best form of
tobacco to use, a cigar or a pipe?   I think a pipe has the
advantage of more certain strength; cigars vary so much,
even the same sort.   The tobacco that I generally employ
is bird's-eye, as being a mild tobacco, and one by which you
run little risk of inducing alarming collapse.   *Shag*, or any
other of the strong tobaccos, should not be used by the uninitiated, as the collapse they produce is apt to become pro-

tracted and unmanageable. For ladies and young children, a few whiffs of a mild cigarette are quite sufficient.*

Of ipecacuanha, I think the powder is better than the wine. I never give a very small dose, it is uncertain and teasing. I would say, always give such a dose as will be certain to secure its own prompt rejection. I never give less than twenty grains, however young the patient may be: it never does harm.

But ipecacuanha is a nauseous thing, and to those who have frequently taken it as an emetic it becomes almost intolerable. I have lately discovered that it may be taken very pleasantly and very efficaciously in the form of some strong ipecacuanha lozenges made by Messrs. Corbyn, of 300, Holborn. They are about four times the strength of ordinary ipecacuanha lozenges; three of them will produce prompt vomiting. They are very convenient, too, for keeping up a slight nausea; and for children they are invaluable. If vomiting is desired, they should be bitten and ground up in the mouth and swallowed at once.

---

* In an old number of the Lancet (vol. ii. 1837) I have met with the following notice of the beneficial administration of tobacco in asthma in the form of a tincture :—

" In disordered respiration tobacco obtained the well-merited confidence of the older physicians in cases where no organic alteration had occurred. It has, however, nearly fallen into neglect, from which state it will most probably revive, for it has lately been tried to a very great extent, and with no small success, under a false name. At the time that the *Lobelia inflata* was the subject of great panegyric, and that clinical lectures appeared in the periodicals, extolling its virtues in asthma, there was not a particle of it in the drug market. One firm, at the head of which was a shrewd, intelligent, practical man, had formerly had great experience of tobacco, and he proclaimed that his house was the sole mart for Lobelia; he made a spirituous tincture of the tobacco, which he supplied to the trade, pretty freely, and it became a great favourite of the profession. My own experience led me to its frequent employment; nor did I discover for some time the artifice which had been practised. It, however, induced me to place great reliance on an æthereal tincture of tobacco to mitigate the paroxysms of spasmodic asthma."

176   TREATMENT BY DEPRESSANTS.

There is one circumstance that greatly detracts from the utility of tobacco in the treatment of asthma, that practically indeed almost destroys it. Our adult male population have so habituated themselves to its use, that they have lost the susceptibility to its full influence, and cannot induce complete collapse by any amount of smoking. Now adult males constitute by far the majority of the subjects of spasmodic asthma; and thus the habit of smoking has rendered powerless, in a large number of cases, what I think may, without any qualification, be called its most potent remedy.

To the practical I need not apologize for these trifling hints, of which I know they will recognise the value.

177

CHAPTER IX.

TREATMENT OF THE ASTHMATIC PAROXYSM (*continued.*)—
TREATMENT BY STIMULANTS.

Theory of the *modus operandi* of stimulants.—Illustrated by coffee.—
Curative influence of violent emotion.—Its action analogous to that of
stimulants.—It acts also as a " nervous derivative."—Cases.

ONE of the commonest and best-reputed remedies of asthma,
one that is almost sure to have been tried in any case that
may come under our observation, and one that in some cases
is more efficacious than any other, is strong coffee. To the
question, " Have you tried strong coffee?" the asthmatic is
pretty sure to answer, " Yes ;" and he is also pretty sure to
add that it gives him relief.

About the *modus operandi* of this remedy I was long
puzzled ; I could not make it out; and it is only lately that
I think I have stumbled upon it. The *rationale* of its efficacy is, I think, to be found, on the one hand, in the
physiological effects of coffee,—the particular nervous condition that it produces,—and, on the other, in a feature
in the clinical history of asthma which I have long observed,
and of which I think the efficacy of coffee is highly
corroborative.

This fact is, that *sleep favours asthma*—that spasm of the
bronchial tubes is more prone to occur during the insensibility and lethargy of sleep than during the waking hours
when the senses and the will are active. I have already referred to this in the chapter on the Clinical History of

N

178   TREATMENT BY STIMULANTS.

Asthma, in describing the phenomena of the paroxysm, and in explaining why the attack invariably (or almost invariably) chooses the hours of mid-sleep for its onset. Let me just refer to this subject again ; for it is both interesting and important, as it explains a curious and very constant phenomenon in asthma—the hour, namely, of the attack,—is highly illustrative of its pathology, and furnishes the key to some of its treatment.

I think, then, that sleep favours the development of asthma in two ways—

1. By producing insensibility to respiratory arrears.

2. By exalting reflex action.

That sleep *does* exalt reflex nervous action there can be no doubt. It is a fact so abundantly inculcated by the history of disease as hardly to require illustration or proof. The phenomena of epilepsy, cramp, lead tremors, and other examples of deranged muscular action, all teach it. It is just as sleep comes on, just as the will is laid to rest, or during sleep, that these different forms of involuntary muscular contraction most commonly occur. Any one, to convince himself of it, has only to fall asleep sitting on the edge of his chair, in such a position that it shall press on his sciatic nerves. As long as he is awake his legs will be motionless ; but the moment he falls asleep they will start up with a plunge and suddenly wake him. As soon as he is awake they are quiet and still again, with no disposition to start, till he again falls asleep, and that moment they start again and wake him; and so he may go on as long as he likes. He changes his position, sits back in his chair, and they start no more. I need not explain what so clearly explains itself. I heard, some years ago, of a case of what might be called chronic traumatic tetanus, in which the source of irritation—the excito-motory stimulant—was extensive disease of the hip-joint. The moment the patient fell asleep he was seized with opisthotonos, which, of course, immediately awoke him. On awakening the tetanus vanished; on again falling asleep it re-appeared; and this alternation of falling asleep and waking continued for weeks, if not for months, the patient getting no continuous rest, till he was quite worn out. As long as he was broad awake the tetanus never appeared.* Hosts of similar facts, illustrative of the same truth, might be cited.

Anything that exalts reflex nervous action increases, of course, the potency of reflex stimuli. Now, I have elsewhere endeavoured to show that the phenomena of asthma are, in almost every case, those of excito-motory action, and that the exciting causes of asthma are, in the great majority of instances, such as act by a reflex circuit. They would, therefore, on the asthmatic's falling asleep, immediately acquire a potency they did not before possess, just as the pressure on the sciatic nerve did in the illustration I have given. Thus it is we see that the asthmatic may gorge himself with unwholesomes, and yet, as long as he keeps himself awake, suffer no consequential asthma;—the irritant is there, the undigested food is in the stomach, but as long as he is awake, as long as the will is dominant, it is inadequate to the production of reflex phenomena. But let him fall asleep, and in an hour or two the paroxysm will be established.

And not only will *sound sleep* determine, by this exaltation of reflex susceptibility, the production of asthma by its exciting causes, but a small dose of the same condition— sleepiness, drowsiness—will favour the supervention of asthma

* I was further informed, respecting this case, that, after everything else had failed, sleep was procured, with an immunity from the tetanic spasms, by putting the patient into the mesmeric state. In this way he got rest, and greatly improved; but what was the ultimate issue of the case I do not know.

N 2

180　　　TREATMENT BY STIMULANTS.

in a proportionate degree. Not only is drowsiness a pre-monitory sign of an attack, but a powerful predisposer to it; and the asthmatic knows that he yields to it at his peril. I have often noticed in asthmatics that the sleepiness that is so apt to come on after dinner will be accompanied by a slight asthmatic oppression and wheezing : as the drowsiness deepens, so does the asthma, and in this way it may settle down into an attack; but if the patient rouses himself, or if anything occurs to engross his attention so as to wake him up, broad awake, the asthma quickly vanishes. It is in this way, I think, that is to be explained the fact, that asthmatics can dine out late and unwholesomely with impunity, while if they dine at the same time and in the same way at home, asthma is sure to come on. At home they want that excite-ment which at a dinner-party keeps the animal functions in a state of exaltation and the mind vividly awake, and effectually banishes the least approach to drowsiness. Of the fact there is not the slightest doubt. I know an asthmatic who can with impunity dine out at seven o'clock, as dinner-eaters of the nineteenth century are apt to dine—shirk nothing from soup to coffee—walk home at eleven o'clock, a distance perhaps of four miles, with the wind of a deer-stalker—go straight to bed, and get up the next morning scathless; but if he were to dine at home at six, or even at five o'clock, he would be wheezing at nine, and by four the next morning downright asthmatic.

I believe a certain amount of the curative influence of fright, or other strong mental emotion, is to be explained in the same way.

" But why," it may be asked, " all this round-about digres-sion ? What has all this to do with the curative influence of coffee?" I believe it is simply its explanation. For, what are the physiological effects of coffee? They consist in the production of a state of mental activity and vivacity, of acuteness of perception and energy of volition, well known to those who have experienced it, and to a certain extent very pleasurable, and which is the very reverse of that abeyance of will and perception which, in drowsiness or sleep, so favours the development of asthma. In sleep, will and sense are suspended ; after taking strong coffee, they are not only active, but exalted. It produces rapidity of thought, vivacity of spirits, clearness of apprehension, greatly increases the working powers, and altogether intensifies mental processes. Not only is there no disposition to sleep, but sleep is impossible : the thoughts hurry one another through the mind ; the bodily movements are energetic and rapid ; and if the effects of the drug are pushed far, a very unpleasant condition is produced, something like that of delirium tremens, *minus* its hallucinations. Now, if the suspension of the will, or its depression, favours the production of excito-motory phenomena, and thus favours the development of asthma, is it unreasonable to suppose that its exaltation should prevent or cure it ? It *must* do so—if not positively, at least negatively, by removing the predisposing condition. And bearing in mind this marked physiological effect of coffee—that this exaltation of the animal nervous functions is exactly what it produces—it certainly does seem to me reasonable to suppose that this is its *modus operandi*. And if of coffee, then of strong tea, and alcohol, and ammonia, and Indian hemp, and ether, and other stimulants of undoubted value in asthma.

To show that this is the *rationale* of the cure of asthma by stimulants I do not think it is necessary to show that it is only when the asthmatic is drowsy, or has been sleeping, that they do good. If anything that rouses the asthmatic to a state of wakefulness will put a stop to asthma that was creeping on him while he was sleeping or sleepy, *à fortiori* anything that carries him beyond a state of mere wakeful-

182   TREATMENT BY STIMULANTS.

ness—that gives him an active, not a mere passive wakefulness—will be still more efficacious, and will be adequate to
the checking of an attack that, in spite of his being broad
awake, was gaining on him.

The very frequency with which coffee gives relief makes
it hardly worth while for me to narrate the history of any
cases.   I should think, from my own experience, that coffee
relieves asthma in two-thirds of the cases in which it is tried.
The relief is very unequal, often merely temporary, and sometimes very slight : sometimes it is complete and permanent.
It is often taken in the morning ; and patients will tell you,
that previous to taking their coffee they are not fit for anything, can hardly move about ; but that taking it is immediately followed by freedom of breathing, and an ability to
enter at once on their daily occupations.

There are two or three practical hints with regard to the
administration of coffee that are worth bearing in mind.

1. It cannot be given too strong.   Unless sufficiently
strong to produce its characteristic physiological effects it
does no good, but rather harm ; moreover, if given very
strong it need not be given in much bulk, and quantity is a
disadvantage—its effect is less rapid, and it oppressively
distends the stomach.

2. I think it is best given without sugar and milk—pure
café noir.

3. It should be given on an empty stomach ; if given on
a full stomach it often does great harm, by putting a stop to
the process of digestion : indeed, so much is this the case
that I consider coffee accompanying a meal, especially late
in the day, so peculiarly apt to induce asthma, that it
deserves to be classed among its special provocatives.   I
have mentioned elsewhere the case of an individual who
never dared to take the usual after-dinner cup of coffee—it
would make the simplest dinner disagree with him.   But

EMOTION A STIMULANT. 183

the same asthmatic found in strong coffee, on an *empty stomach*, one of his most valuable remedies.*

4. For some reason or other, I do not know why, it seems to act better if given hot—very hot.

I adverted just now to the influence of mental emotion on asthma, and stated my belief that its *modus operandi* was, like that of coffee and other stimulants, by producing an exaltation of sense and will—an intense activity of the intellectual part of nervous action—and proportionately lessening the tendency to excito-motion; and this it does to a much greater degree than stimulant remedies, and its effects are, therefore, proportionately more sudden and complete. It was, indeed, the curative influence of violent emotion, and the observation that it and coffee-taking alike banish that condition in which asthma is most prone to come on, that first suggested to my mind the theory of the action of stimulants on asthma that I have just endeavoured to propound. I think, too, that mental emotion acts, if I may so express it, as a nervous derivative. There are many phenomena,

* Since writing the above I have received the following account, from an asthmatic gentleman, singularly confirmatory of my own observations.— " I used to think," writes my informant, " strong coffee the best of all remedies. I remember one instance especially, only a pattern of many others, but more striking when told. With bent back, high shoulders, and elbows fixed on the chair-arms, I had been labouring for breath all the afternoon. About five o'clock I had two breakfast-cups of strong coffee. The hard breathing disappeared rapidly and completely. My sisters were dancing in the next room, and in less than an hour I was dancing with them, quite free from asthma. Of late, coffee has often had an opposite effect upon me. The after-dinner cup of coffee, to which I have been for several years habituated, now produces a sensation of stuffing of the chest, and incapacity of moving about. I believe this is because it stops digestion; and the reason I did not suffer for some years I take to be, that my originally most excellent and enduring stomach could stand it so long, and no longer. Coffee, on an empty stomach, I still deem a most valuable remedy. I do not share the prejudice against putting milk and sugar into coffee that is used as a medicine, provided that it remain *café noir*, and be not made *café au lait*."

184   TREATMENT BY STIMULANTS.

both in health and disease, that seem to show that only a
certain amount of nervous activity can be in operation at a
certain time, and that if a nervous action of one kind comes
into operation, another that had been previously going on is
immediately depressed or arrested.   Such is the explanation
of the well-known experiment of the two dogs, one of which
was taken hunting immediately after a meal, while the other
was allowed to sleep.   In the one that was taken hunting,
digestion, on its return, was found hardly commenced; in
the other, it was completely over, and the stomach empty.
In the sleeping dog the whole vital dynamics, not being
otherwise employed, were appropriated by the function of
digestion; while in the hunting dog they were entirely taken
up by its energetic locomotion, and drafted away, as it were,
from that nervous superintendence of digestion without which
the function cannot be carried on.*   The power of strong
emotion, or hard study, in retarding digestion, is an analogous
fact.   Just in the same way, I think, the extraordinary
activity and exaltation of thought and perception, that
characterise the state of mind that the taking of coffee,
ether, Indian hemp, and other stimulants produces, act as a
nervous derivative in asthma, and divert from the nervous
system of the lungs that morbid activity which engenders the
spasm of the bronchial tubes.

The cure of asthma by violent emotion is more sudden
and complete than by any other remedy whatever; indeed, I
know few things more striking and curious in the whole
history of therapeutics.   The remedy that stands next in
speed and efficacy—tobacco pushed to collapse—takes time, a
few minutes at leàst: but the cure of asthma by sudden

* See Dr. John Reid's experiments, in Todd's *Cyclopædia of Anatomy*,
vol. iii. p. 899; also those of Bernard and of Bischoff, in Müller's *Archiv.*
1843.

alarm takes *no* time; it is instantaneous, the intensest paroxysm ceases on the instant. This is a fact so little known, as far as I can see, and yet so practically important and theoretically interesting, that I think it will not be unprofitable if I endeavour to impress it more deeply by the narration of some cases of its occurrence.

CASE I.—A gentleman suffering an unusually severe attack, so bad that he had been unable to speak or move all day, was suddenly alarmed by the illness of a relative: he ran down two flights of stairs and up again, and administered the restoratives he had procured, and then observed, to his astonishment, that his asthma was gone. This gentleman tells me, that on many other occasions different forms of mental emotion have cured his asthma.

CASE II.—C. R., a confirmed asthmatic, states that when he was suffering from an unusually severe attack a fire occurred just opposite his house. Previous to the occurrence of the fire he was in bed, breathing with the greatest difficulty, and unable to move. When the excitement of the fire was over, he found that he had been standing in his nightshirt, looking with others out of the window, and that he had forgotten all about his asthma. His breath was not quite well the rest of the day, but nearly so. On another occasion, when he was suffering from an attack, some sudden anxiety arose about two of the members of his family being out late: the alarm from which he suffered relieved his asthma, but not so suddenly as in the case of the fire. On another occasion, a sister of his was seized with sudden illness that seemed to threaten suffocation: he was suffering severely from asthma at the time, and was in bed; he jumped out of bed in great alarm, and found then that his asthma was perfectly cured. He was sufficiently well to run for a doctor, and continued well throughout the day.

186   TREATMENT BY STIMULANTS.

CASE III.—Not long ago I was informed by a patient at the hospital, who had suffered greatly for many years, that however severe an attack might be, venereal excitement would almost invariably cure it. He told me also, that, when a youth, he had been guilty of the practice of onanism, and that the unnatural excitement thereby produced had just the same curative effect on his asthma. Indeed, he pleaded this effect of it as a sort of excuse for the practice; and assured me that when his breath was very bad at night he used to resort to it for the purpose of curing it.

I have known two or three cases in which sexual excitement has had just the same effect.

CASE IV.—The following account of the curative influence of mental excitement I have received from a medical friend, who has suffered from asthma all his life:—" On one occasion I was sitting with fixed elbows on a sofa, breathing hard: a lady came into the room whom I knew very well, and whom I had not seen for several years. I got up to receive her, and sat down again on a music-stool; with no especial purchase, therefore, for the respiratory muscles, and yet with comparative ease of breathing. This ease lasted for about an hour, and then the difficulty of breathing came on again. I attribute the temporary amendment to the diversion of nervous energy. Just the same thing has happened to me more than once.—On another occasion I was suffering a good deal at a farm-house. I got on horseback with some difficulty, and an anxious hope that the horse would go quietly, to fetch myself an emetic from a town three miles off. The horse ran away with me. I pulled in, at first weakly and almost despairingly, but the need of exertion brought the power: after a run of about a mile I succeeded in pulling up, and was delighted to find my asthma gone.— Another time I was breathing very hard, and a friend engaged me in an argument. At first I could only get out

SUMMARY CONCLUSIONS. 187

a sentence in successive gasps ; but gradually, as I got excited, the hard breathing went off, and I could talk fluently."*

From the foregoing observations, then, I think we may conclude—

That, since the abeyance of the will favours, in proportion to the degree of that abeyance, the development of asthma, and since the effect of strong coffee is to dispel such suspension or depression of volition and restore the will to its wonted (or even an unwonted) activity, it is by thus exalting the will, and so disfavouring the development of excito-motory action, that this remedy relieves asthma.

That the same interpretation applies to the relief of asthma by all other stimulants whatever.

That thus strong coffee and mental excitement, although apparently so different, belong to the same category of remedies for asthma.

* For additional cases of the cure of asthma by mental emotion, I must refer the reader to Chapter II. on the Pathology of Asthma.

1S8

CHAPTER X.

TREATMENT OF THE ASTHMATIC PAROXYSM (*continued.*)— TREATMENT BY SEDATIVES.

Their number and value.—Tobacco.—Chloroform : its varying efficacy.—
Caution with regard to its use.—Opium.—The objections to it.—Stramonium : its unequal value.—Cases.—Its various preparations and
modes of exhibition.— Practical rules.—Lobelia.—Indian hemp.—
Ether.

THE recognition of the nervous nature of asthma; of the paroxysmal character of its symptoms ; of the fact that the air-
passages were in a state of spasm ; that a part at least of its
essential pathology appeared to be a morbid susceptibility to
certain stimuli ; that many of its exciting causes were such as
exalted nervous irritability ; that the subjects of it were commonly individuals of quick and mobile nervous systems ;—
these, and analogous considerations, long ago suggested the
use of sedatives both for the prevention and alleviation of
the asthmatic paroxysm.

The *modus operandi* of sedatives, both in the cure and
prevention of asthma, is doubtless by allaying nervous irritability ; destroying for the time that morbid sensitiveness of
the pulmonary nervous system that constitutes so essential a
part of the disease.   And whilst, on the one hand, it is the
nervous theory of asthma that has suggested the use of
sedatives, their efficacy on the other,—the immediate and
perfect relief that follows the use of some of them,—is among
the best proofs we have of the correctness of this nervous interpretation of the phenomena of the disease.

TOBACCO. 189

Of all the classes of remedies used in asthma, I think that sedatives constitute the most numerous. I wish I could say that they excelled others in efficacy as much as they do in numbers. But they are of very unequal power; for while one or two of them are of very great value, others appear to be of little worth, and some even prejudicial. Chloroform, for example, is, in my opinion, one of the most valuable remedies for asthma that we possess; the inhalation of its vapour putting a stop to the asthmatic paroxysm more speedily and more certainly than anything else I know. Opium, on the other hand, I have found, as far as my experience has gone, positively worthless.

Moreover, with regard to sedatives, asthma exhibits very strongly its characteristic caprice;—stramonium smoking is, to some patients, an infallible cure, while others might just as well smoke so much sawdust, and not only receive no benefit, but experience no result of any kind from it.

The principal remedies of this class are :—

I. Tobacco, in sedative doses; II. Chloroform; III. Opium; IV. Stramonium; V. Lobelia; VI. Indian Hemp; VII. Ether, in sedative doses.

Of some of these I have had very little practical experience. I will speak of those of which I have, and first of—

I. Tobacco.—I have, in a previous paper, spoken of tobacco as a depressant. But tobacco as a sedative is quite another thing. The dose is different; the physiological effects are different; the principle of the cure is entirely different. In smoking with the view of producing depression, the individual must be unaccustomed to the drug, or the tobacco very strong, or the dose very large; in smoking for sedation none of these is necessary. For tobacco to cure asthma as a depressant it must produce collapse; as a sedative it merely produces that composing and tranquillizing con-

On Asthma: its Pathology and Treatment. *Salter HH*

190   TREATMENT BY SEDATIVES.

dition with which smokers are so familiar. As a depressant it renders spasm impossible by knocking down nervous power (doubtless by poisoning the nervous centres); as a sedative, by temporarily effacing a morbid sensitiveness to certain stimuli, and inducing a normal indifference and tolerance of them. Any one may experience the sedative effects of tobacco, and all smokers do habitually; but the production of its full depressant action is almost impossible in those who have long accustomed themselves to its use; in others, however, as in women and children, it is so easy, that the difficulty is to prevent sedation from running into depression. It is for this reason that it is necessary, in administering tobacco as a sedative only, to the uninitiated, the delicate, or the young, to give the very mildest form, in carefully measured quantities, and to insist on its slow and deliberate exhibition.

It is of the sedative use alone of tobacco that I am now speaking.

Asthmatics are very commonly smokers, and many of them find in the habit an almost unfailing antidote to their disease. But in almost all the cases that I have met with, it is rather as a prophylactic that it is used,—to secure immunity when under dangerous circumstances, or to meet the first threatenings of an attack,—than as a veritable curative to cut short spasm.

II. Chloroform.—One of the most powerful and speediest remedies which we possess for asthma, to which I should, perhaps, give the first place of all, is chloroform. It is, of course, a comparatively recent remedy; but its marked physiological effects early suggested its appropriateness, and the result has fully justified the trial. I have not had many opportunities of witnessing its effects personally, because when asthmatic patients consult one they are generally not

CHLOROFORM. 191

suffering from the disease at the time; but in the cases in which I have witnessed it I have been very much struck with the completeness of the control which it exercises over the asthmatic condition, and with the absence of all danger in its administration, provided the asthma is of the uncomplicated spasmodic form. If the only source of dyspnœa is bronchial spasm it seems to me that it may be as safely given to an asthmatic in the height of a paroxysm as to a healthy person.

I shall not easily forget the first case in which I administered it. A poor woman was brought into King's College Hospital at the time that I was house-physician there, supposed to be dying by those who brought her in. She was quite unable to move, and could barely speak; but it was easy to perceive, from the violent action of the respiratory muscles and the loud wheezing that accompanied it, that the suffocation from which she was suffering was of the asthmatic kind. I at once administered chloroform. After a few whiffs the spasm began to yield, and before I had given her enough to make her insensible it had quite subsided and her breathing was free. In ten minutes after entering it she left the hospital—well.

Even in asthma with bronchitis I have known it, if carefully administered, of great service, by getting rid of the asthmatic element of the dyspnœa, and so putting a stop to one of the sources of suffering, and one of the causes of pulmonary congestion and bronchial exudation; and at the same time, by relaxing the constricted air-passages, facilitating the discharge of the accumulated mucus. In chronic bronchitis I have seen at least half of the dyspnœa vanish on its administration, showing how much of the symptoms were due to spasm. I think its usefulness in these cases has been overlooked, and that if carefully and tentatively given it

On Asthma: Its Pathology and Treatment. *Salter HH*

192   TREATMENT BY SEDATIVES.

might be tried in them without risk. Certainly for the time the patient is placed under much better circumstances, even as far as the bronchitis goes.

The sooner it is given after the commencement of an attack the better, for if the spasm has existed for some time it is apt to recur as soon as the influence of the chloroform passes off. The plan recommended by Dr. Russell Reynolds, of recurring to it at the first indications of an attack, is, I think, a very good one, for the spasm yields with much greater facility, and is cut short while it is in so incipient a state that the treatment is virtually preventive. He mentions the case of a young lady (Lancet, October 29th, 1853) who, by inhaling a few drops on her handkerchief whenever an attack threatened, at once averted it, and was thus virtually cured of her troublesome complaint.

Dr. Walshe says he has seen three results of chloroform inhalation, administered during a fit of asthma, and pushed to narcotism;—" Total relaxation of the spasm during the continuance of insensibility, with the immediate return of dyspnœa on the restoration of consciousness; gradual return of the difficult breathing as consciousness is restored; and suspension, or at least mitigation, of the paroxysm for the time being." The last effect he has found the rarest of the three; but, on the other hand, the temporary relief afforded by chloroform is sometimes more complete and more rapid than that afforded by any other agent.

As in all other cases, so in asthma, the patient should never administer the chloroform himself. Dr. Todd's remarks on this point are so judicious, and enforced by so striking an example, that I cannot forbear quoting them. "In the administration of chloroform," he says, "I would give you this twofold caution;—First, to give it gradually and cautiously, and not in a full dose, not to produce insen-

OPIUM. 193

sibility, especially if there be anything like blueness of the surface ; because, though remedial to asthma, it will tend to increase the very consequences which are most to be feared from the circulation of venous blood. Secondly, to impress on your patient that he must never give it to himself, nor without the presence of a medical man. The following case was related in the papers the other day :—A person who was in the habit of curing his attacks of asthma by inhaling chloroform, when administering it to himself one day, and when in a state of half subjection to its influence, in order to produce the full effect placed his handkerchief on the table and buried his mouth in it ; his insensibility became deeper and deeper, till at last he was too far gone to raise his head. He therefore continued inspiring it ; his coma became more and more profound ; and, a short time after, he was found in that position quite dead." (Medical Gazette, Dec., 1850.)

III. OPIUM.—To opium in asthma I have myself a great objection. I do not mean to impugn the correctness of those who profess to have seen benefit derived from it ; all I would say is, that I am not certain I have ever seen it do good, that I have often seen it do harm, and that I should have antecedently expected, from its known physiological action, that it would be prejudicial, and tend to increase the very condition for which it is given. I have endeavoured to show that sleep favours asthma ; that it does so on account of the ascendancy that excito-motory action then acquires ; that the heavier and more oppressed the patient is the intenser does the asthmatic spasm become ; and, on the other hand, that the wider awake and more vigilant he is—the more exalted sense and will—the more readily does it yield, so that often simple rousing is enough to stop an attack that was gradually creeping on the sleeper.

Anything, therefore, that soporises aggravates the asth-

o

194   TREATMENT BY SEDATIVES.

matic tendency. Now this is exactly what opium does.
What we want in asthma is a sedative that, like stramonium,
sedates but does not narcotise ; or one that, like chloroform, goes much further, and produces universal muscular
relaxation. And not only does opium act prejudicially by
tending to exalt reflex action in proportion to the drowsiness
and lethargy it produces, but, by lowering sensibility, it
prevents that acute and prompt perception of respiratory
arrears which is the normal stimulus to those extraordinary
breathing efforts which are necessary to restore the balance.

But, beyond this, opium seems to have a specific tendency
to excite involuntary muscular action, and induce a tendency
to spasm. The exact explanation of this will depend upon
the theory of muscular contraction that is adopted ; and
into this at present disputed physiological question I will
not enter. If, then, I had been asked, antecedently to all
experience, whether opium would be useful in asthma, I
should have replied, on the strength of the spasm-theory of
the disease, that it would not.

But I would not let any theoretical objection run counter
to clinical evidence ; and if experience said " give opium,"
no theory should prevent my recommending it. My own
experience, however, coincides with these objections ; and I
am disposed to think that the frequency with which it is
given in asthma depends upon an unthinking following of
routine and a want of close and exact observation. Not
only have I often seen asthma worse for it when given
during the fit, but I have seen it brought on when it did not
previously exist. An asthmatic gentleman, in whom I have
often watched this, and who is frequently obliged to resort to
opium on account of colic, never takes it without being
rendered more or less asthmatic by it, however free from the
disease he may have previously been.

I would say, then, prefer any other sedative to opium ;

STRAMONIUM. 195

and, unless there is some special complication that indicates it, never give it at all.

IV. STRAMONIUM.—The smoking of the datura as a remedy for asthma was introduced in 1802, from India, by General Gent, and soon obtained, as new remedies are apt to, the reputation of being specific and infallible ;—everybody with any shortness of breathing was smoking stramonium. Its use, however, has illustrated the general inapplicability of any one remedy to all cases of a disease, and the special caprice of asthma ; and time has shaken it into its proper place, and assigned it its true worth ;—that its original reputation greatly exaggerated its merits, but that it has undoubted though very unequal value, and will probably always maintain its place amongst the real remedies of asthma.

Perhaps no drug has been given with more contradictory results, and perhaps in no way is the caprice of asthma better illustrated than by its effects in different cases. In some it is *the* remedy ; in the majority of cases, as ordinarily used, it seems utterly inoperative, and in some positively injurious.

" Sometimes," writes Dr. Watson, "it calms the paroxysm like a charm. The late Dr. Babington told me of a patient of his, who had been grievously harassed by asthma for a series of years, but who declared to him, after he had made a fair trial of stramonium, that he no longer ' cared a fig' for his asthma, which he could always stop in a moment. So, a Mr. Sills, in a collection of communications relative to the *Datura stramonium*, published in London in 1811, states that he had been a great sufferer from asthma; that the fits continued, with short interruptions, from thirty-six hours to three days and nights successively, during which time he had often, in the seeming agonies of death, given himself over, and even wished for that termination to his miseries. But, having at length discovered the virtues of stramonium, he uses this strong language. ' In truth, the asthma is de-

o 2

196   TREATMENT BY SEDATIVES.

stroyed. I never experience any ill effects whatever from
the use of the remedy ; and I would rather be without life
than without stramonium.' "

Among several striking cases of the efficacy of stramonium,
communicated by Dr. Gooch of Croydon, I will quote the
following :—" Mr. L., 22 years old, for the last four years
has had great difficulty in breathing, attended by wheezing
and cough, which attack him suddenly, when in bed or at
meals, disabling him from his business, and sometimes continuing more than a week. It occasionally seizes him so
violently that he is unable to speak, and appears to be
threatened with instant suffocation. He has had much
medical advice, without receiving material benefit. He now
smoked the thorn-apple, swallowing the saliva and smoke;
by these means the fit terminates in a few minutes. He
smokes every day, even when the fit does not occur. Sometimes it attacks him while dining in company ; in which
case he retires, smokes a pipeful, and returns to his friends
breathing freely." I might go on quoting cases *ad libitum*,
but must content myself with referring the reader to many
very interesting and striking ones in the seventh and eighth
volumes of the Edinburgh Medical and Surgical Journal, the
twenty-sixth volume of the Medical and Physical Journal, and
the various medical periodicals published at the early part of
the present century.

In most of the cases that I have personally witnessed, it
has given only temporary relief—mitigated rather than cured
the spasm ; but, in a case recently communicated to me, its
effects appear to be nearly as striking as in the cases I have
just quoted. The patient was what is commonly termed a
" martyr to gout," and suffered most severely from asthma.
He could not walk, in consequence of the gouty state of his
legs and feet ; and one of his amusements was to pick the
chalk out of his fingers with a knife ! " I remember," writes

UNCERTAINTY OF STRAMONIUM. 197

my informant, " one day, when I was at his house, he came home in his little hand-carriage, in which it was his wont to be wheeled about, and, on being helped into the parlour, he was in such a state from a violent attack of his asthma that he could not speak, but made signs to his daughter, by pointing to a cupboard, that she should reach him his pipe of stramonium. She lighted it, and, after he had taken a few whiffs, the breathing became relieved, and he was able to speak ; and, after a few more, the spasm and oppression so completely vanished that he could converse as well as usual."

On the other hand, one is always being disappointed with it ; in a large per-centage of cases it does no good at all, and in some has been said to prove injurious, and in a few instances fatal. Dr. Bree tried it in eighty-two cases ; in fifty-eight of these it had no permanent effect, and in the remaining twenty-four it acted injuriously. General Gent, who was instrumental in introducing the practice, is said to have fallen a victim to it. Aggravation of the dyspnœa, paralytic tremblings, epilepsy, headache, and apoplexy, are some of the evils said to have been induced in some of the cases above referred to.

To what are these contradictory results to be attributed ? Partly, doubtless, to the caprice of the disease, which behaves in the most irregular way to all remedies ; but partly, I think, to the mode of preparation and drying of the drug. An asthmatic patient of mine informed me that while he received great benefit from stramonium grown and dried by a relative of his, that which he gets at the shops does him no good whatever. He sent me a specimen of this home-prepared stramonium, and certainly it was a very different thing, both in appearance and smell, from what one commonly sees : it had not lost its fresh greenness, nor the genuine solanaceous smell. I think, therefore, asthmatics would do wisely to grow and prepare their own stramonium. Part, too, may depend on the time at which it is administered ; stramonium, like other remedies, will cut short an incipient spasm, while over one that has been long established it has but little power. The great thing is to give it in time ; and for that purpose, since the patient in general is awoke from his sleep by the paroxysm, he should put his pipe, already filled, with the means of lighting it, by his bedside over-night, so that on awaking with the dyspnœa he might immediately use it.

My friend Dr. Buller of Southampton tells me that he has seen benefit from the inhaling (not the mere smoking) of stramonium smoke. "A year ago," he writes, "I met with an old asthmatic, who had cured himself and relieved many others by using *cold* stramonium-smoke. He smoked the stramonium as you do tobacco, then puffed the smoke into a tumbler, and then inhaled the cold smoke into his lungs. I am now attending an asthmatic lady, who could not inhale the hot smoke, but who inhales the cold smoke in this way with great relief."

The same plan of *inhaling* I find mentioned in a very interesting case in the Edinburgh Medical and Surgical Journal, as far back as 1811. The patient says :—" The way in which I employ this remedy is thus : I fill a common tobacco-pipe with the stramonium cut in small pieces, and inhale the smoke as much as possible into the lungs, which causes heat and pain about the fauces and throat, and I am obliged to breathe once or twice before I can inhale it again, when I draw in the smoke ; and so on alternately till the herb is consumed, which occupies about half an hour, once a day. The saliva I swallow." Now this is introducing the drug in a different way, and certainly a more powerful one, than by simply smoking it, and one well worth trying. By ordinary smoking absorption takes place by the oral surface

VARIETIES OF STRAMONIUM. 199

only ; here it is introduced into the lungs themselves and absorbed by the respiratory surface, whose absorbent powers exceed those probably of any other surface of the body. Besides, it has the advantage of being applied to the very part affected.

There are several species of datura in use, of which that commonly employed in this country, the *Datura stramonium*, appears to be the least powerful. The *Datura ferox*, which was first introduced by General Gent, seems to be much stronger. The *Datura tatula*, from which what are called stramonium cigars are made, appears also to be stronger.

The seeds are much more powerful than the other parts of the plant; their analysis yields more than three times as much of the active principle, *daturia*. My friend Dr. Alexander of St. Helena, where spasmodic asthma appears to be rather common, informs me that, while he has found the smoking of the leaves almost worthless, he finds the smoking of the seeds a most efficient and powerful remedy ; and that whereas he was disposed before he tried the seeds to regard the reputation of stramonium as a myth, he has since their employment come to the conclusion that it is one of the most satisfactory of the remedies of asthma. He states, however, that the effects of the seeds are so powerful, that great care is necessary in their administration : they should be smoked in very small and gradually increasing quantities, and their effects closely watched. He has seen, on two or three occasions, alarming symptoms supervene on their use. I have not yet tried the remedy of smoking the seeds, but I shall certainly do so. I do not see why the leaves should not be steeped in a decoction of the seeds, dried, and then smoked, so as to administer by smoking a reliable preparation of an uniform strength.

Exhibition by smoking certainly appears to have some advantages ; absorption by the oral surface, especially if com-

200   TREATMENT BY SEDATIVES.

bined with inhalation, is sufficiently rapid, and at the same time gradual and more easily regulated than by the stomach. One would rather either take or give any preparation of the *Solanaceæ* by smoking than by swallowing. One feels, with regard to such ticklish remedies, the full force of the *facilis descensus* and its alternative. Nevertheless, I frequently give the extract, and often with marked benefit. It should be commenced, I think, in quarter-grain doses, gradually increased to a grain, or a grain and a half. The Edinburgh preparation—an alcoholic, and not a watery extract—is the best and most reliable, the active principle, *daturia*, being very soluble in alcohol, but very sparingly so in water. The tincture may also be given in from ten-minim to twenty-minim doses every four hours, gradually increased till it occasions some obvious effect on the system.

I may say, in conclusion, with regard to this drug, that its great value in some cases would, in spite of its too frequent impotence, always induce me to give it a trial in cases in which it had not been tried; that I do not believe it is attended with any danger except from the most egregious over-dosing; that, since the common fault is want of power, I should prefer the stronger forms, the *ferox* and *tatula*, giving them tentatively and carefully; that inhalation of the smoke and swallowing the saliva may be advantageously combined with the ordinary method of smoking; and that it cannot be given too early in an attack. I think it does more in the way of prevention than cure; I think I have seen better results from the long-continued practice of smoking a pipe of it the last thing at night, whether an attack of asthma is threatening or not, than by waiting until a paroxysm comes on. I have seen this nightly pipe, the last thing before going to bed, apparently keep the disease at bay for an indefinite time, as long as it was continued, but followed by its immediate reappearance as soon as it was left off. The stramonium seems to leave for some hours a state of nervous system in which the asthma is not likely to come on; and, since the attack is almost always at night, the use of the stramonium at bedtime conducts and guards the patient through the critical time. I should say, then, let this always be one part of its administration; and keep up the practice of smoking it the last thing at night for some months after the disease appears to have yielded, so as to completely break through the habit.

V. LOBELIA.—Of lobelia I can say but very little, and the reason I can say so little is, that, being doubtful of its really doing any good, I have for some time ceased to prescribe it. But I have lately heard of some successful cases of its employment by medical friends; and I am inclined to think that my want of success, and the want of success that has generally attended its use in this country, has depended upon not giving it in sufficiently large doses. I have never given it in larger doses than from fifteen minims to half a drachm; but I find that in America, where it is much more used than in this country, and has a high reputation as an almost unfailing specific in spasmodic asthma, they give it in vastly larger doses; they consider half an ounce a full dose, but recommend two drachms every two or three hours till some decided effect is manifested. In many successful cases on record it has been given in small antispasmodic doses;* but I believe, as I have said, its great success among the Americans, and in Dr. Elliotson's hands, and in many cases which I find scattered about in the journals, depends upon its having been given in doses producing the charac-

---

* "I have, for upwards of two years past, been afflicted with inveterate asthma, which deprived me of natural rest, and the spasmodic effects of which were frequent and most distressing. When I found these paroxysms coming on I took fifteen drops of tincture of lobelia, which invariably gave me immediate relief, although previously to my using this remedy the violent fits often lasted for hours." (London Medical Gazette, vol. iii.)

teristic depressant action of the drug. In fact, that condition that a large dose produces is such as I should think no asthma could resist; it is almost identical with tobacco-poisoning— giddiness, faintness, sickness, cold sweat, and complete muscular relaxation. I should have the most perfect faith in its value in asthma when producing such symptoms as these; but they are not the symptoms one likes to produce in one's patients, and cannot be considered devoid of danger. I see no objection, however, to Dr. Elliotson's plan of giving frequent small and gradually increased doses. He recommends ten minims every quarter or half hour, increasing each dose a minim till the disease yields, or the drug seems to disagree with the patient. If this last should be the case, and vomiting and headache come on, the medicine must be left off for a time, and continued when the headache, &c., is removed, not increasing the dose beyond the last given.

One circumstance that makes it the more necessary to be careful of overdosing a patient, and that strongly inculcates commencement with small doses, is that different individuals tolerate it in such different quantities. Dr. Elliotson states that in some instances a single minim produced sickness, while in other cases, on the contrary, sixty or even ninety drops were taken for a dose. He mentions a young lady who, being subject to spasmodic asthma, always carried with her ninety drops of the tincture in a small phial; this dose she swallowed whenever an attack of the disease came on. He mentions, also, the following extraordinary and almost incredible case :—"A medical man, suffering from asthma, having failed to obtain his usual relief from his usual dose of the tincture, increased it to fifty-minim doses, which he took every hour for twenty-four hours. Experiencing but little relief he added a minim to each dose till it reached seventy-five minims; this he took for forty-eight hours, and the disease

INDIAN HEMP. 203

was relieved. His pulse was becoming intermittent, perspiration broke out over the body, and he became languid; small doses of ammonia soon restored him to his usual state. In the last four days this man must have taken twelve ounces of the tincture." (Lancet, vol. ii. p. 144.)

Another circumstance that makes it the more necessary to be careful not to administer this drug in undue quantities is, that different specimens of it differ so much in strength. Dr. Elliotson complains of this, and assigns it to faulty preparation. But the Americans say that the plant itself varies very much in strength, this difference depending chiefly upon the situation in which it has grown; that which has grown in damp situations being rank and strong, while that which has grown in dry places is almost inert. But I must not say any more on a medicine about which I began by saying I could say nothing.

VI. INDIAN HEMP.—The Indian hemp, *Cannabis sativa*, is much given in India as an anti-asthmatic, and among the natives has a great reputation. I can easily imagine from its physiological action that its reputation is well deserved. It is at once a stimulant and a sedative. I should be inclined to think it would act best in small stimulant doses. Given in this way it produces the same effects as coffee, only in a more marked degree—it exhilarates, imparts great activity and intensity to the intellectual faculties, and exalts the functions of animal life. In any case in which coffee is useful I should expect that Indian hemp would be so in a greater degree. I think in large doses it might even do harm, from its hypnotic tendency. In this respect there is the same objection to it as to opium. I can say nothing of it from my own personal experience; I have never given it, nor seen a case of asthma in which it has been given.

VII. ETHER.—Ether is mentioned as a remedy for asthma

204   TREATMENT BY SEDATIVES.

by almost all writers on the disease. I have never seen but one case in which it did any good, though I have given it in scores of cases. In that case it acted, and always had acted, like a charm. I cannot say that in any other case I ever saw it do a particle of good, and think I have often seen it produce a disagreeable oppression, and even increase the spasm. Others speak well of it; but the result of my experience is as I have stated it.

scribing; and not only get into the habit of employing certain remedies, but get *out* of the habit of employing others. I must confess to this fault myself, and feel at a loss to explain on other grounds how it was I went on so long without giving belladonna a fair and thorough trial in asthma. For the last two years, however, I have used it extensively, and am so satisfied with the results that I think it worth while to publish a few of my cases, in illustration of its value and of my method of employing it.

If I were to express what appears to me to be the peculiar excellence of belladonna as a sedative in asthma, I should say it consisted in its power of diminishing reflex irritability—a power which it appears to me to possess in a degree greater, in proportion to its other sedative effects, than any other sedative.

My method of giving it will be best seen in the following cases. I do not know that the tincture has any advantage over other preparations, only it happens to be that which I have tried. I should think that the liquor atropiæ might, from its uniformity of strength, be even preferable.

CASE 1.—R. G——, a lady aged twenty-five, who has been liable to hay fever for eleven years and to asthma for seven, came to me on May 18th, 1868, for the cure of her hay asthma. She had been suffering for nearly a month, and had not had a single night's rest. She was not troubled with her asthma by day, but only with her hay-fever symptoms. As soon, however, as she went to bed on came her asthma, and lasted regularly all night. She was worn out for want of rest, and felt fagged and miserable. I ordered her ten minims of the tincture of belladonna three times a day, telling her to increase the quantity, day by day, till the characteristic effects of the drug were produced. She gradually raised the dose from the ten minims to twenty. She felt better the first night after taking it. She took it for nine days, and had no asthma whatever. She then, thinking herself cured, and feeling her head very uncomfortable, omitted it for one day, and the following night got no sleep from asthma. She then resumed it, and has had no asthma since. She now regularly takes twenty drops three times a day. Her head is slightly affected, and her eyes decidedly so—misty, and she cannot read; but there is not a trace of asthma. She has never found anything else prevent the attacks. The belladonna seems to have no influence whatever over the other hay-fever symptoms; the sneezing, running at the eyes, &c., go on as before.

CASE 2.—Sarah P——, aged forty-six, has had asthma ever since she was nineteen years of age—that is, for twenty-seven years. For the last five months she has been worse than ever, and for some time past has had asthma regularly every night. It begins between two and three o'clock, and after that she gets no rest. I ordered her to take the tincture of belladonna every night on going to bed —to begin at ten minims, and gradually to increase the dose till her head and sight became affected. She came to me on the 29th of last July. On the 14th of August I find the following entry in my note-book:—"This patient came to me a fortnight ago yesterday. She has almost completely lost her symptoms ever since, having had uninterrupted good nights. She has gradually reached thirty drops of the tincture of belladonna, and now takes it every night. She looks wonderfully better, and is able to take long walks." From that time I have not heard anything of her.

CASE 3.—Col. R——, aged forty, has had asthma for sixteen years. For the last few years it has been gradually getting worse, and now he has it almost every night, commencing at from one to two o'clock A.M. He has tried various things without any success—Indian hemp, chlorodyne, ether, the inhalation of chloroform, dry cupping, coffee, iodide of potassium, abstinence, &c. I saw him on Sept. 16th, and ordered him to try the belladonna at night in the usual way. On the 23rd I find the following note:—"He has gradually got the belladonna up to forty minims without any appreciable inconvenience. The nights have been very good. The two last mornings there has been no oppression whatever, nor any sitting up in bed; he has slept right through the night. He walked this morning, directly after breakfast, from his house at Blackheath to the station—a mile—in sixteen minutes, and the same pace up from Charing-cross station here." I have not seen him since.

ON THE TREATMENT OF ASTHMA BY BELLADONNA.

BY HYDE SALTER, M.D., F.R.S.,

FELLOW OF THE ROYAL COLLEGE OF PHYSICIANS, SENIOR PHYSICIAN TO CHARING-CROSS HOSPITAL.

I DO not know any sedative that has more "improved its position" of late years than belladonna. It is certainly given much more extensively, and is much better thought of, than it was twenty years ago. And I think the one is the result of the other: it is better thought of *because* it is more extensively given. There are cycles of therapeutics as well as cycles of disease; and many valuable remedies pass into a temporary desuetude by a common neglect, and then, from some accident, emerge into repute and usefulness. And this is not only true with regard to the medical world in general; it is equally so with regard to the practice of individuals. We are all of us apt to get into a groove in pre-

CASE 4.—Wm. P——, aged thirty-eight, has been asthmatic seventeen years. His attacks come on every morning on rising from bed, but often trouble him throughout the day as well. There is defective respiration at the right base, violent paroxysmal cough, and a good deal of expectoration. This patient came to me on Oct. 13th. A week after I made the following note:—"Since coming to me this patient has taken the belladonna every night—twenty, twenty-five, and then thirty drops, to which last dose he has stuck. The result is that he is quite a different man. He has slept all through the night, dressed himself without any trouble or difficulty, and has walked half over London as quickly and well as ever in his life. When he arrived in town his breath was so bad that he had the greatest difficulty in getting from the Vauxhall station to the church near the bridge. He spits hardly anything. There is now a complete absence of all musical wheezing, and of any adventitious sound whatever: respiratory murmur quite re-established at right base, and indeed perfectly natural everywhere. And this change has taken place in one week."

For the following case, in which liquor atropiæ was used, I am indebted to my friend Mr. Hodson, of Bishop's Stortford.

CASE 5.—"John L——, aged fifty-five, by occupation a gardener, of active and temperate habits, suffered, from the summer of 1864, from frequent attacks of shortness of breath, followed by expectoration. When he first came under my observation (Sept. 2nd) he presented the appearance of a confirmed asthmatic. The respiratory sounds, whenever I saw him, were always more or less characteristic of asthma. At night he generally became worse, so much so that he often found the greatest difficulty in getting up one flight of stairs to his bedroom. I gave him at first iodide of potassium (five-grain doses), then combined it with decoction of senega, afterwards with squills and compound tincture of camphor. He also took lobelia, &c., and burned nitre-paper. With the exception of the last, which always afforded some relief, the frequency and severity of the attacks were uninfluenced by the treatment; indeed he became so bad that his life was a burden to him. I was watching his distress one day, and deploring the inefficiency of treatment, and thinking how the constricted state of his bronchial tubes might be overcome, when the idea of trying a drug that so quickly dilated the pupil occurred to me, and I at once determined to bring him fully under the influence of atropia. He began, Oct. 26th, to take one-sixtieth of a grain in solution every six hours. A few doses produced marked relief, but I pushed the atropia until he took at each dose one-fortieth of a grain. He then became fully under its influence, with greatly impaired vision, entire absence of saliva, and most troublesome strangury. From this time the breathing improved, but he found it necessary to take the medicine two or three times a day up to the middle of the following February. In the spring I sent him for a few weeks for change of air, and upon his return he resumed his full work as a gentleman's gardener, which he has continued without interruption up to the present time (Dec. 1868). When he went away I gave him a supply of his atropia, in case an attack should come on, but he told me yesterday that he has never opened the bottle. During the last three years I have found atropia, in all cases of genuine asthma, quite as useful as in L——'s case, but I have never pushed it with anyone else as I did with him."

I believe one reason why belladonna has not had a greater reputation as a remedy for asthma is that it has not been given in large enough doses. I think that, like lobelia, it must be given in doses sufficiently large to produce its physiological effects, otherwise we have no right to say that it has been fairly tried, or to conclude that it has been a failure if it has not achieved a cure. I think to give ten minims three times a day in some mixture is simply worthless. I have seen now numberless cases in which both belladonna and lobelia have been consigned to the limbo of failures, when a fresh trial of them, on the plan of gradually increasing the doses till an ultimatum has been reached, has proved them to be perfectly successful remedies. Sometimes, but very rarely, belladonna will relieve asthma when given short of a physiological dose; sometimes, but still rarely, it fails to give any relief even when pushed to its full physiological effects; the common thing is for it to fail till so pushed, and then to succeed. When I find belladonna has only been taken in the ordinary small doses, without

any increment, I always regard it as not having been tried at all.

The advantages of administering it in the way I have described are:—

1. That, giving it at night, you bring the full force of the drug to bear upon the disease at the time at which it is most liable to come on, and thus, if you are successful, tide your patient over the critical time.

2. By gradually feeling your way up to the required dose, you are able ultimately to reach without fear a dose which you would be unwilling to prescribe without such a tentative approach.

3. In those cases in which the therapeutical dose is reached before the physiological—that is, in which the asthma yields before the sight or head is appreciably affected,—it enables you to stop short as soon as relief is obtained, and thus spare your patient any of the disagreeable effects of the drug.

4. By giving it only once in the twenty-four hours, you are able to give a larger dose than you would be able to do if oftener repeated.

5. By confining the dose to bedtime, the patient's days are, in spite of a large dose, passed in comfort; for, as the morning advances, the dulness of head, confusion of sight, and drought of mouth pass away.

6. You are thus enabled to find out what is the dose for the individual—a very important point. People differ very much in their tolerance of belladonna. Some of my patients have been unable to take more than twenty minims once in the twenty-four hours without very unpleasant symptoms; while I have known others able to take a drachm three times in the same interval without any inconvenience. And as they differ in their tolerance of the drug, so do they differ in the dose at which their asthma will yield. The only way to ascertain what that dose is, is to make each case a separate experiment, and this can only be done in the way I describe.

7. By giving the remedy three or four hours before the attack is likely to come on, the treatment becomes *prophylactic*. If by taking a dose every night for thirty nights the attacks have been for that time prevented, the patient has ceased to be an asthmatic for a month. This is a very different thing from having had thirty attacks in the same time which have been cut short by the remedy. In all "habitual" diseases, in which the recurrence keeps up the tendency, prophylactic treatment has, in relation to final cure, a pre-eminence it does not possess in diseases in which habit has no place. For such diseases it is *the* treatment. It does more than spare your patient an attack of his malady; it breaks, *pro tanto*, that chain of sequences which is the very life of the morbid tendency.

On the treatment of asthma by belladonna. *Salter HH*

Thorax (1964), **19**, 406.

Variation of drug action on airway obstruction in man

R. E. C. ALTOUNYAN

From the Medical Department, Fisons Pharmaceuticals Ltd., Benger Laboratories Division, Holmes Chapel, Cheshire

Rapid and sustained relief of airway obstruction is a therapeutic aim which is still only rarely achieved in chronic bronchitis or asthma. Although the topical administration of adrenergic smooth muscle relaxants usually affords a rapid symptomatic improvement in these patients, the duration of relief is limited, and the efficacy of this treatment diminishes as breathlessness increases. There is clearly a need for more effective and longer lasting drugs. This communication is primarily concerned with the variations that were observed in the response to aerosols of isoprenaline sulphate and atropine methonitrate after their administration to patients at different phases of airway obstruction. The protective action of some drugs against artificially induced airway obstruction was also investigated.

METHODS AND MATERIALS

ESTIMATION OF AIRWAY RESISTANCE Serial F.E.V.$_1$ and vital capacity values were determined by the author using the same direct writing spirometer throughout. A minimum of three F.E.V.$_1$ recordings were determined for each test before estimating the slow vital capacity, after which a further one to three F.E.V.$_1$ estimations were repeated. The results were plotted to indicate the order of each attempt. When the values progressively diminished, as usually occurred during acute phases of airway obstruction, the F.E.V.$_1$ was calculated as the average of the last three attempts. In the majority of cases, consecutive F.E.V.$_1$ values were similar or increased during the first few attempts; in these circumstances the average of the three highest values was calculated as the F.E.V.$_1$.

DRUG ADMINISTRATION Drug administration was carried out under strict supervision; aerosols were administered in rooms set aside for this purpose, and only one type of drug was administered in each room. Patients received no isoprenaline for three hours, and no atropine for 12 hours, before tests. All aerosol drugs were administered from a Wright nebulizer operating on compressed air, and a different set of

apparatus was used for each type of drug. Aqueous solutions usually contained 5% propylene glycol (0·2% sodium metabisulphite was also included in the stock solutions containing isoprenaline).

AEROSOL DOSE The weight loss from the nebulizer and tubing, operating at 6 and 8 l./min. air flow, was approximately 150 and 220 mg./min. respectively. The maximum calculated dose (referred to below) is an approximate estimate of the dose of drug delivered to the face mask during the inspiratory period. The calculation was based on the total weight loss, and losses due to evaporation were not taken into account.

MINIMUM EFFECTIVE DOSE OF ISOPRENALINE SULPHATE AEROSOL Test doses of isoprenaline were administered during five slow maximal inhalations from a Wright nebulizer operating at 6 l./min. air flow (total inspiratory time approximately 15 seconds). In a given subject, the dose inhaled was altered by varying the concentration of the isoprenaline solution between the ranges of 0·05 and 1·0%. The F.E.V.$_1$ was determined three to five minutes after the test aerosol, after which an inhalation of 1.0% isoprenaline was administered for 60 seconds, and the maximum F.E.V.$_1$ increase from the initial control value was assessed three to five minutes later. The F.E.V.$_1$ improvement after the test aerosol was calculated as a percentage of the maximal F.E.V.$_1$ increase. In the majority of tests the administration of a maximum calculated dose equivalent to less than 0·1 mg. of isoprenaline was sufficient to induce 90 to 100% of the maximum F.E.V.$_1$ response. Similar tests were conducted with a pressurized multidose inhaler which delivered at each dose aproximately 0·075 mg. isoprenaline sulphate as an aerosol. The minimum number of doses required to induce 90 to 100% of the maximum response was estimated to lie between one and two. For the studies reported below, a larger dose of isoprenaline was administered: either five breaths of a 1·0% solution of isoprenaline from the Wright nebulizer (maximum calculated dose 0·37 mg.) or three to four doses from a pressurized multidose inhaler (0·2 to 0·3 mg.).

PROCEDURE FOR ASSESSING DRUG ACTION An increased airway resistance was induced by the aerosol administration of three types of spasmogen: histamine, carbachol or antigen in sensitized patients. The maximum percentage fall in the F.E.V.₁ which followed the selected dose of spasmogen aerosol was calculated (control fall). Subsequently, the prophylactic dose of the drug under investigation was followed at varying time intervals by the standard spasmogen challenge, and the maximum percentage fall in the F.E.V.₁ was determined (test fall). Drug effect was calculated from the formula

$$\% \text{ protection} = \frac{\text{control fall} - \text{test fall}}{\text{control fall}} \times 100$$

Control experiments established that histamine challenge sufficient to induce a 20 to 40% fall in the F.E.V.₁ could be repeated at least twice at hourly intervals without any significant alteration in the magnitude of the response. Carbachol has a slightly longer action, but repeatable results followed challenges at 90-minute intervals. A single antigen challenge led to a variable temporary desensitization, but antigen administered at a minimum of three-day intervals was satisfactory. In order to observe the maximum effect, serial F.E.V.₁ values were estimated at two, five, and 15 minutes after the start of histamine or carbachol challenge, and at five-minute intervals, for a minimum of 30 minutes, after antigen.

CLASSIFICATION OF PATIENTS Ninety-six patients (61 male, 35 female, aged 14 to 73 years, average age 47 years) with spirometric evidence of airway obstruction were investigated as out-patients. The majority were assessed at regular two- to four-week intervals throughout the year; on the average, each patient in this series attended 59 times over a period of 39 months.

The differential diagnosis between chronic bronchitis and intrinsic or extrinsic asthma was difficult to make on the basis of the history and clinical findings alone; moreover, in some patients each condition could have been considered to be present to a variable degree at different periods. In 12 patients (all under 40 years) with seasonal exacerbations, a diagnosis of extrinsic asthma was confirmed by an aerosol provocation test with the appropriate antigen. However, in eight of these 12 subjects a chronic productive cough with frequent infective episodes during the winter months was also present.

In the older age group, it was even more difficult to evaluate the importance of any underlying intrinsic asthma on clinical grounds alone, especially when chronic bronchitis was also evident. A quantitative estimate of the 'allergic' component (intrinsic and/or extrinsic asthma) of the airway obstruction observed in these patients was obtained during corticosteroid therapy. Ninety-three patients received corticosteroid therapy over a total period of 2,720 treatment months. In the majority, prednisone, 20 to 30 mg. daily, was administered initially for seven days, after which the dose was progressively reduced over two weeks to a maintenance level of 7·5 to 15 mg. daily. Basal F.E.V.₁ values were estimated at approximately seven-day

intervals during the first three weeks of each period of corticosteroid therapy. In 87 cases the response was assessed on the basis of the F.E.V.₁ observed during the initial three to six weeks of corticosteroid therapy in comparison with the pre-treatment values. Patients already receiving a maintenance dose of corticosteroids were observed at varying dose regimes in an attempt to establish a dose response relationship. The 96 patients in this study have been divided into two groups as follows.

Group A This group consisted of patients responsive to corticosteroid therapy or suffering from proven extrinsic asthma (60 patients, 32 males, aged 14 to 65, average age 44 years; 28 females, aged 22 to 73, average age 44 years).

The maximum basal F.E.V.₁ increase following corticosteroid therapy was greater than 50% in 36 patients and 10 to 50% in 16 patients. In six cases, corticosteroid therapy could not be withheld altogether owing to the severity of their condition, but evidence of a response to corticosteroids was established at varying dosage. Two patients with proven extrinsic asthma were never sufficiently distressed to justify a trial of corticosteroid therapy.

Group B These patients, 36 in all, were not responsive to corticosteroids (29 males, aged 31 to 67, average age 50 years; 7 females, aged 39 to 60, average age 47 years).

Twenty-eight patients showed no evidence of any improvement after corticosteroid therapy. In seven cases, the improvement was not greater than 10%. One male patient, who was not treated with corticosteroids because of diabetes, has been included in this group as he had no history of allergy and presented with classical chronic bronchitis.

ROUTINE MANAGEMENT Purulent sputum was regarded as evidence of infection. Patients were instructed to examine their sputum daily, and to commence tetracycline therapy on their own initiative (1·5 to 2·0 g. daily for three days followed by 1·0 to 1·5 g. for four days) and report for sputum culture if improvement did not occur within three days. In some cases, frequent relapses of infection necessitated maintenance therapy (0·75 to 1·5 g. daily), particularly during the winter months. Patients who responded to corticosteroids were maintained on the lowest dose consistent with reasonable comfort (5 to 15 mg. prednisone daily). Long-term therapy with oral ephedrine, antihistamines, aminophylline suppositories, and isoprenaline inhalations was continued when a worth-while improvement was claimed by the patient. Chronically dyspnoeic patients were maintained on dichlorphenamide, 25 to 200 mg. daily, when this treatment effected a significant improvement in exercise tolerance, vital capacity, and PCO₂ values.

RESULTS

ISOPRENALINE SULPHATE

Protective action against spasmogen challenge
Figs. 1, 2, and 3 summarize some of the results

408 R. E. C. Altounyan

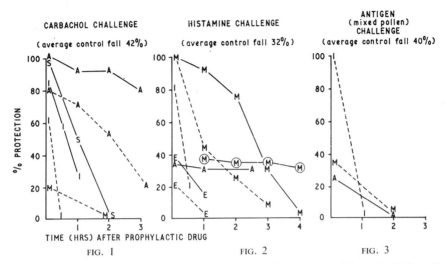

FIGS. 1, 2, and 3. *Protection afforded by prophylactic administration of drugs (as indicated) against spasmogen challenge.*

			max. calculated dose (mg.)					max. calculated dose (mg.)
A——A	Atropine methonitrate	0·2%	0·05		M——M	Mepyramine maleate	0·75%	5·0
A - - - A	,,	0·1%	0·025		M - - - M	,, ,,	0·75%	0·5
S——S	Atropine sulphate	0·2%	0·05		M—M	,, methyl bromide	3·6%	1·8
I——I	Isoprenaline ,,	1·0%	3·0		E——E	Ephedrine HCl	5·0%	15·0
I - - - I	,, ,,	0·1%	0·3		E - - - E	,, ,,	5·0%	7·5

of a series of tests with various bronchodilator compounds which were conducted on the author. Essentially similar results were obtained in a group of volunteer patients although all tests could not be completed on the same individual for accurate comparison. In Figs. 1, 2, and 3, isoprenaline administration at a clinical dose is shown to be effective against all three spasmogens when administered five to 10 minutes before the challenge. The duration of protection was, however, brief and rarely exceeded 60 minutes in any experiment. The administration of a massive dose of isoprenaline, equivalent to 10 times the clinical dose, afforded only a marginal increase in the magnitude and duration of effect, even though serious side effects were induced.

Duration of clinical response After a rest period of at least 20 minutes, the basal F.E.V.$_1$ was determined; isoprenaline was then administered, and the F.E.V.$_1$ was estimated approximately five minutes later and thereafter at intervals of 20 to 60 minutes. The duration of effect was interpolated from these values. The time taken for the F.E.V.$_1$ to decline to a point half way between the basal F.E.V.$_1$ and the maximum F.E.V.$_1$ value was designated the duration of 50% effect.

Whenever possible, the duration of the isoprenaline response was estimated in the same patient at widely different phases of disease. The results from groups A and B patients are shown separately in Figs. 4 and 5 respectively. When the basal F.E.V.$_1$ did not vary more than 20% the results are represented by a single point for each patient. When the basal F.E.V.$_1$ varied more than 20% on different occasions in the same subject, the results representing the widest variation are shown; these are identified as points connected by a continuous line. The results clearly indicate that the duration of relief afforded by isoprenaline was significantly reduced during phases of relatively increased airway obstruction. The duration of 50% effect rarely exceeded 60 minutes in patients of either group, but during the more acute phases it was usually 30 minutes or less. Spasmogen challenge experiments were conducted in a group of selected patients to determine whether the sustained effect of isoprenaline during remissions could be attributed to slower inactivation of the drug. The results from one subject are shown in Figs. 1, 2, and 3, in which little or no protection from the drug is demonstrable 30 minutes after the administration of a clinical dose, although over 50% of the F.E.V.$_1$ increase induced by iso-

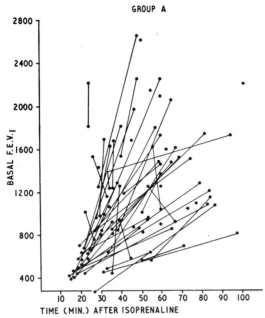

FIG. 4

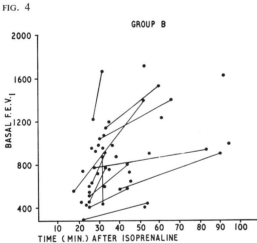

FIG. 5

FIGS. 4 and 5. *Duration of response to isoprenaline inhalations of group A and B patients respectively, in relation to initial airway obstruction.*

antimuscarine (benzhexol), a ganglion-blocking agent (pentolinium) and several antihistamines (*e.g.,* mepyramine) were investigated for bronchodilator activity. Relative potency was assessed from the magnitude and duration of the F.E.V.$_1$ increase, observed over a four-hour period following aerosol administration of the compounds at comparable concentrations, which varied from 0·2 to 1·0%. The tropane class of compounds was found to be the most active. The antihistamines, synthetic anticholinergic, and antimuscarine compounds all showed some transient activity, whereas pentolinium had no detectable action under these experimental conditions. Analogous atropine and hyoscine derivatives were approximately equi-active, homatropine less active, and tropine derivatives almost inactive. Increasing the N-alkyl chain from methyl to ethyl in the atropine series resulted in a significant loss of activity. Similarly, N-butyl hyoscine was less active than N-methyl hyoscine. The duration of effect was significantly prolonged by quaternization (Figs. 1 and 6). The increased duration of topically applied

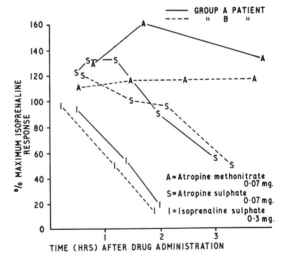

FIG. 6. *Comparison of magnitude and duration of changes in F.E.V.$_1$ after aerosol administration of isoprenaline, atropine sulphate, and atropine methonitrate in two patients.*

prenaline administration was maintained for up to 95 minutes in this subject. The duration of a significant degree of isoprenaline-induced protection against spasmogens did not exceed 60 minutes in any of the test subjects.

Cholinergic blocking agents Seventeen tropane derivatives, three synthetic tertiary and quaternary amine anticholinergic compounds, an

quaternary compounds was also demonstrated by a derivative of mepyramine: mepyramine methyl bromide (quaternary salt) is less active as an antihistamine on a weight basis than mepyramine maleate (tertiary salt), but it has a more prolonged effect when compared with the tertiary salt (Fig. 2).

It was concluded that the potent and sustained

410   *R. E. C. Altounyan*

activity of atropine methonitrate merited further investigation.

ATROPINE METHONITRATE

Protective action against spasmogen challenge
The protection afforded by aerosol atropine methonitrate against carbachol, histamine, and antigen challenge in the same subject is shown in Figs. 1, 2, and 3 respectively.

Atropine is clearly more specific in its action as compared with isoprenaline, and although some protection against both histamine and antigen challenge was demonstrated it is of a low order.
Clinical response to atropine methonitrate aerosol
The approximate minimum dose of atropine methonitrate that could induce a maximum F.E.V.$_1$ increase was investigated by the administration of aerosols containing varying concentrations of the drug. Cartridges with a known quantity of atropine as a finely divided powder were also prepared, so that a predetermined quantity of drug could be dispersed into the inspired air stream.

In the majority of tests, it was found that a maximum calculated dose of between 0·005 and 0·05 mg. of atropine was sufficient to induce a maximum effect.

In some cases the maximum response was not apparent for 30 to 60 minutes after atropine administration. Larger doses, or the administration of tertiary atropine salts, *e.g.,* atropine sulphate, did not significantly affect the time required for the maximum response to develop. The maximum increase in the F.E.V.$_1$ was assessed in 94 patients after five inspirations of a 0·2% aqueous aerosol of atropine methonitrate (maximum calculated dose, 0·07 mg.). The maximum atropine response was compared with the maximum response after a clinical dose of isoprenaline alone. In the majority of tests, each drug was assessed from identical pre-treatment F.E.V.$_1$ values, but where this was not possible, the average of two isoprenaline responses within ±5% of the basal F.E.V.$_1$ value recorded for the atropine test was accepted. When isoprenaline was administered first, both tests could be completed on the same day, and the results obtained in this manner agreed closely with those obtained on different days from similar basal F.E.V.$_1$ values.

Figures 7 and 8 show the results of 60 group A and 34 group B patients respectively. Different symbols indicate the relative degree of basal airway obstruction prevailing in each patient at the time of the test : this assessment was based on the previous records which extended for periods up to five years.

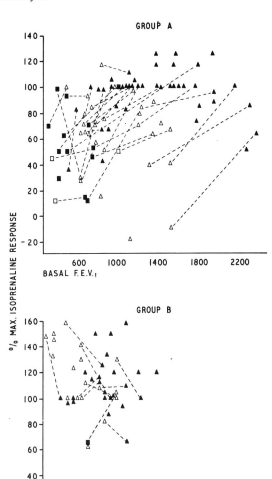

FIGS. 7 and 8. *Magnitude of response in group A and B patients respectively, to inhalations of atropine expressed as a percentage of the maximum response to isoprenaline from similar initial F.E.V.$_1$ values. The phase of airway obstruction in each patient at the time of test is indicated by the following symbols.* ▲ 75 to 100% *maximum recorded F.E.V.;* △ 50 to 74%; ■ 25 to 49%; □ *below 25%. Interrupted lines connect results from the same patient tested at significantly different phases of disease.*

The efficacy of atropine methonitrate clearly differs in the two groups under study.

Group A patients (Fig. 7) showed a variable response. The response to atropine was as great as, or exceeded, that to isoprenaline when these patients were in relative remission. The same

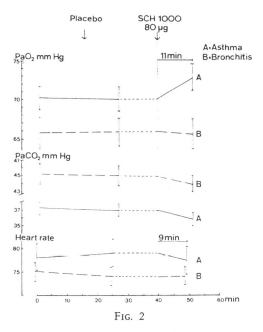

FIG. 2

Change in arterial Po₂, arterial Pco₂ and heart rate following consecutive inhalations of placebo and 80 microgram Sch 1000 in 28 asthmatics (group A) and 21 bronchitics (group B).

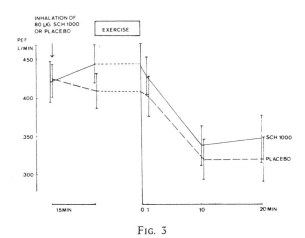

FIG. 3

Effect of pre-exercise inhalation of Sch 1000 on the post-exercise fall of PEF in 22 asthmatics, in whom exercise-induced asthma had been demonstrated in earlier experiments (group E-A).

Inhalation of a new anticholinergic drug, Sch 1000, in asthma and chronic bronchitis, effect on airway resistance, thoracic gas volume, blood gases and exercise-induced asthma. *Poppius H, Salorinne Y, Niljanen AA*

410   *R. E. C. Altounyan*

activity of atropine methonitrate merited further investigation.

ATROPINE METHONITRATE

Protective action against spasmogen challenge
The protection afforded by aerosol atropine methonitrate against carbachol, histamine, and antigen challenge in the same subject is shown in Figs. 1, 2, and 3 respectively.

Atropine is clearly more specific in its action as compared with isoprenaline, and although some protection against both histamine and antigen challenge was demonstrated it is of a low order.

Clinical response to atropine methonitrate aerosol
The approximate minimum dose of atropine methonitrate that could induce a maximum $F.E.V._1$ increase was investigated by the administration of aerosols containing varying concentrations of the drug. Cartridges with a known quantity of atropine as a finely divided powder were also prepared, so that a predetermined quantity of drug could be dispersed into the inspired air stream.

In the majority of tests, it was found that a maximum calculated dose of between 0·005 and 0·05 mg. of atropine was sufficient to induce a maximum effect.

In some cases the maximum response was not apparent for 30 to 60 minutes after atropine administration. Larger doses, or the administration of tertiary atropine salts, *e.g.,* atropine sulphate, did not significantly affect the time required for the maximum response to develop. The maximum increase in the $F.E.V._1$ was assessed in 94 patients after five inspirations of a 0·2% aqueous aerosol of atropine methonitrate (maximum calculated dose, 0·07 mg.). The maximum atropine response was compared with the maximum response after a clinical dose of isoprenaline alone. In the majority of tests, each drug was assessed from identical pre-treatment $F.E.V._1$ values, but where this was not possible, the average of two isoprenaline responses within ±5% of the basal $F.E.V._1$ value recorded for the atropine test was accepted. When isoprenaline was administered first, both tests could be completed on the same day, and the results obtained in this manner agreed closely with those obtained on different days from similar basal $F.E.V._1$ values.

Figures 7 and 8 show the results of 60 group A and 34 group B patients respectively. Different symbols indicate the relative degree of basal airway obstruction prevailing in each patient at the time of the test : this assessment was based on the previous records which extended for periods up to five years.

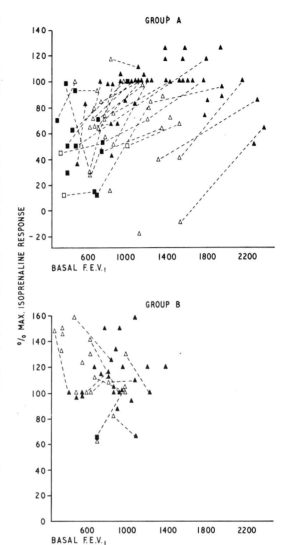

FIGS. 7 and 8. *Magnitude of response in group A and B patients respectively, to inhalations of atropine expressed as a percentage of the maximum response to isoprenaline from similar initial F.E.V.₁ values. The phase of airway obstruction in each patient at the time of test is indicated by the following symbols.* ▲ *75 to 100% maximum recorded F.E.V.;* △ *50 to 74%;* ■ *25 to 49%;* □ *below 25%. Interrupted lines connect results from the same patient tested at significantly different phases of disease.*

The efficacy of atropine methonitrate clearly differs in the two groups under study.

Group A patients (Fig. 7) showed a variable response. The response to atropine was as great as, or exceeded, that to isoprenaline when these patients were in relative remission. The same

Variation of drug action on airway obstruction in man   411

patients tested during periods of increased airway resistance showed a significant and progressive decline of the atropine response compared with the isoprenaline response (assessed from similar basal conditions). Two patients in this group, as well as two similar cases not included in this series, showed a negative response to atropine. The inhalation of an aerosol of distilled water also effected some increase in the airway resistance in these patients.

Group B patients (Fig. 8) showed a more uniform response. In the majority of these subjects, atropine induced an effect equal to or greater than the corresponding isoprenaline response. There did not appear to be any correlation between the prevailing degree of airway obstruction and the relative efficacy of atropine in group B patients.

Duration of response to aerosols of atropine methonitrate combined with isoprenaline sulphate (a) *Administered from the Wright nebulizer* Atropine methonitrate 0.2% and isoprenaline 1.0% were administered at a standard dose (maximum calculated dose of atropine methonitrate, 0.07 mg.; isoprenaline sulphate, 0.37 mg.). The initial increase in the F.E.V.$_1$ approximately five minutes after the aerosol was recorded, and the estimations were repeated at 30- to 60-minute intervals for as long as practicable. The results from 50 group A and 31 group B patients are plotted in Figs. 9 and 10 respectively. The residual effects (expressed as percentages of the maximum increases in the F.E.V.$_1$ recorded during the test day) are plotted as ordinates; the period of observation after drug administration as abscissae. The symbols (see legend to Figs. 7 and 8) signify the relative degree of airway obstruction prevailing in each patient at the time of test; interrupted lines connect results from the same patient when records were obtained at significantly different phases of disease.

Group A patients (responsive to corticosteroids, Fig. 9) showed considerable variation in their responses. The duration of effect was apparently correlated with the relative degree of airway obstruction prevailing in each patient at the time of test. The majority showed a sustained effect, which persisted for several hours when they were well, but the duration of effect was progressively reduced as the relative degree of basal airway obstruction increased. In contrast, in the majority of group B patients (not responsive to corticosteroids, Fig. 10) a sustained response was maintained even during phases of relatively increased airway obstruction.

(b) *Administered from a pressurized multi-dose*

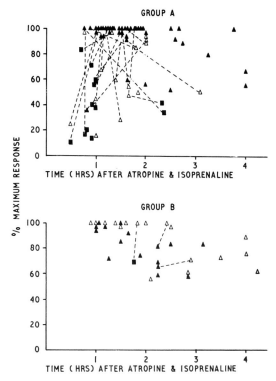

FIGS. 9 and 10. *Rate of decline of the response in group A and B patients respectively to inhalations of isoprenaline and atropine.*

inhaler The inhaler employed delivered an aerosol containing 0.04 mg. atropine methonitrate and 0.1 mg. isoprenaline sulphate at each dose. A valve mechanism was incorporated in the mouthpiece to facilitate the co-ordination of drug release with the commencement of inspiration. In a series of tests on 18 patients (10 group B and eight group A, during a phase of relative remission) the efficacy of this inhaler was compared with that of a similar appliance which delivered isoprenaline alone.

Each type of therapy was administered on a different day, in a random order, over a four-week period. On test days, patients were asked to use isoprenaline alone when relief was necessary in the early morning, and they were requested not to inhale this drug after 8 a.m. Basal F.E.V.$_1$ values were determined at 11 a.m. and were repeated approximately one hour later. When there was more than 10% difference between the two F.E.V.$_1$ values, the test was abandoned on that day. When the difference was less than 10%, the basal F.E.V.$_1$ value was calculated from the

412   *R. E. C. Altounyan*

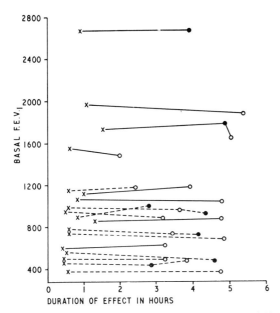

FIG. 11. *Duration of response in eight group A and* 10 *group B patients after inhalations of isoprenaline alone compared with isoprenaline and atropine, administered from a pressurized multi-dose inhaler.* × *Isoprenaline alone (max. calculated dose* 0·2 *mg.);* ○ *Isoprenaline and atropine —one dose (max. calculated dose* 0·1 *and* 0·04 *mg. respectively);* ● *Isoprenaline and atropine—two doses. The results from each group A patient are joined by a continuous line, those of group B patients by interrupted lines.*

second attempt. The test inhalation was then administered by an assistant, and the F.E.V.$_1$ was reassessed after intervals of five minutes, 30 minutes, and thereafter approximately hourly for six hours or until the F.E.V.$_1$ had reverted to pre-treatment values.

A clinically significant residual effect was considered to be equivalent to 50% of the maximum increase in the F.E.V.$_1$ after the administration of isoprenaline alone. The duration of a response which never fell below this value at any period was determined by interpolating the serial F.E.V.$_1$ values obtained after each type of therapy. The results in each patient are shown in Fig. 11.

The administration of the combined drugs clearly afforded a considerably longer period of relief in all the patients tested. There was no evidence that this effect could be significantly prolonged by increasing the dose of the combined drugs. It should be emphasized that atropine offers no advantage during acute phases of airway obstruction in corticosteroid-responsive ('allergic')

patients. This type of patient often inhales isoprenaline every few minutes in an attempt to relieve acute symptoms. In these circumstances, the indiscriminate use of aerosols containing atropine could lead to a serious over-dosage.

PAPAVERINE HCl Papaverine HCl is classed as a non-specific smooth muscle relaxant on the basis of pharmacological tests. It is widely used clinically and included in the National Formulary in Nebula Isoprenalinae Sulphatis Composita B.P.C. as a 2·5% solution. Aerosols of 2·5% papaverine (maximum calculated dose, 1·2 mg.) were administered to 12 patients. An increase in airway resistance occurred in six patients; the remainder showed no significant improvement.

EPHEDRINE HCl Insomnia, palpitation, and urinary retention in elderly male patients precluded effective oral therapy in the majority of cases. Aerosol administration was ineffective at low doses. The low order of protection afforded by higher doses administered by aerosol against histamine challenge is shown in Fig. 2. The combination of ephedrine with isoprenaline by aerosol afforded no significant increase in the magnitude or duration of the isoprenaline response.

MISCELLANEOUS COMPOUNDS In the majority of tests, oral or intravenous aminophylline, intramuscular pethidene or mepyramine maleate, and sublingual glyceryl trinitrate administered at clinical doses were all less effective than isoprenaline and/or atropine.

HISTAMINE AEROSOL CHALLENGE A consistent hypersensitivity to histamine aerosol (maximum calculated dose, 0·017 mg. histamine base) was demonstrated in nearly all group A and B patients tested repeatedly at intervals throughout the year. Patients with seasonal asthma were the exception, as they showed a marked increase in sensitivity coincident with the onset of the asthma season. In two of these cases the increase in the sensitivity to histamine was shown to parallel a corresponding increase in sensitivity to specific antigen ; both forms of hypersensitivity persisted during the asthma season in spite of corticosteroid therapy which was adequate to restore the basal F.E.V.$_1$ to within the normal range. In contrast, in patients with proven grass-pollen sensitivity, who showed evidence of persistent airway obstruction even during the winter months, a high degree of histamine sensitivity was demonstrated throughout the year. Tests with aerosols of carbachol, citric acid, propylene glycol, and other irritants confirm the clinical impression that chronic air flow obstruction is associated with a persistent hypersensitivity to a wide variety of irritants.

DISCUSSION

The short action of isoprenaline reported above confirms the observations of Lowell, Curry, and Schiller (1949), and of Bresnick, Beakey, Levinson, and Segal (1949), who conducted spasmogen challenge experiments after the administration of oral, parenteral, and aerosol isoprenaline.

Rapid metabolic inactivation of isoprenaline can be observed in sputum (expectorated a few minutes after isoprenaline inhalations) in which the pink-brown adrenochrome derivates are sometimes mistaken for blood. This rapid degradation together with diffusion probably accounts for the absence of any significant prolongation of action after the administration of large doses of isoprenaline. By contrast, mepyramine, which is not actively metabolized in the lung, showed a significantly longer duration of action when the dose was increased (Fig. 2). Attempts to block the enzymatic degradation of isoprenaline by the simultaneous administration of ortho-methyltransferase inhibitors have been unsuccessful (unpublished results), but it is possible that this approach can lead to the development of longer-acting adrenaline derivatives.

The prolongation of therapeutic action beyond the period when its presence can be demonstrated by spasmogen challenge tests implies that the factors responsible for airway obstruction are acting slowly. The duration of this 'free wheel' period, during which a reduced airway resistance is apparently maintained in the absence of drug, is an indication of the activity of the noxious processes causing airway obstruction ; when the duration of 50% effect is less than 45 minutes, considerable improvement may be anticipated ; a similar decrease occurring at 90 minutes or later indicates that the patient is in a phase of relative remission.

Atropine, or its analogues, has been used to relieve respiratory distress for over 150 years (Finnegan, 1950), but conflicting reports of its therapeutic value continue to appear (Palmer, 1962 ; Chamberlain, Muir, and Kennedy, 1962). Some of the apparent discrepancies in the literature can be explained on the basis of the results presented above. Hume and Jones (1961) administered atropine as a 4·0% aqueous aerosol but

F.E.V.$_1$ changes were estimated for only 15 minutes after drug administration, so that the maximum effect of atropine may not have been observed in some cases. The side effects which these workers reported were not observed in the present study in which much lower doses were used.

Herxheimer (1959), who administered atropine sulphate as a smoke as well as as a wet aerosol, reported an effective duration of less than three hours. His results with atropine sulphate were confirmed in this study (Fig. 6) ; the quaternary salt, however, was shown to have a longer duration, lasting up to six hours.

It is apparent that a number of factors can influence the outcome of atropine therapy ; failure to recognize these factors has led to conflicting opinions in the past. The selection of patients, the phase of disease, the choice of atropine derivative, the dose and method of administration, and the period of observation can all affect the results.

The mechanism of action of atropine therapy on airway obstruction is of interest. Armitage, Herxheimer, and Rosa (1952) reported that atropine has significant anti-anaphylactic properties when tested by the micro-shock technique on guinea-pigs, but the potent antihistamines were much more effective. The anti-anaphylactic properties of atropine in the guinea-pig can perhaps be attributed entirely to its weak antihistaminic action. In man (Fig. 3), both atropine and potent antihistamines are virtually ineffective against experimentally induced allergic airway obstruction. This suggests that histamine is probably not the major spasmogen released from human lung after anaphylactic challenge (Brocklehurst, 1956). On the other hand, Dautrebande, Lovejoy, and McCredie (1962) have demonstrated that atropine sulphate is as effective as sympathomimetic drugs in preventing the airway changes induced by aluminium powder inhalation in normal and emphysematous patients. Thus the efficacy of atropine depends primarily on the basic aetiology of the airway obstruction. The similar response to atropine of group A patients during a remission and group B patients suggests that the same mechanism underlies the increased airway resistance in these cases. However, during exacerbations of airway obstruction in group A patients, a different mechanism operates, which is resistant to atropine but sensitive to corticosteroid therapy.

The slow onset of the atropine response suggests that its action is not merely due to parasympathetic blockade. A possible explanation of its mode of action is suggested by the work of Vaughan

Williams (1961) on isolated guinea-pig atrial muscle. He reported that the contractility and electrical behaviour of the muscle was altered in opposite directions by acetylcholine and histamine. Most of these effects, he considers, could be attributed to an increase in membrane permeability to potassium and sodium induced by acetylcholine and histamine respectively. It is possible that the contractile properties of human bronchial muscle are also influenced in opposite directions by histamine and acetylcholine. Thus, although atropine is an effective 'competitive inhibitor' at the acetylcholine receptor site, and correspondingly less effective at the histamine receptors, it may also alter the basic tone of the muscle fibre by opposing the permeability changes induced by acetylcholine. The slow onset of the atropine response, as measured by F.E.V.$_1$ increase, in contrast to its immediate effect against carbachol challenge, may be accounted for by the time required to establish a new equilibrium in the muscle fibres after a change in permeability. Absence of effect and, in some cases, an increased airway resistance which follows the administration of atropine to 'allergic' subjects may also be explained on this basis. These subjects liberate excessive quantities of histamine (as shown by eosinophilic sputum), so that under these abnormal conditions the consequences of the permeability changes induced by histamine may be partially held in check by the opposing action of acetylcholine ; the administration of atropine could then enhance the action of histamine and lead to increased airway obstruction.

From the clinical standpoint, estimations of the relative efficacy and duration of action of atropine methonitrate, in comparison with isoprenaline, can help to distinguish between 'allergic' and 'non-allergic' airway obstruction. When a patient is already receiving corticosteroids, a good atropine response implies adequate control ; a poor response to atropine indicates inadequate corticosteroid control, possibly as a result of other factors such as infection.

Quantitative estimations of airway obstruction induced by specific antigen or non-specific spasmogen challenge can be of assistance in the assessment of therapy. It is evident that curative therapy will reduce the abnormally high level of airway irritability which is observed in all patients with 'chronic bronchitis' or asthma.

SUMMARY OF RESULTS

The magnitude and duration of effect of isoprenaline, atropine derivatives, and three types of spasmogen administered as aerosols were estimated in a group of patients at varying phases of increased airway resistance. The type of response was shown to depend on the relative degree of obstruction and the aetiology of the condition.

ISOPRENALINE THERAPY Inhalations of isoprenaline induced some rapid improvement in all forms of spasmodic airway obstruction. The duration of positive effect, as shown by the presence of a significant level of protection against spasmogen challenge, was limited to approximately 30 minutes.

The duration of the F.E.V.$_1$ increase after isoprenaline inhalation served as a useful index of the relative degree of airway obstruction which was present in a given patient at the time of test. No clinically significant prolongation of effect was achieved by increasing the dosage up to the limit of tolerance.

ATROPINE THERAPY Atropine was shown to be a poor antagonist of both antigen and histamine induced airway obstruction.

Compared with isoprenaline, atropine therapy afforded significantly greater relief as well as a more prolonged effect in patients not susceptible to corticosteroids. Patients who benefit from corticosteroids also responded well to atropine during phases of relative remission.

The action of quaternary atropine derivates, *e.g.*, atropine methonitrate, administered topically, was sustained longer than that of the corresponding tertiary salts, *e.g.*, atropine sulphate.

Of the commonly used antispasmodic drugs, isoprenaline and atropine were found to be the most effective.

SPASMOGEN CHALLENGE Histamine and other spasmogen challenge tests have provided precise, quantitative information on the mechanism of action and duration of effect of drugs acting on the bronchial musculature.

Hypersensitivity to irritants was observed in both 'allergic' and 'non-allergic' airway obstructive disease. Fluctuations of the basic level of susceptibility to irritants, induced by therapy or other factors, were assessed quantitatively by determining changes in sensitivity to standard spasmogen challenge.

Measurement of the magnitude of the response to atropine methonitrate compared with isoprenaline alone can be used to identify and assess the progress of patients who will respond to corticosteroid therapy.

Variation of drug action on airway obstruction in man. *Altounyan REC*

Variation of drug action on airway obstruction in man   415

I wish to thank Dr. W. Robinson for permission to study his patients and for his help in providing facilities for this investigation at Monsall Hospital, Manchester. Dr. J. B. L. Howell read the manuscript ; his valuable criticisms are acknowledged with gratitude. I am also deeply indebted to the patients and to Staff Nurse T. Bardsley for their most willing co-operation.

This work was financed by Benger Laboratories Limited. who also manufactured the pressurized multi-dose inhaler containing isoprenaline and atropine (Registered trade mark : Prenomiser Plus). I am grateful for the assistance of Mr. L. Martin and Dr. G. P. Ellis, of the Research Department, and to the directors of the company for permission to publish.

REFERENCES

Armitage, P., Herxheimer, H., and Rosa, L. (1952). The protective action of antihistamines in anaphylactic microshock of the guinea-pig. *Brit. J. Pharmacol.*, **7**, 625.

Bresnick, E., Beakey, J. F., Levinson, L., and Segal, M. S. (1949). Evaluation of therapeutic substances employed for the relief of bronchospasm V. Adrenergic agents. *J. clin. Invest.*, **28**, 1182.

Brocklehurst, W. E. (1956). A slow reacting substance in anaphylaxis "SRS–A." In *Ciba Foundation Symposium on Histamine*, p 175. Churchill, London.

Chamberlain, D. A., Muir, D. C. F., and Kennedy, K. P. (1962). Atropine methonitrate and isoprenaline in bronchial asthma. *Lancet*, **2**, 1019.

Dautrebande, L., Lovejoy, F. W, and McCredie, R. M. (1962). Effects of atropine microaerosols on the airway resistance in man. *Arch. int. Pharmacodyn.*, **139**, 198.

Finnegan, J. K. (1950). Stramonium cigarettes and powders. *Bull. nat. Formulary Comm.*, **18**, 131.

Herxheimer, H. (1959). Atropine cigarettes in asthma and emphysema. *Brit. med. J.*, **2**, 167.

Hume, K. M., and Jones, E. Rhys (1961). The response to bronchodilators in intrinsic asthma. *Quart. J. Med.*, **30**, 189.

Lowell, F. C., Curry, J. J., and Schiller, I. W. (1949). A clinical and experimental study of isuprel in spontaneous and induced asthma. *New Engl. J. Med.*, **240**, 45.

Palmer, K. N. V. (1962). Current Therapeutics 178–. Aerosols in chronic bronchitis. *Practitioner*, **189**, 546.

Vaughan Williams, E. M. (1961). The action of quinidine, acetylcholine and anaphylaxis interpreted from simultaneous records of contractions and intracellular potentials in the heart. *Sci. Basis Med. Ann. Rev.*, p. 302. Athlone Press, London.

INHALATION OF A NEW ANTICHOLINERGIC DRUG, SCH 1000, IN ASTHMA AND CHRONIC BRONCHITIS : EFFECT ON AIRWAY RESISTANCE, THORACIC GAS VOLUME, BLOOD GASES AND EXERCISE-INDUCED ASTHMA *

INHALATION D'UN NOUVEL ANTICHOLINERGIQUE, LE SCH 1000, DANS L'ASTHME ET LA BRONCHITE CHRONIQUE ACTION SUR LA RESISTANCE DES VOIES AERIENNES, LE VOLUME GAZEUX THORACIQUE, LES GAZ DU SANG ET L'ASTHME D'EFFORT

H. Poppius, Y. Salorinne, A.A. Viljanen

Bull. Physio-path. resp., 1972, *8*, 643-652.

ABSTRACT

Inhalation of 80 μg of the anticholinergic drug Sch 1000 (Boehringer Ingelheim) was followed by an equal decrease of airway resistance by one third in asthmatics and bronchitics. Subsequent inhalation of isoprenaline gave a further significant bronchodilation in the asthma group but failed to do so in the bronchitis group. Blood gas values and heart rate were not adversely affected. The drug failed to prevent exercise-induced asthma. It is concluded that the therapeutic value of the drug may be greater in the bronchitic than in the asthmatic type of airways obstruction.

Anticholinergic drugs ; airway resistance ; blood gases ; asthma ; chronic bronchitis.

The anticholinergic drug Sch 1000 ** given by inhalation is reported to have a rapid, longstanding and as strong a bronchodilatation effect as sympathomimetics in patients with chronic bronchitis (ULMER, 1971). The present investigation was undertaken in order to evaluate the acute effect of Sch 1000 on clinically different forms of reversible airways obstruction.

* From the Department of Pulmonary Diseases, University Central Hospital, Helsinki, Finland.

Correspondence to : H. Poppius, Respiratory Function Laboratory, Meilahti Hospital, 00290 Helsinki 29 (Finland).

** N-isopropyl-nortropine tropate bromomethylate, Boehringer Ingelheim.

The study consists of two parts. The first part is concerned with the effect of Sch 1000 on airways obstruction and blood gas values in two patient groups, one with asthma and one with chronic bronchitis. The second part is concerned with the possible preventing effect of Sch 1000 on exercise-induced asthma.

MATERIAL AND METHODS

Part I.

Group A comprised 28 patients with asthma (Ciba Foundation Symposium 1959) with a mean duration of the disease of 12 years (range one month — 40 years). The onset of asthma was before 20 years of age in eight cases, between 20 and 40 years of age in twelve cases and after 40 years of age in eight cases. Positive skin and/or inhalation-provocation tests were obtained in sixteen cases.

Group B comprised 21 patients with chronic bronchitis. Two of the patients had in addition moderately advanced arrested pulmonary tuberculosis. The characteristics of the groups A and B are given in Table I and II.

TABLE I

COMPARISON OF CHARACTERISTICS OF
GROUP A (ASTHMA) AND B (CHRONIC BRONCHITIS)

	A Asthma	B Chronic bronchitis
N	28	21
Men/Women	9/19	17/4
Age, yr, mean	44	56
Age, yr, range	16-65	38-70
Mean height, cm, men	172	172
Mean height, cm, women	162	156
History of hay fever, allergic rhinitis or atopic dermatitis	13	0
Asthma, hay fever or allergic rhinitis in parents or siblings	14	3
Blood eosinophilia (≥ 5%)	17	1

Present cigarette consumption
   1-14 cig./day
   15-24
   25+
	3
	3
	0
		7
		4
		2

Smokers of pipes and / or cigars only	0	1
Non- or ex-smokers	22	7
Cortisone treatment, present	23	0
Cortisone treatment, present or previous	26	0

Inhalation of a new anticholinergic drug, Sch 1000, in asthma and chronic bronchitis, effect on airway resistance, thoracic gas volume, blood gases and exercise-induced asthma. *Poppius H, Salorinne Y, Niljanen AA*

TABLE II

FURTHER CHARACTERISTICS OF GROUP B (CHRONIC BRONCHITIS)

N	21
Persistent sputum (Q. 15-17)*	21
Periods of cough and sputum (Q. 18)*	18
Grade of dyspnoea (Q. 20-24)*	
1	0
2	3
3	6
4	2
5	10
Chest illness (Q. 25)*	18
VC, 1 BTPS, mean ± S.D., men	2.93 ± 0.51
FEV_1, 1 BTPS, mean ± S.D., men	1.24 ± 0.40
VC, 1 BTPS, mean ± S.D., women	2.17 ± 0.60
FEV_1, 1 BTPS, mean ± S.D., women	1.13 ± 0.27
% increase in FEV_1 after isoprenaline	15 ± 11

* Medical Research Council's Questionnaire on respiratory symptoms.

The differentiation between asthma and chronic bronchitis may often be difficult. In the present study, an attempt was made to choose the asthmatics and the bronchitics to represent clearly different areas of the spectrum of obstructive lung diseases. The separation was done on clinical grounds. Only patients with pronounced variability in airways obstruction and no history of chronic bronchitis before the onset of asthma were accepted into the asthma group. Evidence of atopy was not required. No patients with clinical evidence of pronounced variability in airways obstruction were accepted in the bronchitis group. Several patients considered to have a « mixed » type of disease were rejected from the study.

Airway resistance (Raw) and thoracic gas volume at the end-tidal level (Vtg) were determined at a breathing frequency of 30 per minute with a constant-volume body plethysmograph (Siregnost, Siemens) (WOITOWITZ et al., 1967) using an analogue computer for the correction of differences in temperature and humidity between inspired and expired air (MUYSERS et al., 1969). Raw and Vtg are defined as the means of four measurements. Raw was measured as the mean resistance during the whole breathing cycle. In the statistical treatment of Raw values a logaritmic transformation was performed. Arterial P_{O_2} was measured with the Clark oxygen electrode. Arterial P_{CO_2} was measured with the Astrup apparatus (Radiometer), using the interpolation method.

The experiments were made between 10 and 12 a.m. Administration of bronchodilators and disodium cromoglycate was omitted for at least seven and

Inhalation of a new anticholinergic drug, Sch 1000, in asthma and chronic bronchitis, effect on airway resistance, thoracic gas volume, blood gases and exercise-induced asthma. *Poppius H, Salorinne Y, Niljanen AA*

646 H. POPPIUS ET AL.

twelve hours, respectively, before the test. A catheter was inserted into the brachial artery and basal readings of heart rate, blood gas values, Raw and Vtg were taken 30 minutes later. The patient then inhaled two puffs of placebo (propellant only) and the measurements were repeated. After the placebo experiment, the patient inhaled two puffs each of 40 microgram Sch 1000 and the measurements were repeated again. The heart rate was measured nine minutes, the blood gas values eleven minutes, and Raw and Vtg about sixteen minutes after the inhalation of either placebo or Sch 1000. The experiment was concluded with the inhalation of three puffs each of 100 microgram of isoprenaline and the measurements of Raw and Vtg were taken four minutes later. The time interval from the inhalation of Sch 1000 to the last measurement of Raw and Vtg following inhalation of isoprenaline averaged 24 minutes.

Part II.

Group E-A comprised 22 patients with asthma (Ciba Foundation Symposium 1959), in whom previous bicycle exercise tests induced a fall in the peak expiratory flow (PEF) of at least 25 %. Eleven were men, and eleven were women, the mean age being 32 (range 17-60) years.

In the present investigation the patient pedalled a bicycle ergometer (Elema-Schönander) in the supine position, and the load was increased by steps according to the schedule 200, 400, 600, 800, 1000 and 1200 kpm/min., each load being kept up for three minutes. The test was continued up to the subjects limit of exercise tolerance. The heart rate was determined from the ECG. PEF was measured with Wright's peak flow meter. PEF is defined as the mean of the two highest out of five consecutive readings.

Each patient performed two identical exercise tests with an interval of one to three days. Administration of bronchodilators and disodium cromoglycate was omitted for at least seven and twelve hours, respectively, before the test. After determination of the basal value of PEF, the patient inhaled two puffs each of either 40 microgram of Sch 1000 or placebo according to a double-blind cross-over arrangement. Fifteen minutes later the PEF measurement was repeated, the patient performed the exercise test and additional PEF measurements were performed at 1, 10 and 20 minutes after the end of exercise.

RESULTS

Part I. There were only slight changes in the airway resistance, thoracic gas volume, blood gas values and heart rate following inhalation of propellant in the placebo experiment. Subsequent inhalation of 80 microgram Sch 1000 was followed by a pronounced decrease in airway resistance (P < 0.001), the change being almost identical in the asthma group and the bronchitis group (Fig. 1). A subsequent inhalation of 300 microgram isoprenaline was followed by a further decrease in airway resistance in the asthma group (P < 0.001). In the bronchitis group the decrease in airway resistance was much smaller and statistically not significant. The asthma group differed from the bronchitis group (P < 0.01) with regard to the change in airway resistance following of isoprenaline at the end of the experiment.

Inhalation of a new anticholinergic drug, Sch 1000, in asthma and chronic bronchitis, effect on airway resistance, thoracic gas volume, blood gases and exercise-induced asthma. *Poppius H, Salorinne Y, Niljanen AA*

Inhalation of Sch 1000 was followed by a decrease in thoracic gas volume both in the asthma group (P < 0.001) an in the bronchitis group (P < 0.001). The subsequent inhalation of isoprenaline was followed by a further decrease in thoracic gas volume in the asthma group (P < 0.02), but not in the bronchitis group.

Inhalation of Sch 1000 in the asthma group was followed by a small increase in the arterial Po₂ (P < 0.02), a slight decrease in arterial Pco₂ (P < 0.02) and a minor decrease in heart rate (P < 0.01), and in the bronchitis group by a slight decrease in arterial Pco₂ (P < 0.05). Heart rate was not affected (Fig. 2). A few patients reported a slight dryness of mouth following inhalation of Sch 1000. No other side effects were reported.

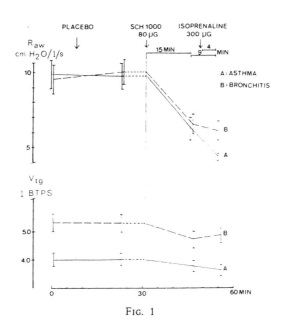

FIG. 1

Change in airway resistance (Raw) and thoracic gas volume (Vtg) following consecutive inhalations of placebo, 80 microgram Sch 1000 and 300 microgram isoprenaline in 28 asthmatics (group A) and 21 bronchitis (group B).

Part II. The results obtained in the exercise experiment are given in Table III and Fig. 3. Inhalation of 80 microgram Sch 1000 was followed by a small increase in PEF. The response was significantly

Inhalation of a new anticholinergic drug, Sch 1000, in asthma and chronic bronchitis, effect on airway resistance, thoracic gas volume, blood gases and exercise-induced asthma. *Poppius H, Salorinne Y, Niljanen AA*

648   H. POPPIUS ET AL.

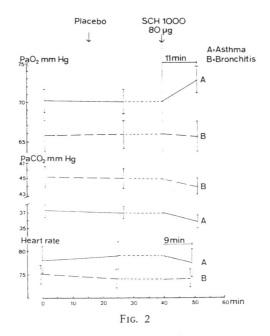

FIG. 2

Change in arterial Po₂, arterial Pco₂ and heart rate following consecutive inhalations of placebo and 80 microgram Sch 1000 in 28 asthmatics (group A) and 21 bronchitics (group B).

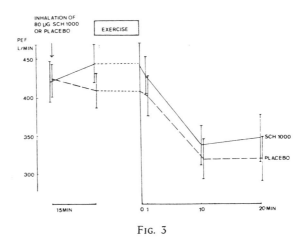

FIG. 3

Effect of pre-exercise inhalation of Sch 1000 on the post-exercise fall of PEF in 22 asthmatics, in whom exercise-induced asthma had been demonstrated in earlier experiments (group E-A).

Inhalation of a new anticholinergic drug, Sch 1000, in asthma and chronic bronchitis, effect on airway resistance, thoracic gas volume, blood gases and exercise-induced asthma. *Poppius H, Salorinne Y, Niljanen AA*

A NEW ANTICHOLINERGIC DRUG 649

TABLE III

SEVERITY OF EXERCISE IN THE BICYCLE EXERCISE TEST
PERFORMED IN 22 ASTHMATICS (GROUP E-A)

	Sch 1000	Placebo
Duration of exercise, min., mean	12.4	12.4
Duration of exercise, min., range	6-20	6-20
Heart rate at end of exercise, mean	156	156
Heart rate at end of exercise, S.E.M.	3.1	3.6

different from the slight fall in PEF obtained after placebo ($P < 0.001$).
The subsequent exercise period was followed by an almost identical
decrease in PEF in the Sch 1000 experiment as in the placebo experiment.
The maximum post-exercise decrease in PEF, expressed in percent of the
PEF value recorded immediately before exercise, was 27 % (S.E.M.
5.2 %) in the Sch 1000 experiment and 28 % (S.E.M. 4.3 %) in the
placebo experiment.

DISCUSSION

The effect of anticholinergic drugs on airways obstruction in asthma
is reported to be variable. In patients with allergic asthma in a relatively
stable clinical state the bronchodilation response to anticholinergic drugs
is slight in comparison to the response to sympathomimetics. Greater
benefit in terms of bronchodilation is seen in asthmatics who need corticosteroid treatment and in patients with chronic bronchitis (ALTOUNYAN
1964 ; CROMPTON, 1968). Using provocation and drug protection tests,
BOOIJ-NOORD et al. (1970) found « bronchitics » to be more sensitive to
the vagal reflex action than « asthmatics » and consequently more likely
to benefit from anticholinergic bronchodilators.

In the present investigation, inhalation of the anticholinergic drug Sch
1000 was followed by a maximum bronchodilation in patients with
chronic bronchitis, i.e. the subsequent inhalation of isoprenaline did not
give any further decrease in airway resistance. In the group of asthmatics,
on the contrary, a further significant bronchodilation was obtained after
the inhalation of isoprenaline in spite of a decrease in airway resistance
of the same magnitude as in the bronchitis group already after the Sch
1000 inhalation.

Inhalation of a new anticholinergic drug, Sch 1000, in asthma and
chronic bronchitis, effect on airway resistance, thoracic gas volume, blood
gases and exercise-induced asthma. *Poppius H, Salorinne Y, Niljanen AA*

D

650   H. POPPIUS ET AL.

The asthmatic patients submitted to the exercise test (group E-A) were in a clinically relatively stable state and most of them did not have a significant obstruction as judged from the PEF values. Accordingly, there was only a slight increase in PEF after the inhalation of Sch 1000. The exercise was followed by airways obstruction demonstrated as a significant post-exercise fall in PEF.

Exercise-induced airways obstruction is a clinically important feature of asthma. Its mechanism has not been clairified, although several hypotheses have been presented. The possibility of a release of broncho-constriction mediators from mast cell stores is compatible with the finding of the preventing effect on the exercise reaction of disodium cromoglycate (DAVIES, 1968 ; POPPIUS et al., 1970), which is thought to stabilize the mast cell membrane. The role of mechanical factors as a possible trigger mechanism is suggested by the observation that running or cycling causes more bronchoconstriction than swimming, the severity of exercise being equal (FITCH and MORTON, 1971), and the finding that gentle massage of a guinea pig lung or stirring of chopped lung tissue causes a release of bronchoconstriction mediators (VANE, 1971). Other authors have stressed the role of vagal reflex mechanisms (SIMONSSON et al., 1971), hypocapnia (REBUCK and READ, 1968) and acidosis (SEATON et al., 1969).

We did not find that Sch 1000 exerted any preventing effect on the increase in airways obstruction following exercise. This finding is in agreement with the observations of MCNEILL et al. (1966), that injection of atropine did not prevent exercise-induced asthma, but somewhat at variance with the results reported by SIMONSSON et al. (1971) who found that inhalation of atropine effectively blocked the exercise reaction. The differences may be due to the selection of patients ; the cases of SIMONSSON et al. were stated to have a non-allergic airways obstruction with increased bronchial reactivity to various non-specific stimuli and the preventing effect of disodium cromoglycate on the exercise reaction was poor, whereas features of atopy and good preventing effect of disodium cromoglycate on the exercise reaction were common findings in our material.

It is concluded that Sch 1000 in a dose of 80 microgram is a powerful bronchodilator without harmful effects on the blood gases or the heart rate. The drug may be of greater benefit for patients with the bronchitic type of airways obstruction than patients with the asthmatic type of obstruction, as the bronchodilation response was submaximal in the asthma group but maximal in the bronchitis group. Exercise-induced airways obstruction was not measurably prevented by the drug. Thus a vagal reflex action did not seem to play a significant role in mediating airways obstruction after exercise in our series.

Inhalation of a new anticholinergic drug, Sch 1000, in asthma and chronic bronchitis, effect on airway resistance, thoracic gas volume, blood gases and exercise-induced asthma. *Poppius H, Salorinne Y, Niljanen AA*

REFERENCES

ALTOUNYAN (R.E.C.). — Variation of drug action on airway obstruction in man.
Thorax, 1964, **19**, 406.

BOOIJ-NOORD (H.), ORIE (N.G.M.), BERG (W.Chr.), DE VRIES (K.). — Results of provocation of human bronchial airways with allergic and non-allergic stimuli and of drug protection tests. In : Bronchitis III. Proceedings of the Third International Symposium on Bronchitis at Groningen, the Netherlands, 23-26 September 1969. Royal Van Gorcum. Assen 1970, 316.

CIBA FOUNDATION SYMPOSIUM. — Terminology, definitions, and classification of chronic pulmonary emphysema and related conditions.
Thorax, 1959, **14**, 286.

CROMPTON (G.K.). — A comparison of responses to bronchodilator drugs in chronic bronchitis and chronic asthma.
Thorax, 1968, **23**, 46.

DAVIES (S.E.). — Effect of disodium cromoglycate on exercise-induced asthma.
Brit. med. J., 1968, **3**, 593.

FITCH (K.D.), MORTON (A.R.). — Specificity of exercise in exercise-induced asthma.
Brit. med. J., 1971, **4**, 577.

JONES (R.S.), WHARTON (M.J.), BUSTON (M.H.). — The place of physical exercise and bronchodilator drugs in the assessment of the asthmatic child.
Arch. Dis. Child., 1963, **38**, 539.

MCNEILL (R.S.), NAIRN (J.R.), MILLAR (J.S.), INGRAM (C.G.). — Exercise-induced asthma.
Quart. J. Med., 1966, **35**, 55.

MUYSERS (K.), SMIDT (U.), BUCHHEIM (F.W.). — Verbesserung ganzkörperplethys-mographischer Unterschungen durch Einsatz eines Analogrechners.
Pflügers Arch., 1969, **307**, 211.

POPPIUS (H.), MUITTARI (A.), KREUS (K.E.), KORHONEN (O.), VILJANEN (A.). — Exercise asthma and disodium cromoglycate.
Brit. med. J., 1970, **4**, 337.

REBUCK (A.S.), READ (J.). — Exercise-induced asthma.
Lancet, 1968, **2**, 429.

SEATON (A.), DAVIES (G.), GAZIANO (D.), OSBORNE HUGHES (R.). — Exercise-induced asthma.
Brit. med. J., 1969, **3**, 556.

SIMONSSON (B.E.), SKOOGH (B.), EKSTROM-JODAL (B.). — Exercise-induced airways constriction.
Scand. J. resp. Dis., 1971, Suppl. No 77, 30.

ULMER (W.T.). — Inhalationstherapie mit Atropinderivaten.
Med. Klin., 1971, **66**, 326.

VANE (J.R.). — Mediators of the anaphylactic reaction. In : Identification of Asthma. Ciba Foundation Study Group No. 38. Churchill Livingstone. Edinburg 1971, 121.

WOITOWITZ (H.J.), BUCHHEIM (F.W.), WOITOWITZ (R.). — Zur Theorie und Praxis der Ganzkörperplethysmographie in der Lungenfunktionsanalyse.
Praxis Pneumol., 1967, **21**, 449.

SUCCESSFUL TREATMENT OF PERSISTENT EXTREME DYSPNEA "STATUS ASTHMATICUS"

USE OF THEOPHYLLINE ETHYLENE DIAMINE (AMINOPHYLLINE, U. S. P.) INTRAVENOUSLY*

GEORGE HERRMANN, M.D., AND M. B. AYNESWORTH, M.D., GALVESTON, TEXAS
WITH THE HELP OF JOHN MARTIN, M.D., AS A SENIOR N. Y. A.
STUDENT ASSISTANT

ACUTE dyspnea is a medical emergency, particularly when persistent and not responsive to epinephrine or morphine. Any preparation which will relieve the acute respiratory distress under such conditions fairly regularly, promptly, and with reasonable safety deserves careful consideration.

The measures generally employed depend to some extent upon the underlying pathologic physiology and the accompanying complications. In general practice as well as in the emergency service of a large metropolitan hospital one is likely to have presented acute dyspneas of various types. The great majority of dyspneic patients suffer from cardiovascular disorders, particularly acute congestive left ventricular failure. However, acute bronchopulmonary conditions are responsible for a large number of the most severe types of acute dyspnea. These at times are not quieted by morphine and have become refractory to epinephrine and adrenalin hypodermatically. Such are often designated as "adrenalin fast status asthmaticus" cases.

Morphine sulfate has long been the drug of choice in most types of dyspnea. It is the most indispensable drug in the physician's possession. The dramatic life-saving effect, the effort-sparing and quieting action of morphine in patients in acute congestive failure, acute pulmonary edema, and paroxysmal nocturnal dyspnea are well known. Cheyne-Stokes breathing may, however, be aggravated, with the apneic periods greatly lengthened, by morphine. In status asthmaticus morphine is palliative at best, may actually depress the respiratory center dangerously and contribute to pulmonary edema if given repeatedly in large doses.

Epinephrine hydrochloride (adrenalin) and ephedrine hydrochloride are, of course, usually most efficacious in bronchial asthma but not infrequently one encounters cases in which the drugs fail to relieve the dyspnea. Such patients are sometimes designated as "adrenalin-fast status asthmaticus" cases. Under such circumstances one must resort to more heroic methods, such as the intravenous injection of small doses of 0.1 to 0.2 c.c. of 1-1,000 adrenalin; 10 c.c. cal-

*From the Department of Medicine of the University of Texas and The Medical Service of the John Sealy Hospital.
Received for publication, April 15, 1937.
Presented as part of a paper on the "Xanthine and Mercurial Diuretics" before the Section on Pharmacology and Therapeutics of the American Medical Association at the Kansas City Meeting on May 13, 1936.

135

Successful treatment of persistent extreme dyspnea, "status asthmaticus" – use of theophylline ethylene diamine (aminophylline, U.S.P.) intravenously. *Herrmann G, Aynesworth MB, Martin J*

136   THE JOURNAL OF LABORATORY AND CLINICAL MEDICINE

cium chloride 10 per cent solution; calcium gluconate 10 per cent solution; or 25 to 50 c.c. of hypertonic 50 per cent glucose solution. All of these have been used with some success.

We have found, however, that theophylline ethylene diamine (aminophylline, U. S. P., euphyllin, metaphyllin, thephyldine) in doses of 0.48 gm. (7½ grains) in 10 c.c. saline injected slowly is most uniformly successful with least serious reactions. We have found aminophyllin effective promptly and totally in fully 75 per cent of the cases of "status asthmaticus" in which we have used it. In some cases the relief afforded has not been immediate and complete but in most of these it has been both delayed and partial. In our hands the drug has rarely been totally ineffectual.

Our interest in this seemingly neglected and apparently important therapeutic action of aminophylline, U. S. P., was aroused during the progress of some clinical investigations (1) on the comparative diuretic effectiveness of various intravenously injected xanthines or purines, and mercurials begun in the Charity Hospital in New Orleans and continued in the John Sealy Hospital in Galveston.[1] We were often struck by the spectacular relief of urgent dyspnea as well as cardiac pain that resulted from the intravenous introduction of aminophylline in 0.48 gm. (7½ gr.) doses. We frequently noted the immediate disappearance of Cheyne-Stokes breathing following the intravenous introduction of aminophylline and have tried to explain the improvement on the basis of increased blood flow through the medulla but the response was so prompt that such could hardly be the case. It may be the result of a direct action of the drug on the cells of the respiratory center. Paroxysmal nocturnal dyspnea, cardiac asthma, have been noted to subside quickly after intravenous aminophylline. Again this may be response to improved circulation but it may also be central effect. Similar subsidence of nocturnal attacks may, however, follow profuse diuresis of salyrgan origin. Some of our patients whom we considered to be suffering from congestive heart failure also had pulmonary signs suggestive of asthmatic bronchitis and sometimes it was difficult to determine which was primary.

In one early series (1931) studied with Dr. Wm. L. Marr, of 5 elderly patients suffering from acute respiratory infection, asthmatic bronchitis and acute vesicular emphysema, 4 were treated with the usual antispasmodics and all died, while the fifth one treated with aminophylline (0.48 gm. diluted to 10 c.c.) intravenously alone survived.

We have found reports of respiratory improvement following the administration of aminophylline. Respiratory stimulating effects pulmonary circulatory augmenting effect, and the smooth muscle relaxing or possible bronchial clearing or effects have, however, not been commented upon in our literature.

Vogl[2] has reported on the value of xanthines, especially aminophylline, in respiratory disorders of central origin, particularly Cheyne-Stokes breathing in patients with general arteriosclerosis; and in central dyspnea resulting from pulmonary congestion and cardiac asthma. These conditions were relieved by the intravenous administration of 0.48 gm. (7½ gr.) of aminophylline.

Successful treatment of persistent extreme dyspnea, "status asthmaticus" – use of theophylline ethylene diamine (aminophylline, U.S.P.) intravenously. *Herrmann G, Aynesworth MB, Martin J*

Freud[3] has used aminophylline successfully, by rectal administration, in infants with periodic breathing of capillary bronchitis, in pneumonias of childhood, and in the periodic breathing of encephalitis, all of which are considered central disturbances of respiration.

Bock[4] demonstrated uniform dilatation of the blood vessels of the isolated dog's lung perfused under constant pressure as well as of the dog's extremity and kidney after the injection of 0.5 to 1.0 gm. of theophylline. The effect appeared within one to five minutes, usually within two minutes and lasted from one-half hour to one and one-half hours. The maximum effect was present in fifteen to twenty-one minutes. The effects of xanthines on the cerebral vessels and on the bronchial musculature have not been experimentally established.

In the report of the referee for the Council on Pharmacy and Chemistry of the American Medical Association (J. A. M. A. 94: 1306, 1930), there is abstracted the important literature up to that time with reference to the therapeutic effects of the xanthine derivatives. It is stated that according to Eppinger and Hess[5] the coronary artery dilated when placed in a weak solution of caffeine. Sollmann and Pilcher[6] found that the vasodilation resulted from peripheral inhibition of vasoconstriction. Meyer,[7] Hedbom,[8] and Loeb,[9] in perfusing isolated hearts with xanthine solutions, noted increased coronary flow which they considered to be due to vasodilation while other investigators, Sakai and Saneyoshi,[10] believed the increased coronary output to be the result of a rise in blood pressure. The latter experimenters[10] found that theobromin gave a greater augmentation of coronary flow. Heathcote[11] added that theophylline, as well as the other preparations, was an active vasodilator for coronary arteries, an action that he concluded was probably muscular in origin. Smith, Miller, and Graber[12] found experimentally that theophylline was the most effective of all the xanthines when given in the minute doses in which it might be found in the blood after administration by mouth. There has been much indirect personal clinical confirmation of this by the relief of angina pectoris following the ingestion and particularly injection of the drug. Blood pressure lowering has not been conspicuous and the value of the xanthines for this purpose has not been established. The council decided that the claims for diuretic action and myocardial stimulation and possibly vasodilating action were permissible. There was no mention of any theophylline effect on respiratory disorders, on the pulmonary circulation, or on the bronchial musculature in the earlier studies.

OUR PRESENT STUDIES

For the past six years we have been using the intravenous injection of theophylline in doses of 0.48 gm. in 10 c.c. of saline for the relief of persistent extreme dyspnea, "status asthmaticus" and "adrenaline fast" asthmatics. We have always given the solution slowly through a very small needle in order to avoid unpleasant reactions. Such reactions, however, have occurred fairly frequently in spite of all precautions but have been only slightly unpleasant and never serious, in our experience. Most of the patients complain of a momentary feeling of heat in the skin, particularly of the face, burning in the eyes, some-

Successful treatment of persistent extreme dyspnea, "status asthmaticus" – use of theophylline ethylene diamine (aminophylline, U.S.P.) intravenously. *Herrmann G, Aynesworth MB, Martin J*

138 THE JOURNAL OF LABORATORY AND CLINICAL MEDICINE

TABLE I

EFFECT OF AMINOPHYLLINE INTRAVENOUSLY IN STATUS ASTHMATICUS IN HOSPITAL PATIENTS

CASE	NAME, COLOR, SEX, AGE, HOSPITAL NUMBER	ADDITIONAL DIAGNOSES	PREVIOUS MEDICATION (EMERGENCY ROOM)	DURATION OF ASTHMA DURATION OF ATTACK	DOSE GM.	RELIEF IMMEDIATE	INTERVAL UNTIL NEXT ATTACK	REACTION TO DRUG	REMARKS
I	W. E. W. M., 79 205449	Chronic emphysema. Fibroid tuberculosis.	Adrenalin, ephedrine, morphine, digitalis. Ca Cl₂, Ca gluconate intravenously, Catarrhal vaccine.	25 years. Hours to 10 days.	0.48	Prompt. As short as eight minutes.	Usually a year. Sometimes only eight months.	Burning sensation in eyes. Headache.	After first treatment, blood pressure fell from 200/130 to 135/75, and remained at the low level. Vital capacity increased as much as 750 c.c.
II	R. L. W. F., 13 39381	Broncho-pneumonia.	Adrenalin, to ♏ L. Atropine, novatropine. Morphine. Glucose I-V. Phenobarbital. Ephedrine pantopon. Oxygen tent.	7 years. Hours to 3 days.	0.24	Sometimes in only ten minutes, other times, definite but not spectacular.	Long enough to be removed to Arizona, away from sensitive zone.	Heat over body. Nausea. Could not sleep for hours.	Subsequently moved to Arizona, where patient has been free from symptoms. Relieved in extremis by aminophylline, when all else had failed.
III	A. G. G. W. F., 37 4981	Urticaria. Diaphragmatic hernia.	Ephedrine, atropine, codeine, adrenalin, morphine, novatropine. Glucose, calcium gluconate.	11 years. Hours to days.	0.24 and 0.48	"Complete before injection was finished."	3 months.	Warmth. Nausea. Vomiting.	After patient had become "adrenalin-fast," aminophylline relieved her many times.

Successful treatment of persistent extreme dyspnea, "status asthmaticus" – use of theophylline ethylene diamine (aminophylline, U.S.P.) intravenously. *Herrmann G, Aynesworth MB, Martin J*

TABLE I—CONT'D

CASE	NAME, COLOR, SEX, AGE, HOSPITAL NUMBER	ADDITIONAL DIAGNOSES	PREVIOUS MEDICATION (EMERGENCY ROOM)	DURATION OF ASTHMA / DURATION OF ATTACK	DOSE GM.	RELIEF IMMEDIATE	INTERVAL UNTIL NEXT ATTACK	REACTION TO DRUG	REMARKS
IV	H. H. T. W. M., 25 (?) 34900	Maxillary sinusitis.	Adrenalin (large amount). Ca. gluconate & glucose. Oxygen tent.	4 years (only when in Galveston). Hours to days.	0.24 and 0.48	"Greatly relieved."	Moved after graduation.	Slight flushing, momentary increased constriction of chest, sensation of warmth and of "something let loose."	Senior medical student. Reported no further distress after graduation.
V	J. C. M. G. W. M., 66 206037	Extensive old bilateral tuberculosis.	Adrenalin.	8 months. Hours to days.	0.24 and 0.48	Complete relief in thirty minutes.	Two weeks.	"Peculiar," precordial feeling.	Loss of 30 pounds in the eight months. Sputum contained tubercle bacilli.
VI	W. E. R. M., 63 46007	Asthmatic bronchitis.	Codeine, novatropine. Phenobarbital. Ephedrine. Atropine, digitalis.	7 years. Several hours.	0.48	Complete symptomatic relief.	3 months (?).	Excitation. Sleeplessness.	While symptoms were relieved, vital capacity, pulse, and blood-pressure were not affected.
VII	B. C. W. 32683	Maxillary sinusitis. Emphysema.	Ephedrine. Adrenalin. Typhoid vaccine.	17 years. Hours to "2½ years, day and night, summer and winter."	0.48	Marked relief at first, but in time, only "improvement."	1 month. Patient moved.	None noted.	Patient first became refractory to adrenalin, after which aminophylline afforded relief, then patient became refractory to latter drug, and adrenalin again became effective.

Successful treatment of persistent extreme dyspnea, "status asthmaticus" – use of theophylline ethylene diamine (aminophylline, U.S.P.) intravenously. *Herrmann G, Aynesworth MB, Martin J*

140   THE JOURNAL OF LABORATORY AND CLINICAL MEDICINE

times there is a sense of constriction in the chest, occasionally nausea and vomiting and in very rare instances cerebral manifestations, twitching, convulsion, and coma. There have not, however, been any fatalities as a result of the injection of this drug in a hundred or more experiments and no report of death from intravenous injection of theophylline has been found in the literature.

We have not kept a cross index of all of our cases of respiratory distress treated with intravenous theophylline and we are certain many injections were given that were not recorded, particularly in the emergency room. We have, however, found the records of 7 of our hospital cases and 9 out-patients that were so treated. Short abstracts of the histories of these will be set down to illustrate our results.

SOME CASES OF STATUS ASTHMATICUS TREATED BY THEOPHYLLINE ETHYLENE DIAMINE

Case 1.—W. E. (Hospital number 205449), a white male, aged seventy-nine years, had suffered from attacks of shortness of breath for twenty-five years. The attacks usually have been associated with respiratory infection during the cold damp months of January, February, March, and April. For about fifteen years he has been having attacks earlier in the fall and winter and later in the spring. Since 1930 he has been admitted to the hospital with severe attacks no less than 20 times, each time with the same symptoms and signs of asthmatic bronchitis with evidences of chronic emphysema and a roentgenologic diagnosis by Dr. J. B. Johnson of fibroid tuberculosis. He had generally been relieved by the use of adrenalin or ephedrine with or without morphine, and occasionally digitalis was used and on rare occasions calcium chloride or calcium gluconate had to be given intravenously to get results.

At times, however, he has been refractory to all this therapy. Early on October 8, 1931 he had, in addition to dyspnea, a very severe attack of abdominal pain with vomiting, a blood pressure rise to 200/130, and electrocardiograms showing defective intraventricular conduction. At this time he was given theophylline ethylene diamine (thephyldine) 0.48 gm. diluted to 10 c.c. with saline intravenously, which promptly and completely relieved him of extreme dyspnea which was considered to be a part of his asthmatic bronchitis. His blood pressure ever after this attack was much lower, usually in the neighborhood of 130 to 140 over 70 to 80. This may have been an attack of coronary thrombosis.

He was given two courses of catarrhal vaccine but this did relatively little good. An exacerbation and exaggeration of the thoracic pulmonary distress followed each acute upper respiratory infection. All sorts of expectorants were used without avail and ephedrine, digitalis, theophylline e. d. (metaphyllin) tablets, 1½ gr. tablets were given regularly thrice daily by mouth. He was kept fairly comfortable on this regime and occasionally adrenalin had to be given hypodermatically.

At times he became refractory even to adrenalin and morphine and then 0.48 gm. of aminophyllin in 10 c.c. of normal saline was administered intravenously with, as a rule, prompt and complete relief with only a momentary burning sensation in his eyes as a reaction to the drug. On Oct. 7, 1932 his vital capacity rose from 1.75 liters, about 49 per cent of normal for him, to 2.2 liters and his blood pressure dropped to 128/60 to 119/58. This therapy was repeated Feb. 12, 1933, Feb. 13, 1934, Sept. 7, 1934, June 9, 1935. Calcium chloride 10 c.c. of a 10 per cent solution intravenously was tried on Sept. 13, 1935 and calcium gluconate 10 c.c. of a 10 per cent solution intravenously on Dec. 3, 1935 but aminophyllin was again resorted to on Dec. 6, 1935, and on May 6, 1936 when he had in addition to his dyspnea a severe precordial pain which was thought to be possibly coronary thrombosis but may well have been an interstitial mediastinal emphysema.

On Dec. 9, 1935, 3 gr. of aminophyllin by mouth t.i.d. kept him comfortable for a few days. He had been taking his regular oral medication of ephedrine and digitalis as

Successful treatment of persistent extreme dyspnea, "status asthmaticus" – use of theophylline ethylene diamine (aminophylline, U.S.P.) intravenously. *Herrmann G, Aynesworth MB, Martin J*

well as aminophyllin. Nevertheless, on Dec. 16, 1935 he came into the emergency room severely dyspneic and cyanosed. Adrenalin failed to relieve him and again 0.48 gm. of aminophyllin intravenously was promptly effective. On Oct. 10, 1936 he came in with an attack that had been persistent for ten days in spite of all medication including adrenalin. In addition to dyspnea and cyanosis, precordial pain and coughing were complained of and again 0.48 gm. of aminophyllin intravenously at 4 P.M. relieved him completely. He always felt the momentary burning sensation following the injection. On Jan. 22, 23, 24, and 25, 1937 the effect of the intravenous injection of 0.48 gm. of aminophyllin in 10 c.c. of saline on the vital capacity, blood pressure, respiration, and pulse were recorded.

During the seizure on Jan. 22, 1937, the vital capacity was 1,500 c.c.; the respiration rate, 24; the pulse rate, 96; and the blood pressure, 130/70. Eight minutes after injection he was completely relieved, had some burning in the eyes and headache, and his vital capacity had increased to 1,750 c.c.; his respirations dropped to 20; and his pulse, to 60 while his blood pressure remained unchanged.

Under similar circumstances on Jan. 23, 1937 with a vital capacity of 2,100 c.c.; respiration, 20; pulse, 64; and blood pressure, 110/60; aminophyllin relieved his distress and his vital capacity rose to 2,200 c.c.; his respirations to 24; and his blood pressure to 120/65.

Likewise on Jan. 24, 1937 in a severe attack his vital capacity was 1,750 c.c.; respiration 20, pulse 60, and blood pressure 110/60, while after relief by aminophyllin his vital capacity rose to 2,100 c.c. but no change was recorded in the respirations, pulse, and blood pressure.

And on Jan. 25, 1937 his vital capacity dropped to 1,500 c.c. with respiration rate 24, pulse rate 60, and blood pressure 120/68, while following aminophyllin the vital capacity rose to 2,250 c.c., the respirations and pulse rates remained unchanged and the blood pressure dropped to 110/60.

CASE II.—R. L. (Hospital number 39381), a school girl, aged thirteen, was first treated when she was eight years old, Oct. 5, 1932, for status asthmaticus. She had been under the care of Dr. Paul Woodard for some time, but he had not been able to find her sensitive to any of the ordinary allergens. Her attacks apparently followed each ''norther'' and were usually accompanied by an infection of the upper respiratory tract. On this day she had become much worse and failed to respond to adrenalin in 1 c.c. doses of 1/1000, atropine, novatropine, and morphine. All had failed to relieve her, and she went into collapse. She was given 20 c.c. of 25 per cent solution of glucose, intravenously and put under an oxygen tent. Then 1 c.c. containing 0.24 gm. of theophyllin e. d. was diluted and given intravenously following which she improved definitely though not spectacularly. She was discharged in a few days, but on Oct. 12, 1932 she again became refractory to all therapy which she was taking and was readmitted to the hospital and put on the same regime which she previously had taken and again 1 c.c. of 0.24 gm. of theophyllin e. d. was the only medication that brought any relief. She improved sufficiently to be moved to the southwest where she was entirely free of symptoms and in good health.

In the fall of 1936 she returned to Galveston. On Jan. 31, 1937 following a sinus infection she had a recurrence of her severe attack of asthma and was given phenobarbital and ephedrine and recovered. On Feb. 13, 1937 following another upper respiratory infection she was admitted to the hospital with fever of 103.8°, respirations 28, pulse 120, and a roentgenogram revealed evidence of bronchopneumonia with diffuse infiltration throughout both lungs, and an interlobar pleurisy between the middle and upper lobe on the right.

She had fever for only three days, and the respiratory distress continued in spite of the counterirritation to the chest, expectorants, sedatives, atropine and adrenalin. On Feb. 11, 1937 she went into a status asthmaticus and was given subcutaneously pantopon, ⅓ gr., atropine, 1/150 gr., and adrenalin minims 10. This was repeated six hours later but between these doses three injections of 15 minims each of adrenalin had to be given. She was most certainly adrenalin-fast. Oxygen therapy was instituted and she was given 20 c.c. of 50 per cent glucose intravenously. As this seemingly did no good and she was in extremis, intravenous aminophyllin administration was ordered but only a half dose of 1 c.c. or 0.24 gm. was diluted and injected. She complained some of a feeling of heat over the body and some nausea but within ten minutes she could breathe with comparative ease. She was

Successful treatment of persistent extreme dyspnea, "status asthmaticus" – use of theophylline ethylene diamine (aminophylline, U.S.P.) intravenously. *Herrmann G, Aynesworth MB, Martin J*

somewhat excited by the drug and although exhausted she could not go to sleep for some hours. Phenobarbital quieted her. The aminophyllin injection was repeated once more in the early morning hours. Improvement was rapid thereafter. Within twenty-four hours she was on her way back to Tucson, Arizona. She cleared up on the trip and remains free of trouble in Arizona.

CASE III.—A. G. G. (Hospital number 4981), a Mexican housewife, aged thirty-seven, first came under observation, Aug. 19, 1931 with a burn on the hand and asthma. She appeared in attacks in the clinic in 1926 and 1927 at which time ephedrine capsules of ¾ gr. each were successful in relieving attacks. In 1928 on one occasion she became refractory but was relieved after many capsules were taken and an injection of atropine and codeine sulphate. Her attacks usually began in the month of August and recurred each fall with greater intensity, particularly when the wind was in the north. After a few years she suffered attacks at other times in the year.

In 1929 a severe attack was relieved by adrenalin. She was seen at this time by Dr. Homer Prince who thought that there was a nervous basis rather than an allergic basis for her attacks since they were always worse during and after pregnancy. She had pain in the left chest on frequent occasions. Ephedrine and adrenalin seemed to relieve her of attacks during 1929 and 1930. In 1931 her attacks became more frequent in the spring as well as the fall. She had severe coughing as well and on one occasion she thought she pulled something loose inside of her chest. She showed the same symptoms, dyspnea and pain and signs as sonorous râles of asthmatic bronchitis and emphysema throughout both lungs on each admission. The roentgenogram revealed lungs that were clear except for considerable fibrosis in and about the hilar regions.

She was operated upon for bilateral salpingitis, appendicitis, and suffered from chronic pleuritis late in 1931. In 1932 she had an attack of rash and urticaria following the eating of raw oysters. On one occasion in the late fall of 1932 ephedrine was ineffectual and adrenalin 15 min. 1 c.c. and morphine 15 mg. relieved the attack. In 1933 0.0025 gm. of novatropine t.i.d. was used with some success to prevent the asthmatic seizures. In 1933 the attacks recurred about every two months. Atropine and morphine were frequently used along with 1.3 c.c. of adrenalin. She became "adrenalin-fast" during a prolonged attack in the autumn of 1933. One cubic centimeter of 0.24 gm. of theophyllin ethylene diamine intravenously was followed by some relief. Afterwards she again responded to adrenalin. During 1934 she was taking ephedrine religiously. Her blood pressure which had previously been normal, rose to 144/78, 187/88, 190/112, and 210/100. She began to have attacks of asthma at least once a month and often every two weeks. In 1935 she was given 1½ gr. of aminophyllin t.i.d. in addition to her previous therapy. Her attacks became less frequent, occurring only about once in three months. The asthma, however, did not clear up entirely. Examination of the lungs always showed râles, even between the severe attacks. The blood pressure continued at high levels. In 1935 it was 190/120, and in a severe seizure on Feb. 21, 1935 she was given intravenously 10 c.c. of calcium gluconate of a 10 per cent solution diluted in 50 c.c. of a 50 per cent solution of glucose which relieved the status asthmaticus. The blood pressure dropped to 148/80.

On Sept. 28, 1935 she came in to the hospital in an attack of status asthmaticus which had been continuous for two weeks in spite of the taking of 50 mg. (¾ gr.) capsules of ephedrine every four hours and an injection of 1 c.c. of adrenalin in the emergency room. Upon admission to the hospital her condition was considered to be grave and theophylline e. d. (aminophyllin) Searle's 0.48 gm. in 10 c.c. of saline was administered intravenously. The attack ceased before the injection was completed. She complained of a momentary feeling of warmth and nausea which was followed by vomiting. She left the hospital the next morning.

She continued to have recurrent minor attacks of dyspnea which were relieved by the ordinary medication. On Jan. 31, 1936 she had a rash with itching, burning, smarting, and swelling of the lower lip after eating eggs and bacon for breakfast. This was relieved by adrenalin. On Feb. 5, 1936 she had a similar attack and was placed on elimination

Successful treatment of persistent extreme dyspnea, "status asthmaticus" – use of theophylline ethylene diamine (aminophylline, U.S.P.) intravenously. *Herrmann G, Aynesworth MB, Martin J*

diet. She has had no recurrences of the rash but the dyspneic attacks have recurred. She was found to have a massive herniation of the stomach through the diaphragm into the left chest.

CASE IV.—H. H. T. (Hospital number 34900), a senior medical student, first came under observation in 1931 with sinusitis which required surgical drainage. He had never had any trouble before coming to Galveston to attend the medical school. Each autumn following each "norther" he would have asthmatic attacks. Various tests for sensitization were tried, and he was found to be slightly sensitive to house dust and marsh elder but not markedly so to either. The asthmatic seizures became longer and more severe each year.

During the latter part of his senior year, May 19, 1934, he began to have an attack following a spring "norther" and unlike most of his attacks he was unable to control this one with adrenalin. He had injected adrenalin in 1 c.c. doses at hourly intervals for about half a day before he sought admission to the hospital. He was extremely tremulous, dyspneic, orthopneic, and cyanotic. The neck veins were distended and auscultation of· the chest revealed high pitched musical râles. Adrenalin injections were continued. Each administration caused him to vomit. Ten cubic centimeters of calcium gluconate of a 10 per cent solution was given in 100 c.c. of 25 per cent glucose solution which helped very little. The oxygen tent seemed to do little good. Finally theophyllin e. d. (metaphyllin 0.24 gm.) was given intravenously. This caused slight flushing, momentary increased constriction of the chest, a feeling of warmth and then "a feeling as though something let loose." He was able to expectorate a thick tenacious mucopurulent sputum and was greatly relieved. He seemed better able to make use of the oxygen tent which was continued for some hours. Dilaudid 1/20 gr. was given and he went off into a peaceful sleep. On awakening he continued to vomit for some hours and developed a mild acidosis. The patient became jaundiced. Dr. D. P. Wall found nasal polyps and a maxillary sinusitis and took steps to shrink the nasal mucosa with adrenalin. The sinuses were drained, the polyps were removed and he improved. Upon graduation he took an internship in a northern hospital. As a result of the climatic change it was reported that he had had very little trouble.

CASE V.—J. M. C. G. (Hospital number 206037), a white painter, aged sixty-six years, complained of attacks of coughing, expectoration of pus, acute shortness of breath, palpitation, pain over the heart and weakness. According to his story the symptoms had appeared only eight months previously, that is in May, 1936. Not until November, 1936 had they progressed to the point of severity necessitating medical attention. He had lost 30 pounds in weight. There was no history of idiosyncrasy or allergy of any type and no history suggestive of previous tuberculosis in himself or in his family.

The peripheral arteries were generally sclerosed. The blood pressure was 130/70. The heart was negative. The pulmonary findings were those of asthmatic bronchitis. The sputum, however, contained a few tubercle bacilli along with myriads of other organisms. The roentgenologist reported extensive bilateral old pulmonary tuberculosis.

On Jan. 19, 1937 he had a severe attack of difficult breathing which was only partly relieved by an injection of 1 c.c. of adrenalin solution. On Jan. 20, 1937 during the night he developed an attack of respiratory distress which was refractory to adrenalin (1 c.c.) treatment but gradually let up after 1 c.c. or 0.24 gm. (3½ gr.) of aminophyllin intravenously. On Jan. 20, 1937 he had severe early morning attacks of dyspnea which were relieved by 0.48 gm. of aminophyllin (7½ gr.) intravenously, and Dr. Peticolas found that the vital capacity rose from 1,200 c.c. to 1,400 c.c. while the respiratory rate of 20 remained unchanged, the pulse dropped from 88 to 80 and the blood pressure remained 120/80. On Jan. 21, 1937 another attack responded to aminophyllin 0.48 gm. (7½ gr.) i.v. but the patient complained of a peculiar sensation over the precordium not a true pain. Its exact nature could not be determined though it persisted for several hours.

At 4 A.M. Feb. 18, 1937 he had another bad spell of coughing and struggling for breath. It passed off thirty minutes after an intravenous injection of 0.24 gm. (3½ gr.) of aminophyllin. On March 4 at about 4:30 A.M. he again became extremely dyspneic and an intravenous injection of 0.46 gm. of aminophyllin relieved him completely. On March 17 he suffered from a status asthmaticus with his vital capacity depressed to 800 c.c., a respiratory

Successful treatment of persistent extreme dyspnea, "status asthmaticus" – use of theophylline ethylene diamine (aminophylline, U.S.P.) intravenously. *Herrmann G, Aynesworth MB, Martin J*

TABLE II

EFFECT OF AMINOPHYLLINE (0.48 GM.) INTRAVENOUSLY IN STATUS ASTHMATICUS IN OUT PATIENTS

NAME, COLOR, AGE, SEX OUT-PATIENT NUMBER	DIAGNOSES	PREVIOUS MEDICINE (IN E. R., ETC.)	DURATION OF ASTHMA / DURATION OF ATTACK	DOSE (OTHER THAN 0.48 GM.)	RELIEF, IMMEDIATE	INTERVAL UNTIL NEXT ATTACK	REACTION (IF ANY)	REMARKS
R. E. B.; W, 27, M. 67382	Br. asthma	Adren., ♏ x-xv; Ephedrine, gr. ¾; Tr. Benz. Co.; Morphine, gr. ¼; Atropine, gr. 1/150; Glucose I-V	11 Years; 11-24 hours	gr. iii; gr. iv	Complete; Complete; Complete	4 hours; 2 months; 4 months	None noted	Has not been to clinic with "Asthma," as chief complaint since Oct. 20, 1936, when he last received aminophylline. The adrenalin, etc., conspicuously failed to relieve him.
H. M.; B, 27, F. 16700	Br. asthma, Syphilis, tertiary Cervicitis	Adren., ♏ x-xv; Ephedrine, gr. ¾; Atropine, gr. 1/75; Ca. gluconate I-V	8 Years; 2-12 hours		Complete; Complete; Complete	One year; 6 days; 4 days	"Hot flash" following injection on one occasion	Has been treated at least once by almost every interne for past three years. Other medicine afforded only irregular relief.
H. S.; B, 33, M. 9060	Br. asthma	Adren., ♏ x-xv; Ephedrine, gr. ¾	"Since childhood"; 4 hours		Partial (delayed)	Two weeks; One week	No reaction noted	Relieved on one occasion when two injections of adrenalin same night had failed. None-to-complete relief with adrenalin.
D. T. M.; B, 41, M. 75023	Br. asthma, Syphilis, tertiary	Adren., ♏ x-xv; Ephedrine, gr. ¾	1½ Years; Minutes—hours		Partial	8 days	Some feeling of oppression over chest	Aminophylline given only one time. Succeeded after ♏ x adrenalin same day had failed.
J. B.; B, 44, M. 61141	Br. asthma	Adren., ♏ x-xv; Ephed., gr. ⅜	20 Years		Complete	5 months	No reaction noted	Was treated with Aminophylline only one time, and on that occasion it succeeded after ♏ x and ♏ xv of adrenalin had failed.

Successful treatment of persistent extreme dyspnea, "status asthmaticus" – use of theophylline ethylene diamine (aminophylline, U.S.P.) intravenously. *Herrmann G, Aynesworth MB, Martin J*

HERRMANN-AYNESWORTH: PERSISTENT EXTREME DYSPNEA 145

TABLE II—Cont'd

NAME, COLOR, AGE, SEX OUT-PATIENT NUMBER	DIAGNOSES	PREVIOUS MEDICINE (IN E. R., ETC.)	DURATION OF ASTHMA DURATION OF ATTACK	DOSE (OTHER THAN 0.48 GM.)	RELIEF, IMMEDIATE	INTERVAL UNTIL NEXT ATTACK	REACTION (IF ANY)	REMARKS
J. B.; W, 51, M. 56101	Br. asthma	Adren., ♏ x	17 Years	gr. viiss gr. ii	Complete Complete	3 months 3 months	No reaction noted after either injection	Periodic attacks for seventeen years. Adrenalin usually relieved attacks during this period.
J. H.; B, 37, M. 58351	Br. asthma Urethral stricture	Adren., ♏ x-xv Ephedrine, gr. ¾ Amyl nitrite Morphine Amytal Autog. vaccine	9 Years Seasonal Minutes to 8 hours		Complete	One month	None noted	Rapid recovery from attack after administration of Aminophylline.
W. H. W.; B, 62, M. 13787	Chr. Br. asthma Hypertensive H. D.	Adren., ♏ x Ephedrine, gr. ¾	About 20 years 2-4-8 hours		Complete	One month	"Hot flash," very transient	Had only one dose of Aminophylline in 1935, that was given with ephedrine. Prompt relief usually followed adrenalin and ephedrine.
B. W.; B, 37, F. 14212	Asthma bronchitis Hay fever Gastro-intestinal allergy	Adren., ♏ x-xv Ephed., gr. ¾ Autog. vaccine Morph. sulf. gr. ¼ Atropine gr. 1/150 Ca. gluconate I-V Adren., ♏ xii Amyl nitrite	12 Years 4-10 hours Not effective		Partial (delayed) Partial (delayed) Very Little	One day 24 days —?—	No reaction noted in any instance	Termed an "adrenalin-fast" case by several internes. All types of medications had failed signally in many of her visits to the emergency room and to the dispensary.

Successful treatment of persistent extreme dyspnea, "status asthmaticus" – use of theophylline ethylene diamine (aminophylline, U.S.P.) intravenously. *Herrmann G, Aynesworth MB, Martin J*

144   THE JOURNAL OF LABORATORY AND CLINICAL MEDICINE

TABLE II

Effect of Aminophylline (0.48 Gm.) Intravenously in Status Asthmaticus in Out Patients

NAME, COLOR, AGE, SEX OUT-PATIENT NUMBER	DIAGNOSES	PREVIOUS MEDICINE (IN E. R., ETC.)	DURATION OF ASTHMA DURATION OF ATTACK	DOSE (OTHER THAN 0.48 GM.)	RELIEF, IMMEDIATE	INTERVAL UNTIL NEXT ATTACK	REACTION (IF ANY)	REMARKS
R. E. B.; W, 27, M. 67382	Br. asthma	Adren., ℳ x-xv Ephedrine, gr. ¾ Tr. Benz. Co. Morphine, gr. ¼ Atropine, gr. 1/150 Glucose I-V	11 Years 11-24 hours	gr. iii gr. iv	Complete Complete Complete	4 hours 2 months 4 months	None noted	Has not been to clinic with "Asthma," as chief complaint since Oct. 20, 1936, when he last received aminophylline. The adrenalin, etc., conspicuously failed to relieve him.
H. M.; B, 27, F. 16700	Br. asthma, Syphilis, tertiary Cervicitis	Adren., ℳ x-xv Ephedrine, gr. ¾ Atropine, gr. 1/75 Ca. gluconate I-V	8 Years 2-12 hours		Complete Complete Complete	One year 6 days 4 days	"Hot flash" following injection on one occasion	Has been treated at least once by almost every interne for past three years. Other medicine afforded only irregular relief.
H. S.; B, 33, M. 9060	Br. asthma	Adren., ℳ x Ephedrine, gr. ¾	"Since childhood" 4 hours		Partial (delayed)	Two weeks One week	No reaction noted	Relieved on one occasion when two injections of adrenalin same night had failed. None-to-complete relief with adrenalin.
D. T. M.; B, 41, M. 75023	Br. asthma, Syphilis, tertiary	Adren., ℳ x-xv Ephedrine, gr. ¾	1½ Years Minutes—hours		Partial	8 days	Some feeling of oppression over chest	Aminophylline given only one time. Succeeded after ℳ x adrenalin same day had failed.
J. B.; B, 44, M. 61141	Br. asthma	Adren., ℳ x-xv Ephed., gr. ⅜	20 Years		Complete	5 months	No reaction noted	Was treated with Aminophylline only one time, and on that occasion it succeeded after ℳ x and ℳ xv of adrenalin had failed.

Successful treatment of persistent extreme dyspnea, "status asthmaticus" – use of theophylline ethylene diamine (aminophylline, U.S.P.) intravenously. *Herrmann G, Aynesworth MB, Martin J*

TABLE II—CONT'D

NAME, COLOR, AGE, SEX OUT-PATIENT NUMBER	DIAGNOSES	PREVIOUS MEDICINE (IN E. R., ETC.)	DURATION OF ASTHMA / DURATION OF ATTACK	DOSE (OTHER THAN 0.48 GM.)	RELIEF, IMMEDIATE	INTERVAL UNTIL NEXT ATTACK	REACTION (IF ANY)	REMARKS
J. B.; W, 51, M. 56101	Br. asthma	Adren., m x	17 Years	gr. viss / gr. ii	Complete / Complete	3 months / 3 months	No reaction noted after injection either time	Periodic attacks for seventeen years. Adrenalin usually relieved attacks during this period.
J. H.; B, 37, M. 58351	Br. asthma / Urethral stricture	Adren., m x-xv / Ephedrine, gr. ¾ / Amyl nitrite / Morphine / Amytal / Autog. vaccine	9 Years Seasonal / Minutes to 8 hours		Complete	One month	None noted	Rapid recovery from attack after administration of Aminophylline.
W. H. W.; B, 62, M. 13787	Chr. Br. asthma / Hypertensive H. D.	Adren., m x / Ephedrine, gr. ¾	About 20 years / 2-4-8 hours		Complete	One month	"Hot flash," very transient	Had only one dose of Aminophylline in 1935, that was given with ephedrine. Prompt relief usually followed adrenalin and ephedrine.
B. W.; B, 37, F. 14212	Asthma / bronchitis / Hay fever / Gastro-intestinal allergy	Adren., m x-xv / Ephed., gr. ¾ / Autog. vaccine / Morph. sulf.. gr. ¼ / Atropine gr. 1/150 / Ca. gluconate I-V / Adren., m xii / Amyl nitrite	12 Years / 4-10 hours / Not effective		Partial (delayed) / Partial (delayed) / Very Little	One day / 24 days / —?—	No reaction noted in any instance	Termed an "adrenalin-fast" case by several internes. All types of medications had failed signally in many of her visits to the emergency room and to the dispensary.

Successful treatment of persistent extreme dyspnea, "status asthmaticus" – use of theophylline ethylene diamine (aminophylline, U.S.P.) intravenously. *Herrmann G, Aynesworth MB, Martin J*

146   THE JOURNAL OF LABORATORY AND CLINICAL MEDICINE

rate of 28, pulse rate of 100, and blood pressure of 128/86. After 0.48 gm. of aminophyllin had been given intravenously his vital capacity rose to 1,400 c.c. his respiration dropped to 24, and his pulse rate to 88, while his blood pressure rose to 142/84, and he was completely relieved. His vital capacity rose to 1,500 c.c. on March 21, and on March 27 it was 1,700 c.c.

CASE VI.—W. E. R. (Hospital number 46007), a male, cook, aged sixty-three, began to have asthmatic attacks in 1930 as a sequence of fall and winter colds with cough and chest pains which had been recurrent and of increasing severity for several years. Exertion would often bring on attacks of wheezing in the chest, choking sensations, vise-like pain in the left chest around the nipple radiating to the left shoulder, followed by a hacking cough with some white mucous expectoration. At times there was sputum. Vertigo usually came on at the end of an attack. Palpitation, weakness, loss of weight had occurred. The pain was vise-like in character brought on by exertion and by lying on the left chest and then arising. The patient had an occasional night sweat.

The chief physical abnormalities were found in the examination of the chest which was barrel shaped with a scar of an old liver drainage at the right base anteriorly and hyperesthesia about the left nipple. The chest was hyperresonant and showed the signs of asthmatic bronchitis. The heart was not enlarged. The blood pressure was normal. The heart rate was 68. The aortic second sound was slightly accentuated. No murmurs were heard. The peripheral vessels were moderately sclerosed. The blood pressure was 128/75 and 135/82. A roentgenogram showed signs of old fibroid pulmonary tuberculosis for the most part in the upper half of the right lung but to some extent throughout both lungs there were multiple pleurodiaphragmatic adhesions. The electrocardiogram showed slurring and low voltage in all leads, some left axis deviation but no pathognomic electrocardiographic signs were present.

On Oct. 12, 1934 his vital capacity was found to be 46.3 per cent of normal. On Feb. 7, 1935 his vital capacity was estimated to be 1,850 c.c. which for his 1.5 square meters body surface was 50 per cent of normal. The blood pressure dropped to as low as 105/65. He had been treated with codeine, novatropine, phenobarbital, ephedrine, atropine, and digitalis. He was maintained on the latter. The coughing spells continued. Tightness in the chest developed and dyspnea increased. Paroxysms of coughing which usually occurred in the early morning hours often developed into status asthmaticus and caused him to struggle for air. At such times piping high pitched musical râles were heard in both chests, particularly on inspiration. There seemed to be an acute vesicular emphysema engrafted upon a chronic emphysema. His vital capacity was reduced to 27 per cent of normal.

On Jan. 21, 1937 at 2:30 A.M. he had a sharp severe attack. His vital capacity was found to be only 700 c.c. with respiration 24, pulse 100, and blood pressure 110/70. He was given 0.48 gm. of aminophyllin intravenously in 10 c.c. of saline and his distress immediately subsided. His respirations dropped to 20 but his vital capacity, pulse, and blood pressure were unchanged in spite of striking symptomatic relief. He was, however, unable to go to sleep because of the excitation produced by the xanthine.

CASE VII.—B. C. (Hospital number 32683), a housewife, was admitted in status asthmaticus in which distressing condition she said she had been more or less constantly for two and one-half years, day and night, summer and winter. Her first attack occurred in 1920, when after recovering from the measles she had a smothering spell and wheezing in the chest. This attack cleared up shortly only to recur at first only after she caught cold or had upper respiratory infection to which she was particularly susceptible. Later sweeping and eating brought on the attack and finally they came on spontaneously. At first she was relieved by ephedrine and adrenalin but the drugs gradually became less and less effective and finally the relaxation lasted only about ten or fifteen minutes. She was worse after the effects wore off. She had lost 38 pounds in eight months before admission. She had been under the care of an allergist and had been tested with all sorts of pollens, emanations, dusts, and foods and was found to be only slightly sensitive to house dust but to nothing else. The patient had one brother who had had asthma but had recovered.

Successful treatment of persistent extreme dyspnea, "status asthmaticus" – use of theophylline ethylene diamine (aminophylline, U.S.P.) intravenously. *Herrmann G, Aynesworth MB, Martin J*

On physical examination she was orthopneic, unable to lie down, cyanotic and in severe distress. She had had frequent attacks of sinusitis and drainage of pus from the maxillary had been accomplished. The accessory muscles of respiration were constantly used and well developed. The chest was somewhat barrel shaped, emphysematous. Hyperresonance was noted on percussion. The signs of severe asthmatic state were present. Whistling, squeaking, sonorous groans and râles were heard on inspiration and on expiration. The heart was not enlarged. No murmurs were heard and no abnormal sounds. The blood pressure was 125/90. Scars, the result of numerous hypodermic injections were found on the extremities.

The roentgenologist reported extensive fibrosis in the right lung and, to a slightly less extent, the left. There was chronic bronchitis with an old pleuropneumonic disease of the right base. The left antrum and ethmoids were clouded.

The left antrum had been radically operated upon and upon subsequent puncture yielded a tablespoonful of mucopurulent exudate.

Records were unfortunately not kept of the early emergency treatment of this case. However, the progress note of Sept. 11, 1926 stated that 0.48 gm. (7½ gr.) of aminophyllin in 10 c.c. of saline intravenously had had a marked effect at the beginning of her hospitalization but had become less effective. Aminophyllin 0.1 gm. or 1-gr. doses t.i.d. p.o. was also tried in this case without any apparent benefit. Aminophyllin solution containing 0.6 gm. or 10 gr. per rectum was successful in one instance. Nevertheless, the patient was noted to have improved generally and was reported as sleeping better. The asthmatic attacks recurred but she had relatively long free periods such as she had not enjoyed for two or three years and adrenalin again became useful. There were few changes in her chest signs.

She was submitted to a course of typhoid vaccine intravenously which gave her a severe chill and temperatures that rose to 104° F. after which she felt better. After this adrenalin again became more effective as it did following the aminophyllin therapy. On Oct. 16, 1936 she was up and about the ward and while walking she became warm and suffered a most severe asthmatic attack. She, however, responded immediately to adrenalin. Because of the climatic conditions she was advised that she would probably continue her improvement more certainly in a higher drier climate and was therefore discharged home.

It is indeed unusual for a patient to become refractory to the effects of aminophyllin intravenously as this patient apparently did. Aminophyllin did not cause in her any more excitement or feeling of anxiety than adrenalin. It was effective longer, was not followed by a letdown, such as followed adrenalin, and seemed to restore the desirable reactivity to adrenalin.

SUMMARY AND CONCLUSIONS

Sixteen clinical cases of asthmatic bronchitis or chronic bronchial asthma presenting attacks of status asthmaticus are recorded, in which 41 injections of theophylline ethylene diamine (aminophyllin) had been administered intravenously as emergency therapy, usually with success after adrenalin had been ineffectual. Of these 41 injections 31 afforded prompt, complete, and persistent relief, but at least 6 of these were of the half dosage of 0.24 gm. or 3¾ gr.

In two instances the full dose of 0.48 gm. (7½ gr.) seemingly failed. There was one failure to accomplish relief and even in this instance posttheophylline e. d. adrenalin injections became effective. In one instance the patient was made slightly more uncomfortable.

In practically all cases that had become adrenalin fast theophylline e. d. seemed to restore the sensitiveness to adrenalin.

In only one instance was there the development of anything that might be considered a refractoriness to theophylline e. d.

Reactions to the intravenous injection of 0.48 gm. (7½ gr.) of theophylline e. d. were common but as a rule quite mild and innocuous and rarely very dis-

Successful treatment of persistent extreme dyspnea, "status asthmaticus" – use of theophylline ethylene diamine (aminophylline, U.S.P.) intravenously. *Herrmann G, Aynesworth MB, Martin J*

148 THE JOURNAL OF LABORATORY AND CLINICAL MEDICINE

turbing. The precautions of diluting the 2 c.c. containing 0.48 gm. of theophylline e. d. to 10 c.c. with saline or glucose solution and injecting it slowly through a fine 22 gauge needle were always taken.

Theophylline e. d. in 0.48 gm. doses diluted to 10 c.c. and introduced slowly intravenously seems to be a most effective, prompt, reliable and safe therapeutic procedure for the combating of status asthmaticus even after there has developed a refractoriness to adrenalin.

REFERENCES

1. Herrmann, George and associates: Proc. Soc. Exper. Biol. & Med. 28: 263, 1930; Trans. Assn. Am. Phys. 46: 360, 1931; South M. J. 25: 934, 1932; Trans. Assn. Am. Phys. 47: 279, 1932; J. A. M. A. 99: 1647, 1932; J. LAB. & CLIN. MED. 18: 902, 1933; Proc. Soc. Exper. Biol. & Med. 30: 1315, 1933; Trans. Assn. Am. Phys. 48: 364, 1933; Texas S. J. Med. 29: 240, 1933; J. LAB. & CLIN. MED. 22: 767, 1937.
2. Vogl, A.: Erfahrungen uber Euphyllin bei Cheyne-Stokes und anderen Formen zentraler atmenstorung, Med. Klin. 28: 9, 1932.
3. Freud, P.: Bekämfung zentraler Atemstörungen im Kindesalter mit Euphyllin, Deutsche med. Wchnschr. 61: 277, 1935.
4. Bock, H. E.: Zur Gefasswirking des Strophanthins, Theozins und Caffeine, Arch. f. Exper. Path. u. Pharmak., 1932.
*5. Eppinger and Hess: Ztschr. f. Exper. Path. 5: 622, 1909, quoted by Rabe: Ibid. 11: 175, 1912.
6. Sollmann and Pilcher: The Actions of Caffeine on the Mammalian Circulation, J. Pharm. & Exper. Therap. 3: 19, 19-11-1012.
7. Meyer: Arch. f. Anat. u. Physiol. p. 223, 1912, quoted by Heathcote.
8. Hedbom: Skand. Arch. f. Physiol. 9: 1, 1899, quoted by Smith, Miller and Graber.
9. Loeb: Arch. f. Exper. Path. u. Pharmakol. 51: 64, 1903-1904, quoted by Smith, Miller and Graber.
10. Sakai and Saneyoshi: Arch. f. Exper. Path. u. Pharmakol. 78: 331, 1914-1915, quoted by Smith, Miller and Graber.
11. Heathcote, R. St. A.: The Action of Caffeine, Theobromine and Theophylline on the Mammalian and Batrachian Heart, J. Pharmacol. & Exper. Therapy 16: 327, 1920-1921.
12. Smith, F. M., Miller, G. H., and Graber, V. C.: The Effect of Caffeine Sodiobenzoate, Theobromin Sodiosalicylate, Theophylline and Euphylline on the Coronary Flow and Cardiac Action of the Rabbit, J. Clin. Investigation 2: 157, 1926.

*5 to 12 Quoted from Report of Council on Pharmacy and Chemistry. Therapeutic claims for theobromine and theophylline preparations, J. A. M. A., 94: 1306, 1930.

Successful treatment of persistent extreme dyspnea, "status asthmaticus" – use of theophylline ethylene diamine (aminophylline, U.S.P.) intravenously. *Herrmann G, Aynesworth MB, Martin J*

THE ACTION OF THEOPHYLLINE
WITH ETHYLENEDIAMINE

ON INTRATHECAL AND VENOUS PRESSURES IN
CARDIAC FAILURE AND ON BRONCHIAL
OBSTRUCTION IN CARDIAC FAILURE
AND IN BRONCHIAL ASTHMA

JAMES A. GREENE, M.D.

W. D. PAUL, M.D.

AND

A. E. FELLER, M.D.

IOWA CITY

It has been definitely established that theophylline with ethylenediamine has a favorable influence on the dyspnea of cardiac failure.[1] These results have been attributed in part to the effect on the coronary and cerebral circulation. The present investigation was undertaken in the hope that further information might be obtained relative to the action of the drug in cardiac failure. We are concerned with the effect of the intravenous administration on the intrathecal and venous pressures and on bronchial obstruction.

In the study of the intrathecal pressures the patient was placed on the side in a horizontal position with the head supported by two pillows. The puncture was made in the lumbar region and the pressure recorded by a water manometer. Pressure applied to the cervical veins before and after each study always produced a temporary increase in pressure.

The venous pressure was measured by a modification of the method described by Hussey.[2] The apparatus consisted of a three way stopcock with a 22 gage needle attached to one opening, a glass manometer to another and a 30 cc. syringe to the other. The needle, manometer and syringe were filled with 3 per cent sodium citrate solution. The system can be kept practically free of blood by proper manipulation of the stopcock and accurate measurements obtained for long periods. The pressures were obtained from the median basilic vein with the patient in the supine position and were

From the Department of Internal Medicine, State University of Iowa College of Medicine.
Read before the Section on Pharmacology and Therapeutics at the Eighty-Eighth Annual Session of the American Medical Association, Atlantic City, N. J., June 9, 1937.

1. Smith, F. M.; Rathe, H. W., and Paul, W. D.: Theophylline in the Treatment of Disease of the Coronary Arteries, Arch. Int. Med. **56**: 1250-1262 (Dec.) 1935. Vogl, A.: Erfahrungen über Euphyllin bei Cheyne-Stokes und anderen Formen zentraler Atemstorungen, Med. Klin. **28**: 9-11 (Jan. 1) 1932. Guggenheimer, H.: Ueber die Wirkungsweise des Euphyllins bei kardiovascularem Cheyne-Stokes und Asthma Cardiale, Ztschr. f. Kreislaufforsch. **25**: 98-109 (Feb. 1) 1933. Greene, J. A., and Heeren, R. H.: Observations on Cheyne-Stokes Respiration: The Effect of Drugs and Mechanical Measures Which Produce Vasodilation and Vasoconstriction, Medical Papers Dedicated to Dr. Henry A. Christian, Baltimore, Waverly Press, 1936, pp. 51-59.
2. Hussey, H. H.: Clinical Application of Venous Pressure Measurement, M. Ann. District of Columbia **5**: 232-237 (Aug.) 1936.

recorded in millimeters of 3 per cent sodium citrate solution. The arm remained at the same relative position to the heart during the period of study, but it was not always at the level of the right auricle.

The vital capacity was measured by the usual method before and at fifteen and thirty minutes after injection of the drug.

These studies include observations on the intrathecal pressure alone in five normal subjects, fifteen patients with hypertension and arteriosclerosis without evidence of cardiac failure, six with congestive heart failure due to arteriosclerosis and hypertension, and four with intracranial lesions producing elevation of intrathecal pressures but with normal cardiovascular systems. Observations on the venous pressure alone were made in five normal subjects and in nine patients with congestive cardiac failure. In six patients with cardiac failure the effect on the venous and intrathecal pressures were measured simultaneously. Finally the effect of intravenous administration of the drug was observed on the bronchial obstruction in five patients during an acute attack of bronchial asthma associated with chronic pulmonary disease and in eleven cases in which the asthma was on an allergic basis.

The drug was given in doses of 0.48 Gm. diluted to 30 cc. with physiologic solution of sodium chloride and from three to five minutes was required for the injection. Frequent measurement of arterial pressures showed no significant alteration in either systolic or diastolic pressures and no change in cardiac rate was noted in frequent electrocardiograms.

RESULTS

The results of the study on intrathecal pressure alone are summarized in tables 1, 2, 3 and 4. It is to be noted that a reduction in the pressure occurred in each

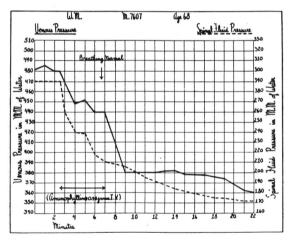

Time of onset and degree of reduction of venous and intrathecal pressures in a patient with congestive cardiac failure and Cheyne-Stokes respiration. It is to be noted that restoration of normal breathing coincided approximately with the maximum decline in the pressures.

instance. The effect reached its maximum after the injection of from 20 to 25 cc. of the solution and coincided with the onset of the relief of dyspnea (cases 2, 4 and 6, table 3), and with restoration of regular breathing in those with Cheyne-Stokes respiration (case 5, table 3, and case 3, table 4). It is to be noted from tables 5 and 6, which summarize the results of the study on venous pressure alone, that the pressure fell in all cases of cardiac failure. The maximum effect also coincided with injection of from 20

The action of theophylline with ethylenediamine on intrathecal and
venous pressures in cardiac failure and on bronchial obstruction in
cardiac failure and in bronchial asthma. *Greene JA, Paul WD, Feller AE*

VOLUME 109
NUMBER 21
CARDIAC FAILURE—GREENE ET AL.   1713

to 25 cc. of the solution and with onset of relief of dyspnea (cases 2, 4, 6 and 7, table 6) and restoration of regular rhythm (cases 2, 5 and 9, table 6).

The observations on the simultaneous measurement of intrathecal and venous pressures are summarized in table 7. These show a close correlation as to the extent of the effect. The relation of time of onset and the character and degree of reduction of the two pressures are illustrated in the accompanying chart. In five of the six patients there was a very obvious relief from dyspnea. One remarked, "The position and needles

TABLE 1.—*Reduction in Intrathecal Pressure After the Intravenous Injection of Aminophylline (Theophylline with Ethylenediamine) in Patients with Normal Cardiovascular Systems*

Case	Arterial Pressure	Intrathecal Pressure	
		Before Aminophylline, Mm.	After Aminophylline, Mm.
1	114/70	80	64
2	134/70	105	86
3	120/64	145	110
4	130/70	125	67
5	130/70	160	135

TABLE 2.—*Reduction in Intrathecal Pressure Which Occurred After Intravenous Injection of Aminophylline in Patients with Arteriosclerosis and Arterial Hypertension*

Case	Arterial Pressure	Intrathecal Pressure	
		Before Aminophylline, Mm.	After Aminophylline, Mm.
1	160/ 80	85	15
2	200/110	170	150
3	228/120	155	117
4	218/138	247	198
5	180/110	260	217
6	260/118	234	135
7	190/100	175	116
8	230/150	230	115
9	230/140	180	155
10	204/110	140	116
11	200/110	170	150
12	170/110	280	160
13	240/120	245	165
14	208/110	286	180
15	170/116	185	135

TABLE 3.—*Reduction in Intrathecal Pressure After the Intravenous Injection of Aminophylline in Patients with Severe Congestive Cardiac Failure*

Case	Arterial Pressure	Intrathecal Pressure	
		Before Aminophylline, Mm.	After Aminophylline, Mm.
1	200/114	136	112
2	224/148	254	235
3	250/100	180	155
4	160/100	260	160
5	200/130	320	240
6	140/ 80	270	250

were very uncomfortable but it was worth it"; another, "I have not been able to breath so easily in weeks." In the one case presenting Cheyne-Stokes breathing regular rhythm was restored. The respiratory distress was ameliorated in these patients from four to twenty-four hours.

Symptomatic relief occurred in all cases of asthma, as will be noted in tables 8 and 9, and the vital capacity increased in nine of eleven instances.

COMMENT

These studies show that the improvement in dyspnea and the conversion of periodic breathing to a regular rhythm in cardiac failure are related to the decline in intrathecal and venous pressures produced by the intravenous administration of theophylline with ethylene-

TABLE 4.—*Reduction in Intrathecal Pressure Following the Intravenous Injection of Aminophylline in Patients with Intracranial Lesions*

Case	Arterial Pressure	Intrathecal Pressure	
		Before Aminophylline, Mm.	After Aminophylline, Mm.
1	92/58	210	180
2	108/58	276	150
3	142/92	645	555
4	130/80	225	130

TABLE 5.—*Effect of Intravenous Injection of Aminophylline on the Venous Pressure in Patients Without Cardiac Failure*

Case	Venous Pressure	
	Before Aminophylline, Mm.	After Aminophylline, Mm.
1	113	103
2	45	45
3	138	110
4	57	43
5	125	110

TABLE 6.—*Reduction in Venous Pressure After the Intravenous Administration of Aminophylline in Patients with Cardiac Failure*

Case	Venous Pressure	
	Before Aminophylline, Mm.	After Aminophylline, Mm.
1	155	129
2	340	180
2	310	185
2	280	245
3	125	85
4	350	300
5	218	188
6	225	175
7	205	128
8	175	125
9	245	171

diamine. Harrison[3] noted a temporary improvement in respiratory distress in cases of heart failure following removal of cerebrospinal fluid. He also observed a parallel decline in venous and intrathecal pressures which corresponded in general to the extent of recovery from cardiac failure. Loman and Myerson[4] report a reduction in intrathecal pressure in normal subjects following the administration of caffeine.

There is a difference of opinion regarding the importance of the elevation of cerebral venous and intrathecal pressures in the production of dyspnea and orthopnea in cardiac failure. Harrison[3] found that the intrathecal pressures measured from the cistern were greater in the horizontal than in the sitting position and sug-

3. Harrison, W. G.: Cerebrospinal Fluid Pressure and Venous Pressure in Cardiac Failure, and Effect of Spinal Drainage in the Treatment of Cardiac Decompensation, Arch. Int. Med. 53: 782-791 (May) 1934.
4. Loman, Julius, and Myerson, Abraham: The Action of Certain Drugs on the Cerebrospinal Fluid and on the Internal Jugular Venous and Systemic Arterial Pressure of Man, Arch. Neurol. & Psychiat. 27: 1226-1244 (May) 1932.

The action of theophylline with ethylenediamine on intrathecal and venous pressures in cardiac failure and on bronchial obstruction in cardiac failure and in bronchial asthma. *Greene JA, Paul WD, Feller AE* gested that the increased pressure in the former position is a factor in the production of orthopnea. Ernstene and Blumgart [5] called attention to the parallelism between orthopnea and the elevation of venous pressure. They concluded that the latter reduces the circulation to the respiratory center and thus contributes to the production of orthopnea. Calhoun, Cullen, Harrison, Wilkins and Tims,[6] on the other hand, doubt that the increase in cerebral venous pressure is a factor in the production of dyspnea or orthopnea. They were unable to produce respiratory distress in normal subjects or to increase it in cases of cardiac failure by an elevation of the cerebral venous pressure by partial obstruction of the cervical veins.

Our observations confirm those of Harrison [3] relative to the close relationship of the increased venous and intrathecal pressures in cardiac failure and the observation that a reduction in these pressures has a favorable influence on the dyspnea. They show also that this effect may be produced by the intravenous administration of theophylline with ethylenediamine. Moreover, this drug ameliorates the bronchial obstruction in both bronchial asthma and cardiac failure.

These results provide further information regarding the effect of theophylline with ethylenediamine in cardiac failure, but the mechanism of the action, except for that on the heart, is not clear. It is hoped that the studies now in progress may throw additional light on the subject.

TABLE 7.—*Reduction in Venous and Intrathecal Pressures When Measured Simultaneously Following the Intravenous Injection of Aminophylline in Patients with Cardiac Failure*

Case	Venous Pressure		Spinal Fluid Pressure	
	Before Amino-phylline, Mm.	After Amino-phylline, Mm.	Before Amino-phylline, Mm.	After Amino-phylline, Mm.
1	195	175	163	132
2	532+	440	400+	261
3*	428	416	185	155
4	195	153	390	321
5	175	125	270	250
6	480	360	300	171

* Patient did not cooperate satisfactorily.

TABLE 8.—*Change in Vital Capacity and the Subjective Relief Obtained in Patients with Asthma Associated with Chronic Pulmonary Disease When Aminophylline Was Injected Intravenously During an Acute Attack*

Number	Vital Capacity Before Aminophylline, Liters	Vital Capacity 15 Minutes After Aminophylline, Liters	Subjective Relief
1	1.4	2.2	Yes
2	3.1	4.2	Yes
3	*	1.5	Yes
4	2.2	2.2	Yes
5	...	...	Yes, temporarily

* Patient too dyspneic to be measured.

SUMMARY

The effect of the intravenous administration of theophylline with ethylenediamine on the intrathecal and venous pressures, measured separately and simul-

taneously, has been studied in normal subjects, in patients with cardiac failure and in patients with cerebral lesions. The effect on bronchial obstruction has been studied in patients with bronchial asthma associated with chronic pulmonary disease and in patients in whom the asthma was on an allergic basis.

TABLE 9.—*Change in Vital Capacity and the Symptomatic Relief Obtained in Patients with Allergic Asthma When Aminophylline Was Injected Intravenously During an Acute Attack*

Number	Vital Capacity Before Aminophylline, Liters	Vital Capacity 15 Minutes After Aminophylline, Liters	Subjective Relief
1	0.2	0.6	Yes
2	4.6	5.6	Yes
3	0.8	0.8	Yes
4*	0.6	2.4	Yes
5*	0.4	2.0	Yes
6*	1.8	2.0	Yes
7	1.0	2.2	Yes
8	...	...	Yes
9	...	...	Yes
10	...	...	Yes
11	...	...	Yes

* These patients also had pulmonary emphysema secondary to allergic asthma of many years' duration.

The results show a correlation between elevation of venous and intrathecal pressures in cardiac failure. Furthermore, relief of dyspnea or restoration of regular rhythm in Cheyne-Stokes breathing is related to the decline observed in intrathecal and venous pressures following intravenous administration of theophylline with ethylenediamine.

Finally, theophylline with ethylenediamine has a favorable action on bronchial obstruction both in bronchial asthma and in cardiac failure.

———

5. Ernstene, A. C., and Blumgart, H. L.: Orthopnea: Its Relation to the Increased Venous Pressure of Myocardial Failure, Arch. Int. Med. **45**: 593-610 (April) 1930.

6. Calhoun, J. A.; Cullen, G. E.; Harrison, T. R.; Wilkins, W. L., and Tims, M. M.: Studies in Congestive Heart Failure: XIV. Orthopnea: Its Relation to Ventilation, Vital Capacity, Oxygen Saturation, and Acid Base Condition of Arterial and Jugular Blood, J. Clin. Investigation **10**: 833-855 (Oct.) 1931.

The action of theophylline with ethylenediamine on intrathecal and venous pressures in cardiac failure and on bronchial obstruction in cardiac failure and in bronchial asthma. *Greene JA, Paul WD, Feller AE*

THE ACTION OF EPHEDRINE, THE ACTIVE PRINCIPLE OF THE CHINESE DRUG MA HUANG

K. K. CHEN AND CARL F. SCHMIDT

From the Laboratory of Pharmacology of Peking Union Medical College, Peking, China

Received for publication July 10, 1924

Ma Huang, identified as Ephedra vulgaris var. helvetica Fam. Gnetaceae (1), is described by the Pentsao Kang Mu (2) as a diaphoretic, circulatory stimulant, antipyretic, sedative in cough, etc., and is an ingredient of many famous Chinese prescriptions. It was one of the medicinal herbs tasted by Emperor Shen Nung some 5100 years ago and was placed by him in the "medium class" (3). It is sold by Peking drug shops in the form of brownish green sticks about 1 mm. in diameter and 10 to 15 mm. long.

The drug was investigated by Nagai (4) who isolated from it an alkaloid which he named ephedrine. With this alkaloid he later conducted various physiological experiments (9). Merck (5) obtained from the European variety of E. vulgaris an isomeric alkaloid which he called pseudoephedrine. The empirical formula of these alkaloids is $C_{10}H_{15}ON$. Their chemical structure has been repeatedly studied (6) (7) (8) and is most probably phenyl 1-ol 1-methyl 2-methyl-amino 2-ethane, $C_6H_5OH \cdot - CH \cdot CH \cdot CH_3 \cdot NHCH_3$.

Concerning the physiological effects of ephedrine, Miura (13) first observed mydriasis and Amatsu and Kubota (10) described relaxation of intestinal muscle and a rise in blood pressure from vasoconstriction in dogs, while the frog's heart was depressed by the drug. The effects of pseudoephedrine are apparently very similar; the mydriatic effect of these alkaloids is attributed to an action like that of cocaine (11).

As far as we know the effects of Ma Huang have never been completely investigated. Our first experiment, in which a decoc-

339

340   K. K. CHEN AND CARL F. SCHMIDT

tion of the drug was injected into a vein of an anesthetized dog, showed a sharp and prolonged rise in blood pressure accompanied by cardiac acceleration and vasoconstriction.

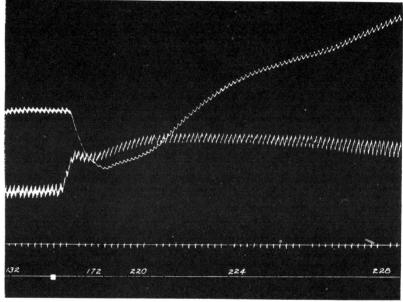

FIG. 1. SHOWING THE EFFECT OF AN INTRAVENOUS INJECTION OF EPHEDRINE ON KIDNEY VOLUME AND BLOOD PRESSURE AFTER PARALYTIC DOSES OF NICOTINE. FROM EXPERIMENT 27, JANUARY 19, 1924

Dog, 7 kilos; anesthetized with phenobarbital sodium (0.15 gram per kilo intramuscularly). Tracing follows injection of a total of 70 mgm. of nicotine intravenously, by which respiratory center was paralyzed; artificial respiration; stimulation of vagus by strongest tetanizing current caused slight slowing of heart.

Records from above down are: Kidney volume; carotid blood pressure; time in five-second intervals; signal tracing which is abscissa for blood pressure and is set at 0 mm.; the figures indicate pulse rate per minute.

At the signal mark 5 mgm. of ephedrine hydrochloride were injected intravenously. Blood pressure rose from 94 to 148 mm. of mercury, and remained above normal for thirty minutes. Note that the cardia cacceleration outlasts the kidney constriction.

All tracings to be read from left to right.

These effects were soon found to be due to an alkaloid which has been identified as ephedrine by its melting point (base 210°C., hydrochloride 214°C., sulphate 242°C.) and specific rotation (hydrochloride in aqueous solution [a]_D 25–35°). It is present in 0.018 to 0.072 per cent in the crude drug. Chemical and pharmacognostic studies of the drug and alkaloid are to be published elsewhere. This paper is concerned with the physiological effects of ephedrine, the active principle of Ma Huang.

Experiments on dogs, cats, and rabbits have shown uniformly that the effects of ephedrine on circulation, smooth muscle, and secretions are analogous to those of sympathetic stimulation and are qualitatively similar to those of epinephrine.

I. THE ACTION ON THE CIRCULATION

The outstanding result of an injection of 0.25 to 20 mgm. of ephedrine hydrochloride or sulphate into a vein of a dog, cat, or rabbit was a prolonged rise of blood pressure, accompanied by cardiac acceleration and usually but not always by vasoconstriction (fig. 1). After pithing the brain and cord of the animal the effects of ephedrine were the same, so that its action was obviously peripheral.

a. The action on the heart

Experiments with the myocardiograph in dogs and cats showed an increase in strength as well as rate of cardiac contractions following an intravenous injection of ephedrine (fig. 2). The effect was not prevented by vagotomy or atropine and threshold electrical stimulation of the vagus caused cardiac inhibition during the acceleration which followed ephedrine (fig. 2).

In an effort to localize the effect, a solution of ephedrine was applied directly to the stellate ganglion; this caused a prolonged increase in rate and strength of cardiac contractions and a slight rise in blood pressure (fig. 3). After nicotinization of the ganglion, local application of ephedrine had no effect; the stimulant effect of local application, before the ganglion was paralyzed by nicotine, must therefore be attributed to actual stimulation of the ganglion and not to absorption from the pleura. After ephedrine had produced maximal effects upon one ganglion it produced further stimulation when applied to the ganglion of the other

The action of ephedrine, the active principle of
the Chinese drug Ma Huang. *Chen KK, Schmidt CF*

342   K. K. CHEN AND CARL F. SCHMIDT

side. When maximal stimulation had been obtained by local application to both ganglia, either electrical stimulation of the preganglionic accelerator fibers or an intravenous injection of ephedrine caused further acceleration and augmentation. Nico-

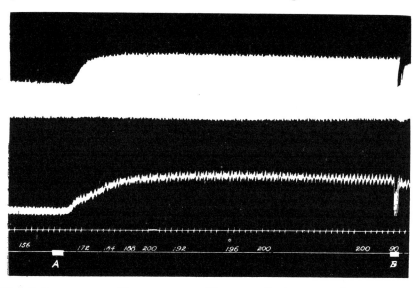

FIG. 2. SHOWING THE EFFECT ON THE HEART OF INTRAVENOUS INJECTION OF EPHEDRINE. FROM EXPERIMENT 13, DECEMBER 13, 1923

Dog, 9 kilos; anesthesia by morphine sulphate (2 mgm. per kilo subcutaneously) and urethane (0.75 gram per kilo by stomach tube). Artificial respiration by compressed air interrupted by rotating valve. Right vagus intact, left cut; no atropine.

Records from above down are: Myocardiogram of right ventricle, the lever moving up in systole; carotid blood pressure; time in five seconds; signal tracing, which is abscissa for blood pressure and is set at 0 mm. The figures indicate pulse rate per minute.

At A, 10 mgm. of ephedrine hydrochloride were injected intravenously, blood pressure rising from 52 to 97 mm. At B peripheral stump of the left vagus was stimulated with the weakest current (secondary at 8 cm.) which caused cardiac inhibition before ephedrine.

tine applied to a ganglion or injected intravenously at this stage also produced marked accelerator stimulation. It was evident that the stimulant action of ephedrine on accelerator ganglia was not followed by depression or paralysis.

The action of ephedrine, the active principle of
the Chinese drug Ma Huang. *Chen KK, Schmidt CF*

ACTION OF EPHEDRINE 343

The fact that, after ephedrine had produced maximum cardiac stimulation by local application to the stellate ganglia, an intravenous injection caused further stimulation, suggested that ephedrine also stimulated other parts of the accelerator mechanism.

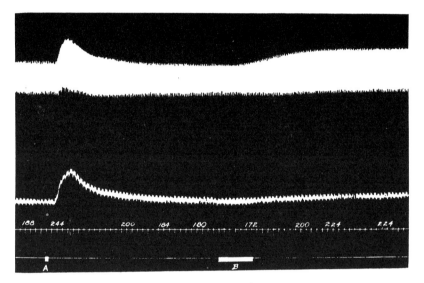

FIG. 3. SHOWING THE COMPARATIVE EFFECT ON THE HEART OF INTRAVENOUS INJECTION OF EPINEPHRINE AND OF APPLICATION OF EPHEDRINE TO THE STELLATE GANGLION. FROM EXPERIMENT 17, DECEMBER 20, 1923

Dog, 10.2 kilos; anesthesia by phenobarbital sodium (0.15 gram per kilo intramuscularly). Atropine, 1 mgm., injected at start of experiment.

Tracings from above down are: Myocardiogram of right ventricle; carotid blood pressure; time in five seconds; signal tracing, abscissa for blood pressure, set at 0 mm. figures indicate pulse rate per minute.

At A, 0.3 cc. of 1:10,000 solution of epinephrine was injected intravenously. At B, a pledget of cotton soaked in 0.5 per cent solution of ephedrine hydrochloride was applied to the right stellate ganglion. Blood pressure was raised only from 73 to 75 mm. of mercury in spite of the indicated cardiac effects. The cardiac effect lasted indefinitely.

After both ganglia had been paralyzed by local application of nicotine, or after intravenous injection of nicotine in dosage sufficient to prevent cardiac inhibition by any but the strongest electrical stimulation of the vagus (10 mgm. per kilo in dogs) an intravenous injection of ephedrine caused a marked increase in

The action of ephedrine, the active principle of
the Chinese drug Ma Huang. *Chen KK, Schmidt CF*

344   K. K. CHEN AND CARL F. SCHMIDT

rate and strength of heart beats. Hearts of rabbits perfused by Langendorff's method showed a marked and prolonged acceleration and augmentation of contractions when exposed to dilute solutions (1:100,000) of ephedrine. The drug therefore stimulated accelerator endings as well as ganglia.

The cardiac acceleration produced by one injection of ephedrine commonly persisted for more than fifteen minutes, and sometimes indefinitely. The degree and duration of the effect were not proportional to the dose, for 0.5 mgm. sometimes caused more marked stimulation than 10 mgm., especially if the blood pressure was above 100 mm. of mercury before the injection. Upon repeated injections cardiac stimulation reached a maximum after the second or third dose as a rule, but further injections caused a progressive rise in blood pressure, due apparently to vasoconstriction. By repeated small injections it was possible to raise the blood pressure to a sustained level of over 200 mm. of mercury in a dog whose brain and cord were destroyed.

After repeated injections, a stage was finally reached at which further doses of ephedrine not only failed to raise blood pressure but caused a temporary fall, accompanied by a decrease in rate and strength of heart beats. That the apparent reversal was not due to depression or paralysis of the nervous mechanisms was shown by the fact that electrical stimulation of the splanchnic or accelerator nerve brought out typical effects at this stage, and an injection of nicotine or adrenaline caused marked stimulation. The reversal was therefore to be attributed to depression of the heart. This was confirmed by experiments with the isolated rabbit's heart in which stronger solutions of ephedrine (1:20,000) caused pure depression, accompanied by increased coronary flow; adrenaline caused prompt stimulation at this stage. Only depression was observed in the hearts of frogs and turtles irrigated with ephedrine solutions of any strength.

The action of ephedrine on the heart therefore appears to be a threefold one: (a) Stimulation of accelerator ganglia; (b) stimulation of accelerator endings; (c) direct depression of heart muscle, not due to coronary constriction.

The action of ephedrine, the active principle of
the Chinese drug Ma Huang. *Chen KK, Schmidt CF*

ACTION OF EPHEDRINE   345

b. *The action on blood vessels*

The usual effect of an injection of ephedrine in dogs and cats was sharp constriction of kidney vessels (fig. 1). Sometimes the first injection caused a rise in blood pressure accompanied by dilatation of kidney, intestinal, and limb vessels, cardiac effects apparently overcoming vasoconstriction. Subsequent doses, however, always caused constriction of kidney and intestinal vessels, for maximum cardiac effects followed the first few injections, but the volume of a denervated or intact limb was

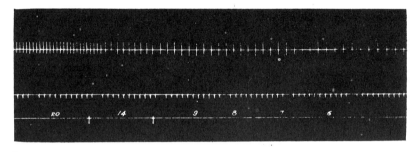

Fig. 4. Showing the Effect of Ephedrine on the Venous Outflow from a Perfused Kidney. From Experiment 26, January 15, 1924

Kidney of dog; cannulae in renal artery and vein; Ringer's fluid at 40°C. perfused through arterial cannula, recording outflow from renal vein in drops.

Records from above down are: Outflow from renal vein in drops; time in five seconds; signal tracing. The figures indicate rate of venous flow in drops per minute.

Between the signal marks, 0.5 cc. of a 0.1 per cent solution of ephedrine was injected into the arterial cannula. The effect persisted indefinitely.

increased whenever blood pressure rose, whether splanchnic vessels were dilated or constricted.

The vasoconstriction was apparently not concerned with ganglia, for it was even sharper after nicotine (fig. 1) and local application of ephedrine to the thoracic ganglia had no effect on kidney volume. Vessels of a dog's kidney perfused with Ringer's solution were definitely constricted by ephedrine (fig. 4), the effect persisting indefinitely after the first application and further injections having no further effect.

The action of ephedrine, the active principle of the Chinese drug Ma Huang. *Chen KK, Schmidt CF*

346   K. K. CHEN AND CARL F. SCHMIDT

Vasoconstriction appeared to be due to stimulation of nerve endings rather than to a direct muscular effect, for coronary flow in the perfused mammalian heart was increased and the rate of flow through the vessels of perfused lungs of dogs was not definitely affected by ephedrine. Constriction was apparently more powerful in the splanchnic vessels than in those of the skin and muscles (leg); the dilatation of cutaneous vessels when there was constriction in those of kidney and intestine must have meant an altered distribution of blood.

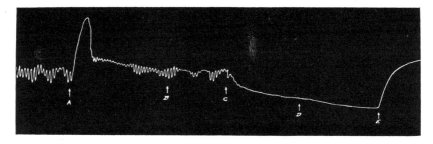

FIG. 5. SHOWING THE EFFECT OF EPHEDRINE ON THE ISOLATED INTESTINE. FROM EXPERIMENT OF JANUARY 21, 1924

Strip of ileum of rabbit suspended in Locke's solution at 38°C.

At A, 6 drops of 1 per cent solution of nicotine were added; at B, 6 drops of nicotine had no effect; at C, 0.5 cc. of 0.5 per cent solution of ephedrine hydrochloride (total concentration 1:140,000); D, 6 drops of nicotine; at E, 10 drops of 0.5 per cent pilocarpine hydrochloride. The effect of pilocarpine was not affected by subsequent addition of ephedrine, but was promptly removed by atropine.

II. THE ACTION ON SMOOTH MUSCLE

Intestine in situ or isolated was relaxed and its movements were inhibited by ephedrine. Isolated rabbit's intestine was inhibited by ephedrine after nicotine but pilocarpine caused the usual spasm (fig. 5), which was overcome by atropine but not by ephedrine. The effects of ephedrine on the intestine were therefore analogous to those of adrenaline and were not concerned with intrinsic ganglia.

The uterus of the dog showed an increase in tone or a tonic contraction after intravenous injection of ephedrine. Strips of rabbit's uterus suspended in Tyrode's or Locke's solution underwent one or more powerful contractions when ephedrine was added; virgin and pregnant organs have similar results, but the uterus of one recently delivered rabbit was relaxed by ephedrine —the only instance of pure relaxation observed.

The effect on bronchical muscle was observed in one experiment on a pithed dog in which the degree of bronchial dilatation was estimated by the changes in intrathoracic pressure during constant artificial respiration. At first ephedrine had no effect, but after an injection of physostigmine had produced marked bronchial spasm ephedrine caused prompt dilatation. The effect was not well sustained and subsequent doses did not cause dilatation, though epinephrine continued to be effective.

The pupils of dogs, rabbits, and cats were dilated by ephedrine, whether the drug was injected intravenously or applied to the conjunctival sac. The mydriasis following local applicacation of a 0.5 per cent solution came on in about ten minutes, lasted over an hour, and was limited to the corresponding side. The light reflex was retained and physostigmine caused prompt miosis. After atropine ephedrine produced further dilatation of the pupil. The mydriasis was slower in onset but more powerful than that of cocaine. There was no definite constriction of conjunctival vessels, no sign of local irritation or tissue damage, and no local anesthesia after ephedrine.

The mydriatic effect was wholly peripheral, as indicated by its limitation to the side to which the drug was applied. Application of ephedrine solution to the superior cervical sympathetic ganglion in anesthetized rabbits or anesthetized or decerebrated cats failed to produce dilatation of the corresponding pupil. After degeneration of the long ciliary nerves following extirpation of the superior cervical sympathetic ganglion of one side in rabbits ephedrine caused definite dilatation of the denervated pupil in every 1 of 6 animals; cocaine failed to cause mydriasis of the denervated eye in all of these animals.

III. THE ACTION ON SECRETIONS

Incomplete information has been obtained regarding the action of ephedrine on urine, saliva, sweat, and lymph flow.

The action of ephedrine, the active principle of
the Chinese drug Ma Huang. *Chen KK, Schmidt CF*

348   K. K. CHEN AND CARL F. SCHMIDT

Urine flow was usually increased after the vasoconstrictor effect of the injection had disappeared in anesthetized dogs; the cardiac effects outlasted the vascular action and kidney vessels were usually dilated after primary constriction (fig. 1). After repeated doses urine was suppressed though blood pressure was higher than before; this corresponded to the period of maximum vasoconstriction. An intact rabbit which received daily intravenous injections of ephedrine showed a well-marked diuresis. The effects on urine appeared to be bound up with the vascular effects of the drug, though renal irritation may also have been a factor, as shown by the presence of degeneration of kidney cells in the rabbit after daily injections of ephedrine. These changes will be described below.

Flow of saliva from submaxillary glands of anesthetized dogs was never greatly changed by an intravenous injection of ephedrine. In one experiment ephedrine caused a definite increase in secretion after atropine when chorda stimulation was ineffective. Its effects were therefore analogous to those of stimulation of the sympathetic nerve to the gland.

Sweat secretion in the paw of an anesthetized cat was not increased when ephedrine was injected into the paw, estimating its effect by the number of droplets visible under a hand lens and by changes in weight of a filter paper applied to the part. Profuse sweating is said by the Chinese to be a constant result of Ma Huang. One of us took a decoction of the drug in the doses usually prescribed in Chinese medicine; there was slight perspiration after ninety minutes. After taking 60 mgm. of ephedrine by mouth there was very slight sweating. In no case was there any nausea. The effect on lymph flow was investigated in 6 experiments on anesthetized dogs, lymph being collected from a cannula in the thoracic duct and measured in a graduated cylinder or in drops. Ephedrine regularly caused an increase in lymph flow which reached its maximum about fifteen minutes after the injection. This effect was comparable to that of epinephrine, the increased flow being parallel and apparently due to a rise in arterial blood pressure.

The action of ephedrine, the active principle of
the Chinese drug Ma Huang. *Chen KK, Schmidt CF*

IV. OTHER EFFECTS

The effect on body temperature was investigated in experiments on anesthetized dogs, but no constant change was noted in rectal temperature. One of us, after taking a decoction of Ma Huang, noted a fall of 0.4°F. in oral temperature in fifty minutes, and temperature remained 0.2°F. below the previous normal (98.6°F.) for two hours. This slight change was accompanied by some sweating.

The effect on glycogenic functions was investigated in two anesthetized dogs but the results were inconclusive. Further experiments were required to determine if the similarity of ephedrine to epinephrine extends to a similar effect on glycogen metabolism.

V. ABSORPTION AND EXCRETION

An intravenous injection of 0.25 to 0.5 mgm. of ephedrine hydrochloride or sulphate always elicited definite effects in anesthetized dogs and cats. The same dose by subcutaneous or intramuscular injection had no effect, and even 10 mgm. was not constantly effective when so given to anesthetized dogs. In adult human beings an intramuscular injection of 40 to 100 mgm. of ephedrine sulphate was constantly followed by a definite rise in systolic and diastolic blood pressure and a decrease in pulse rate, but no mydriasis or other effects were seen.

Given by stomach tube to an anesthetized dog, a dose of 25 mgm. of ephedrine was apparently not absorbed, but when injected into the lumen of the duodenum the same dose was followed by a gradual rise in blood pressure and prolonged cardiac acceleration. After swallowing, in a capsule, 60 mgm. of the alkaloid, one of us experienced a rise in blood pressure from 128–60 to 150–68 mm. of mercury, slowing of pulse from 74 to 60 per minute, throbbing of the head and slight headache, palpitation, and slight sweating. The effect began within thirty minutes and persisted for more than two hours. There was no mydriasis and the only symptoms noted were obviously due to the circulatory effects. There can be no doubt therefore that ephedrine is effectively absorbed from the intestinal tract.

The action of ephedrine, the active principle of
the Chinese drug Ma Huang. *Chen KK, Schmidt CF*

350   K. K. CHEN AND CARL F. SCHMIDT

The mode of excretion is obscure. A rabbit which was given daily intravenous injections of ephedrine showed no trace of alkaloid in the urine. As the effects are more persistent than those of epinephrine, if ephedrine is destroyed in the body the process must be a relatively slow one.

VI. TOXICITY

Miura (13) has shown that the toxicity of this alkaloid is relatively low. Whilst the following experiments confirm this general observation, they show that the kidneys and contents of the urine are seriously affected by large doses.

A frog showed no symptoms after an injection of 0.3 mgm. of ephedrine per gram of body weight. Rabbits receiving 20 mgm. per kilo by intravenous injection showed temporary mydriasis but no other symptoms. The minimum lethal dose for rats lay between 100 and 145 mgm. per kilo by intravenous injection, these doses causing restlessness, salivation, lachrymation, and finally epileptiform convulsions followed by collapse and death; doses too small to produce convulsions had no apparent effect, the animals surviving indefinitely. The cause of death appeared to be paralysis following stimulation of the central nervous system. The doses required were enormously excessive, for 0.05 mgm. per kilo always stimulated the circulation when injected into a vein of an anesthetized dog or cat, and 0.6 mgm. per kilo by intramuscular injection or less than 1 mgm. per kilo taken by mouth was effective in man.

A rabbit which was given 20 mgm. of ephedrine per kilo by vein every day for nine days showed no symptoms of any sort except brief mydriasis after each injection and diuresis with intermittent glycosuria and albuminuria. During twelve days after the last injection the animal remained in perfect health and gained 240 grams in weight. It was then sacrificed and the organs were examined histologically.

Heart muscle, coronary vessels, and aorta were normal, and none of the parenchymatous organs showed any change except the kidney, where there were signs of degeneration; the convo-

The action of ephedrine, the active principle of
the Chinese drug Ma Huang. *Chen KK, Schmidt CF*

luted tubules showed some cloudy swelling, the glomeruli remaining relatively unaffected. Dr. R. G. Mills was kind enough to examine these tissues; he felt that the renal degeneration was probably due to the drug.

The kidney changes furnish a probable explanation of the albuminuria and glycosuria as well as a possible factor in the diuresis. They also suggest that the drug is eliminated by the kidney in some form, the nature of which we have been unable to determine. It should be noted, however, that the doses of ephedrine given to this animal were enormously in excess of the effective dose. Further studies on the effect of the drug on body tissues are being made.

VII. STABILITY OF SOLUTIONS

Compared with epinephrine, ephedrine is much more stable in solution. One aqueous solution was kept, without any preservative, exposed to light and air, and after forty-five days it was clear and colorless; on injection into anesthetized animals it was as effective as a fresh solution. Other solutions were sterilized by immersion in boiling water, and their effects were unaltered. The crystalline alkaloid and salts are apparently stable indefinitely. Solutions of ephedrine are therefore very stable, are not decomposed by heat, air or light, and are not subject to the growth of microörganisms from the air.

VIII. CLINICAL USES

We have tried ephedrine in patients in the wards of the Hospital of Peking Union Medical College, as well as on ourselves, with uniformly favorable results; no untoward symptoms of any kind have been observed.

As a circulatory stimulant in normal persons, an intramuscular injection of 40 to 60 mgm. always caused a rise of 20 to 30 mm. of mercury in systolic blood pressure while pulse rate was simultaneously decreased. The effects came on within fifteen minutes and persisted at a maximum for over an hour. Mydriasis did not occur, the only symptoms noted being slight throb-

The action of ephedrine, the active principle of
the Chinese drug Ma Huang. *Chen KK, Schmidt CF*

352			K. K. CHEN AND CARL F. SCHMIDT

bing in the head.   There was no pain at the site of injection and
there were no local reactions.   Taken by mouth, 60 mgm. caused
a rise in blood pressure and slowing of pulse rate as great as the
effects produced by intramuscular injection—a rise of systolic
blood pressure from 124 to 150 mm., a slowing of pulse rate from
74 to 60 per minute, the effects persisting for more than two hours.
In one patient in moderate shock following a surgical operation
intramuscular injection of 40 mgm. of ephedrine raised systolic
blood pressure to normal and recovery was prompt and complete.   The most striking effects have been obtained in a patient
with symptoms of marked adrenal insufficiency (Addison's disease); intramuscular injections of 100 mgm. of ephedrine twice
daily have raised blood pressure from 70–42 to 110–68 mm., the
pulse being reduced from 90 to 72 per minute; the effects of one
injection on circulation persist for about two hours, and attempts
are now being made to secure more lasting effects by oral administration; this patient's condition has been greatly improved—he
feels stronger, appetite has returned, and the symptomatic effects
are quite remarkable.

Attempts at relieving bronchial asthma or anaphylaxis by
ephedrine are awaiting suitable material.   In view of the similarity of the effects of ephedrine to those of adrenaline and the specific effects of adrenaline on bronchial spasm, there is reason to
expect beneficial results from ephedrine, though what little
experimental evidence we have obtained indicates that it is a
weaker bronchodilator than epinephrine.   The greater persistence
of the effect and the possibility of securing effects by oral administration are theoretical advantages of ephedrine over adrenaline
in the relief of asthma.

The mydriatic action of ephedrine has long been known (13)
and is certainly of the order of cocaine rather than that of atropine.   In animals ephedrine mydriasis was less rapid but more
marked and prolonged than that of cocaine.   In human subjects ephedrine sulphate, in 2 or 4 per cent solution, causes
complete mydriasis in dim light in twenty to thirty minutes, the
light reflex being retained.   Simultaneously there is an incomplete cycloplegic effect, amounting to 3 or 4 diopters.   Intraocu-

The action of ephedrine, the active principle of
the Chinese drug Ma Huang. *Chen KK, Schmidt CF*

lar tension is not altered. Examination of the cornea by means of the slit lamp and corneal microscope shows no loosening of epithelium—an effect which may follow cocaine. Ephedrine is therefore of little or no value when complete paralysis of accommodation is required, but for examination of the fundus it is more powerful than cocaine, though rather less rapid in action. The dilatation of the pupil produced by ephedrine can be readily overcome by pilocarpine or physostigmine in animals, though this has not been tested in man. No local irritant effects have been observed. These observations for the most part confirm those made by Miura (13), who obtained mydriasis after forty to sixty minutes by introducing into the eye 1 or 2 drops of a ten per cent solution of ephedrine.

DISCUSSION

It is evident that the physiological effects of ephedrine are qualitatively almost identical with those of epinephrine and tyramine. The chemical relation of the three bases is therefore of some interest.

Epinephrine   Tyramine   Ephedrine
((6); (7))

Compared to epinephrine ephedrine differs in that it contains no phenolic hydroxy group but has an extra methyl radical; in contrast with tyramine, ephedrine lacks a phenolic hydroxy radical, but contains two methyl radicals and one alcoholic hydroxy group which are not present in tyramine. In view of its physiological effects it seems proper to include ephedrine in the group of natural amines which possess "sympathomimetic effects" (12).

The action of ephedrine, the active principle of the Chinese drug Ma Huang. *Chen KK, Schmidt CF*

354   K. K. CHEN AND CARL F. SCHMIDT

While the effects of ephedrine are qualitatively analogous to those of epinephrine, there are several quantitative differences which appear to be important. These are: the more persistent but less intense effects of ephedrine, its more marked action on the heart than on the peripheral vessels in animals, though apparently not in man, and the apparent loss or reversal of effect upon repeated doses of ephedrine. These differences from epinephrine seem to be bound up with a firm combination of ephedrine with receptor substances and a slow rate of destruction or elimination of the drug, as a result of which maximal effects are produced by relatively small doses; the apparent reversal seems to depend entirely on depression of cardiac muscle by excessive concentrations after maximal stimulation has been reached. We have tried to detect actual depression or paralysis of the receptor substance by excessive doses of ephedrine but have consistently found that electrical or chemical stimulation of the sympathetic system was perfectly effective at all stages of ephedrine action. The apparent reversal is therefore to be attributed entirely to cardiac depression. The relative predominance of cardiac over vascular effects in animals and the greater susceptibility of the accelerator mechanism than the vasoconstrictor endings to ephedrine may be bound up with the stimulant action of ephedrine on accelerator ganglia as well as endings, a feature which is apparently unique in the action of ephedrine as compared to that of epinephrine or tyramine; as far as we have been able to determine, ephedrine does not stimulate any other ganglia. The prominence of cardiac acceleration in the circulatory effects of ephedrine appeared to limit the usefulness of the drug as a circulatory stimulant, but we have always found the heart slowed when blood pressure was raised by ephedrine in human subjects; the circulatory action of ephedrine in man is therefore more vascular than cardiac, probably because of the more perfect cardioinhibitory mechanism of man.

Other than its effect on accelerator ganglia, the action of ephedrine is apparently exerted only through stimulation of sympathetic endings. A direct muscular action is negatived by such diverse effects as contraction of the uterus or constriction of

The action of ephedrine, the active principle of
the Chinese drug Ma Huang. *Chen KK, Schmidt CF*

ACTION OF EPHEDRINE 355

splanchnic blood vessels and inhibition of the gut or dilatation of the bronchi. The fact that ephedrine always caused mydriasis after degeneration of the sympathetic innervation of the pupil, when cocaine was ineffective, points to an action on some receptor substance peripheral to the point of action of cocaine. The drug has no effects that are not analogous to those of sympathetic stimulation other than the convulsant action of toxic doses and possibly the irritant effect of excessive concentrations on the kidney.

These findings, together with the apparently low toxicity of the drug, suggest that ephedrine may be of value clinically in conditions in which epinephrine would be useful. Ephedrine has the obvious advantages of more persistent if less intense effects, the possibility of securing effects when the drug is given by mouth, and the greater stability of its solutions.

Our experiments have failed to explain the reputed antipyretic and diaphoretic effects of Ma Huang on any basis other than a diversion of blood to the cutaneous circulation because of increased cardiac output and more marked constriction of blood vessels in the splanchnic region than in the skin. No traces of active principles other than ephedrine have been found, and ephedrine has no nauseant or true diaphoretic action.

SUMMARY

1. Ma Huang—Ephedra Vulgaris var. helvetica—contains an alkaloid which is its active principle. This alkaloid is identical with ephedrine and isomeric with pseudoephedrine.

2. The physiological effects of ephedrine are very similar to those of epinephrine but are much more prolonged. All of its effects are comparable to those of sympathetic stimulation.

3. The outstanding effect of ephedrine is circulatory stimulation, which is due largely to stimulation of the cardiac accelerator mechanism, exerted simultaneously on ganglia and endings. Large doses depress heart muscle and cause a fall in blood pressure. Constriction also occurs in blood vessels supplied with vasoconstrictor nerves, and is more marked in the splanchnic

The action of ephedrine, the active principle of the Chinese drug Ma Huang. *Chen KK, Schmidt CF*

356　　　　K. K. CHEN AND CARL F. SCHMIDT

area than in a limb. Maximal cardiac effects are elicited before vasoconstriction is marked, and subsequent doses cause further constriction until a maximum is reached, beyond which further doses depress the heart muscle and lower blood pressure. In man vasoconstriction is apparently more prominent, for pulse rate is always decreased as blood pressure rises.

4. The other effects are analogous to those of epinephrine: the intestine is inhibited and relaxed, the uterus is stimulated, the bronchi are dilated and mydriasis occurs after local or systemic exhibition of ephedrine; salivary secretion is sometimes increased by ephedrine after atropine, but there is no definite effect on secretion of sweat; diuresis occurs after the vasoconstrictor effect diminishes due apparently to more prolonged effects on heart than on vessels and possibly also to irritation of the kidney by the drug.

5. Ephedrine is not very toxic, the minimum fatal dose being 100 to 145 mgm. per kilo in rats, death following convulsions. Smaller doses are apparently harmless, though repeated intravenous injections of large doses produced kidney degeneration in a rabbit.

6. The drug is effectively absorbed from the intestines or following subcutaneous or intramuscular injection. Its solutions are stable indefinitely when exposed to light and air and are not decomposed by boiling.

7. Ephedrine has been tried clinically as a circulatory stimulant, with favorable results. A patient with Addison's disease has been markedly improved by it. Its efficiency as a bronchodilator has not been tested. Its mydriatic effects are of the cocaine order, but are more intense than those of cocaine.

8. Should ephedrine prove valuable clinically, its advantages over epinephrine lie in the greater persistence of ephedrine effects, the greater stability of its solutions, and the possibility of securing effects when the drug is given by mouth.

We wish to express our deep appreciation of the cooperation of Dr. Mokichi Kayumi, of the Pharmacological Institute of Yokyo Imperial University, in testing the action of ephedrine on lymph flow in the course of another investigation; of Drs. A. S. Taylor

The action of ephedrine, the active principle of
the Chinese drug Ma Huang. *Chen KK, Schmidt CF*

and H. E. Meleney in trying the drug on patients in the wards of this hospital; of Drs. T. M. Li, H. T. Pi, and T. Y. Lai in investigating its effects on the human eye; and of Dr. R. G. Mills in examining tissues of animals injected with large doses of ephedrine.

REFERENCES

(1) Botanical Nomenclature, Commercial Press, Shanghai, 1917, p. 1004.
(2) Pentsao Kang Mu, a revision of Pentsao by Li Shih Cheng in 1596 A.D., greatly enlarged, containing 1871 drugs under 62 orders and 16 classes, in 52 chapters.
(3) EMPEROR SHEN NUNG, 3217–3077 B.C., father of Chinese Agriculture, tasted many medicinal plants. It is believed that he wrote Pentsao, containing 360 drugs, divided into "superior," "medium" and "inferior" classes.
(4) NAGAI: Pharm. Zeit., 1887, xxxii, 700.
(5) Merck's Ber., 1893, p. 13.
(6) LADENBURG, A., AND OELSCHAGEL, C.: Ber. Deutsch. Chem. Ges., 1889, xxii, 1823.
(7) RABE, P.: Ibid., 1911, xliv, 824.
(8) SCHMIDT, E.: Arch. Pharm., 1915, ccliii, 52.
(9) NAGAI: Chem. Zeit., 1888, p. 755.
(10) AMATSU, H., AND KUBOTA, S.: Kyoto Igaku, Zasshi, 1917, xiv, 77, through Chem. Abs., 1918, xii, 2019.
(11) MEYER, H. H., AND GOTTLIEB, R.: Exp. Pharmakol., Vienna, 1922, p. 198.
(12) BARGER, G., AND DALE, H. H.: Jour. Physiol., 1910, xli (i), 19.
(13) MIURA, K.: Berlin. Klin. Wochens., 1887, xxxviii, 707.

The action of ephedrine, the active principle of the Chinese drug Ma Huang. *Chen KK, Schmidt CF*

ON THE HYPODERMATIC USE OF ADRENALIN CHLORIDE IN THE TREATMENT OF ASTHMATIC ATTACKS.*

BY JESSE G. M. BULLOWA, M.D.,

AND

DAVID M. KAPLAN, M.D.,

OF NEW YORK.

(*A Preliminary Communication.*)

THERE are among the patients at Montefiore Home many cases of asthma that differ in their mode of onset, and in the variety and frequency of their seizures. These patients have afforded the material for the observations in this paper.

Before the use of adrenalin chloride hypodermatically the attacks were treated by the following methods. Fumes were inhaled from the various powders the bases of which are stramonium, belladonna or hyoscyamus with potassium nitrate. Opium and morphine were given by mouth, rectum and hypodermatically. In some cases relief was afforded in one-half to one hour, but only when doses large enough to produce stupor were administered. Frequently when the narcotic effect wore off the attack would return. Chloral and the bromides were given, but their action was not prompt and not always satisfactory. Nitroglycerin and hyoscine were administered. Camphor and ether were given hypodermatically. A combination consisting of antipyrin, antifebrin and caffeine was used. Chloroform anesthesia was resorted to in some obstinate cases in order to produce general relaxation; often the attacks would return with the wearing off of the anesthetic. Inhalations of oxygen were tried. Emetics were exhibited, cupping and mustard footbaths were resorted to. Silver nitrate injections into the vagus region were used. Adrenalin chloride was given by mouth but it had no effect on the attack. Adrenalin chloride was sprayed into the pharynx without satisfactory results. In fact, almost all the text-book methods were exhausted without much benefit to the patient.

As may be seen, the methods enumerated did not readily break up the attacks of asthma. They ought to be cut short as quickly as possible when one considers the sequelæ of a succession of asthmatic seizures. Although in some cases the patient's distress alone may cause anxiety to the physician it is what follows repeated prolonged attacks which gives him concern. Asthma itself has no known pathology; the repeated recurrences of asthmatic attacks, however, lead to the well-known changes characteristic of emphysema. Though there is no accepted pathology of asthma, during the asthmatic attack the pneumatic conditions in the lungs are presumably the following: There is an obstruction to the escape of air from the air vesicles and the air vesicles are overdistended. As a result of the obstruction the walls of the air vesicles are forced to expend their elastisity upon an air-cushion, so that, finally, they are overstretched, thus losing part of their elasticity. With the frequent recurrence of the above conditions the walls of a great many of the air vesicles lose their power to contract and remain distended. The passive hyperemia depending upon the vasoparesis results in an impairment of the vitality of the lung tissue and the walls of the vesicles atrophy. The many distended vesicles with their non-elastic walls enlarge the lungs to such an extent that they cause an increased intrathoracic pressure, producing an enlargement of the thorax and the characteristic barrel-shaped chest. In view of these consequences of the asthmatic seizure, and the obstructive explanation of the attack, the therapeutic attempt is properly directed toward relieving the obstruction and allowing the free egress and ingress of air. In order to remove the obstruction it is necessary to consider its nature first. It was such a consideration which led logically to the hypodermatic use of adrenalin chloride in asthma.

There are two chief theories accounting for the obstruction in an asthmatic attack. First, that the bronchial obstruction is brought about by a spasm of the circular muscles of the bronchi; second, that the obstruction is caused by a turgidity of the bronchial mucosa. The former theory is upheld by the majority of the medical profession, and is the one recently supported by the experimental studies of Brodie and Dixon,* in England. The data for the latter, or angioneurotic theory, have been presented by Goodhart in the chapter on Hay-fever and Asthma in Allbutt's "Practice of Medicine." The recent experimental studies on hay-fever by Dunbar† also seem to be in conformity with this second theory, as well as the article by Norman Bridge on Asthma, Bronchitis and Whooping-cough, in Hare's "System of Practical Therapeutics." The repeated failures of antispasmodics, to cut short the asthmatic attack, suggested the employment of adrenalin chloride hypodermatically, as a general vasoconstrictor, in conformity with the second hypothesis. The satisfactory result in one instance led to the repetition of the procedure and to the making of the following clinical observations:

Case I.—Female, aged seventeen years; Russian, admitted, 1900. Family history.—Mother has heart disease and hemoptyses. Father T. B. Personal history.—Until present illness personal history is negative. In 1898 patient caught cold while bathing. Two weeks later she had a typical asthmatic seizure lasting two days and three nights. One month later she had another attack lasting three days. Another spell, which was observed at the New York Hospital, lasted three days. Since then attacks of asthma recurred at intervals of from one day to two months. These attacks are usually preceded by malaise, pallor of the face and a few wheezing râles upon deep inspiration. Then the dyspnea becomes more and more marked, the mucous membranes become congested, the face and extremities cyanotic and cold, the wheezing and noisy breathing is heard at some distance from the bed, and the patient's

---

* From the Montefiore Home for Chronic Invalids, New York City, presented for publication, Sept. 22, 1903.

* The American Journal of the Medical Sciences, Sept. 19, 1903. "The Pathology of Asthma."
† Deutsche medicinische Wochenschrift, No. 9, Feb. 26, 1903.

distress is evident. These attacks return at irregular intervals and are apparently influenced by various conditions, such as atmospheric changes, dust, smoke, physical or mental exertion, menstruation, constipation, and, at times, without any evident cause. No constant pathological change in any of the organs has been found which would account for the origin of the attack. Some of these seizures were so severe as to leave the patient almost exhausted. Respiration would go up to 50 per minute and the pulse to 160.

These attacks were treated in various ways. Three years ago suprarenal extract in 5-grain doses was given by mouth and soon abandoned. The bromides, morphine, and digitalis, and at times atropine were used. On a few occasions the attacks were so severe that chloroform anesthesia was resorted to in order to relax the spasm. Adrenalin sprays into the pharynx were employed but they did not relieve the attack. Finally, after the patient's weight was reduced twenty pounds in two months, by a succession of attacks, the hypodermatic use of adrenalin chloride was suggested in agreement with the angioneurotic theory.

After the patient had been suffering for twenty-four hours and the attack was still in full force, the first dose of 7½ minims of an old solution of adrenalin chloride was administered. Half an hour later the patient was enjoying a quiet sleep. The attacks have taken place as frequently as before, but owing to the promptness with which they are cut short the patient has regained 8 pounds in the first month and 12 pounds in the second. During an attack the blood condition is as follows: Hemoglobin, 80 per cent.; red blood corpuscles, 4,800,000; white blood corpuscles, 8,600; differential count of white blood corpuscles gave polynuclear neutrophiles, 38 per cent.; transitionals, 8 per cent.; small lymphocytes, 6 per cent.; large lymphocytes, 8 per cent.; mononuclear leucocytes, 10 per cent.; eosinophiles, 26 per cent.; basophiles, 4 per cent.

While treating the patient by this method, the following observations were made: On one occasion after being awakened suddenly during the night by the advent of an attack and having suffered for several hours intensely, the patient was again seen at 7.10 A.M. after several antispasmodics had been given and 10 minims of adrenalin chloride had been administered by mouth without effect. At this time the patient was found sitting up in bed with her face cyanotic and her extremities cold. The breathing was loud and typically asthmatic, with the chest muscles overacting in a futile effort to aerate the lungs. At 7.11 respiration was 42 per minute, pulse 126. At 7.15 four minims of adrenalin chloride were injected into the arm. At 7.18, or three minutes after the injection, the patient's dyspnea was suddenly and completely relieved and the chest ceased to labor. At this time her face was pale and she could converse with comfort. Her respiration was 48 and her pulse 132; at 7.26, respiration 36, pulse 120; at 7.33, respiration 32, pulse 96 and the patient was quietly dozing.

An attack was recently observed (Sept. 6, 1903). Patient having visited her relatives during bad weather, came back suffering from malaise. Next morning, after several hours of increasing dyspnea, the patient was suffering considerable discomfort, her respiration being 40, pulse 128, of poor tension. At 12.38 P.M., one minute after the above observation, four minims of adrenalin chloride were injected into the arm. At 12.41 P.M. her respiration was 37, pulse 144, of good tension. At 12.46 all the subjective symptoms as well as the râles were gone. Breathing was comfortable—38 per minute—pulse 114. At 12.50 P.M. respiration 35, pulse 110. This patient's pulse normally ranges between 90 and 100.

On some occasions we had the opportunity to study the effects of the drug upon the pulse, as the following sphygmographic tracings indicate. In order to eliminate the psychical element the following experiments were performed:

Fig. 1.

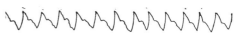

Usual tracing between attacks. Dudgeon's Sphygmograph.

Fig. 2.

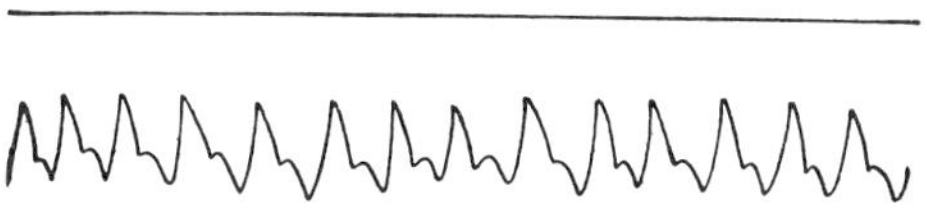

During an attack before adrenalin chloride was injected.

Fig. 3.

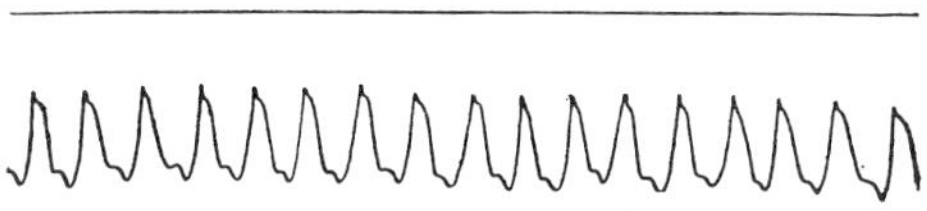

During an attack one minute after adrenalin chloride was injected.

Fig. 4.

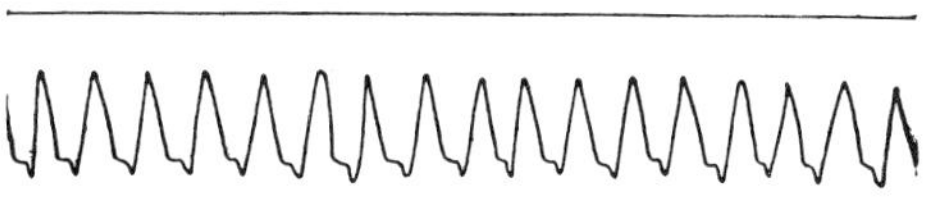

Four minutes after adrenalin chloride was injected.

Fig. 5.

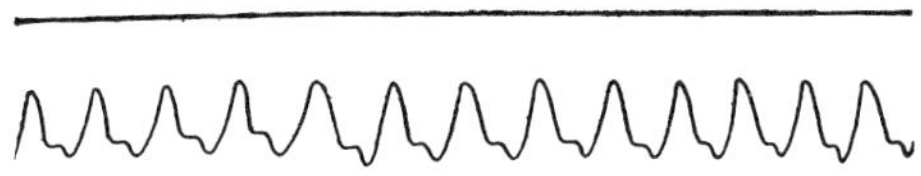

Seven minutes after adrenalin chloride was injected.

Tracings 2, 3, 4 and 5 were taken without changing the adjustment of the instrument, so that their distance from the horizontal lines approximately indicate the relative blood-pressure.

During an attack the respiration at 10.30 A.M. was 40, pulse 125. Breathing labored and wheez-

On the hypodermatic use of adrenalin chloride in the treatment of asthmatic attacks. *Bullowa JGM, Kaplan DM*

ing. Ten minims of water withdrawn from an adrenalin bottle were at once injected.

At 10.38 her respiration was 40, pulse 128; breathing unchanged. At 10.40 A.M. 3 minims of adrenalin chloride were injected into the arm. At 10.43 her respiration was 27, pulse 125, breathing practically normal. No râles. Recently (Sept. 9, 1903) the same experiment was repeated with the same results.

Case II.—Male, aged sixty-three years; tailor; Hungarian; admitted 1900. The salient features in this history are the following: He is an excessive smoker and moderately alcoholic. For thirteen years he has had severe attacks of bronchial asthma, which usually lasted for several days and nights. He suffers from emphysema and his customary dyspnea varies in intensity from time to time. The asthmatic seizures are typical, though sometimes they are associated with hiccough; sometimes they alternate with attacks of hiccoughing.

During a severe attack, the patient was seen at 12.19 A.M., his respirations were 22, pulse 108. His breathing was wheezing and could be heard all over the ward. Three minims of a fresh adrenalin chloride solution were immediately injected into the arm. At 12.22 there was no improvement, so that another two minims were administered. At 12.25 his respiration was 30 and his pulse 84, with increased tension. The breathing became quiet and a few râles could be heard, only when the ear was closely applied to chest. The patient was comfortable. Ten minutes later the patient shivered, as if in a chill, for about two minutes—and felt cold for a few minutes longer. One hour later the patient was resting quietly, the hiccough being relieved as well as the other symptoms. Following this attack the blood condition was: Hemoglobin, 70 per cent.; red blood corpuscles, 4,200,000; white blood corpuscles, 8,000. Differential count showed polynuclear nuetrophiles, 54 per cent.; small lymphocytes, 3 per cent.; large lymphocytes, 17 per cent.; mononuclear leucocytes, 3 per cent.; transitionals, 6 per cent.; basophiles, 2 per cent.; eosinophiles, 15 per cent.

Case III.—Female, aged thirty-seven years; housewife; Russian. She had grip in 1889, coughing very much and was very weak. Since then she has had moderately severe attacks of asthmatic dyspnea, which lasted for a week or ten days. After an injection of 5 minims of adrenalin chloride the condition is promptly relieved in about three minutes, and she feels better for several days. Following one such injection when the blood pressure had been increased by excitement and a fresher solution had been used, she experienced pain in the heart and a sensation of coldness. She shivered, her extremities were cold, cyanosed and tremulous and the visible mucous membranes were pale. These symptoms were considerably relieved by one-half ounce of whisky.

Case IV.—Female, aged sixteen years; seamstress. In May, 1902, she caught cold, vomited and had dyspnea. Inhaling some "smoke" re-

lieved her a little. Worked for one week and got another attack, compelling her to stay in bed. She came to this institution after a stay for some weeks in Gouverneur and Mt. Sinai hospitals. The attacks usually come on at night, causing considerable distress to patient. August 23, 1903, patient had an attack at night, 7½ minims of adrenalin chloride were injected and the seizure was cut short in two minutes. The patient said that later in the night she had a slight recurrence.

Case V.—Male, aged sixty years; peddler; moderate drinker; heavy smoker. Fourteen years ago had a cough for five months. Now he has all the physical signs of an emphysema and frequently gets typical asthmatic attacks at night. During one of these attacks, at 10.30 P.M. respiration was 35, pulse 102. Wheezing and sonorous râles all over the chest. Five minutes after the injection of 6 minims of adrenalin chloride, the respiration dropped to 30, and the pulse to 100; all râles disappeared and the patient slept quietly.

A number of other cases were treated with adrenalin chloride hypodermatically with precisely the same results.

It has been noticed that during an attack of asthma the pulse tension is diminished. This fact furnishes an additional indication for the hypodermatic use of adrenalin chloride, which has an accepted vasoconstrictor effect. Excessive vasoconstriction, however, is followed by a short rigor or chill without pyrexia, a sensation of pain and palpitation of the heart, a feeling of light headedness or headache as well as coldness and general shivering with a feeling of tingling and numbness of the extremities. A general blanching of the skin and visible mucous membranes is observed, together with tremors of the extremities.* These sensations never lasted longer than ten minutes and have never been noticed to any marked degree when the drug has been administered in the proper dose. This effect has been noticed in persons with stiff arteries from a smaller dose, and more often than in other patients. It is conceivable that patients with brittle arteries might be injured by an overdose; in such cases the drug must be given cautiously and the dose must be divided. There were no harmful effects observed in any of the patients, though some of them had marked arteriosclerosis.

In conformity with the angioparetic theory of the asthmatic attack, a dose sufficient to cause general vasoconstriction is necessary to cut short the seizure. Doses too small to bring about this result did not relieve the patient. Doses which are large enough to cause too marked constriction of the capillaries, such as will be followed by muscular fatigue and consequent loss of vascular tone, are sure, though the attack may be stopped temporarily, to be followed by a return of the symptoms, when the vasodilation manifests the muscular fatigue. No matter how large the dose, time sufficient for it to traverse the lesser circulation must elapse before the drug can act.

---

* In four patients who presented these symptoms, urinalysis showed no glycosuria.

On the hypodermatic use of adrenalin chloride in the treatment of asthmatic attacks. *Bullowa JGM, Kaplan DM*

With fresh preparations of the drug 3 to 6 minims of the 1 in 1,000 solution, hypodermatically, cut short the asthmatic attack, usually without disagreeable sequelæ. It is worth while mentioning the fact that solutions of adrenalin chloride deteriorate from exposure to light and air, and that the dose must ·be increased accordingly.

The immediate vasoconstriction necessary to cut short an attack can only be obtained by the hypodermatic method of administration.   Much larger doses by mouth do not cause the above effect; sprays into the throat are likewise inefficient. Adrenalin chloride used externally has only a local constricting on the capillaries, for which reason it is poorly absorbed when applied to the mucous membranes, therefore, in order to produce a constricting effect on the capillaries in the lung it must be introduced into the circulation. These facts are in accordance with Simonowitch's observations on the "Action of Adrenalin" in *Roussky Vratch,* June 14, 1903, who mentions among other things, the slow absorption of the drug by mucous membranes.

The hypodermatic administration of adrenalin chloride is not painful. In some cases there is a blanching of the tissues about the puncture with a reddened areola. This can be obviated by a deeper injection.

From these observations the following preliminary conclusions suggest themselves: (1) Given hypodermatically, adrenalin chloride is capable of cutting short attacks of asthma in from two to twenty minutes. (2) In conformity with the angioparetic theory of an attack, the dose must be such as will cause prompt general vasoconstriction, three to six minims of the 1 in 1,000 solution, in a single or divided dose, being used in adults.

In closing, the authors wish to express their sincere thanks to the House Physician, Dr. Siegfried Wachsmann, for his generosity, encouragement and advice during the progress of their work.

On the hypodermatic use of adrenalin chloride in the treatment of asthmatic attacks. *Bullowa JGM, Kaplan DM*

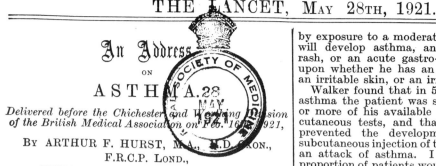

THE LANCET, May 28th, 1921.

An Address
ON
ASTHMA.

*Delivered before the Chichester and Worthing Division
of the British Medical Association on Feb. 16th, 1921,*

By ARTHUR F. HURST, M.A., M.D. Oxon.,
F.R.C.P. Lond.,

PHYSICIAN AND NEUROLOGIST TO GUY'S HOSPITAL.

LIKE Sir John Floyer, who published the first book in the English language on asthma in 1698, I myself suffer from asthma, so I have the advantage, which few writers on the subject possess, of 27 years of observation on my own corpus vile. The subject is one of special interest at present, as recent research in England, America, and France, has led to the explanation of many problems connected with asthma which had previously been obscure.

DEFINITION.

I would define asthma as the reaction of an over-excitable bronchial centre to blood-borne irritants and to peripheral and psychical stimuli. One part of the vagal nucleus in the medulla controls the activity of the bronchi. Normally it is in a certain degree of tonic activity. When over-active the broncho-motor fibres of the vagus cause the bronchioles to contract and the broncho-secretory fibres cause the secretion of bronchial mucus to be excessive. This general over-activity is associated with congestion of the bronchial mucous membrane, analogous to what occurs in all other organs when in a condition of functional activity. The engorged mucous membrane adds to the bronchial obstruction caused by the spasm of the circular muscle fibres, and consequently the mucus cannot be easily expelled. It is retained so long that it undergoes a process of coagulation, similar to the change which occurs in the formation of fibrin from fibrinogen, this being due to the activity of a ferment, mucinase, which is present in the bronchial mucous membrane. As the coagulated mucous casts of the bronchioles are slowly expelled along the spiral bronchi they assume the characteristic features of the spiral mucous filaments described by Curschmann, of Leipzig, in 1883. An exactly similar process occurs in the bowel in muco-membranous colitis ; mucus is secreted in excess, and owing to the associated spasm it is retained abnormally long, so that there is time for the characteristic membrane to form as a result of the action of the mucinase of the intestinal mucous membrane

ASTHMA AND ANAPHYLAXIS.

Our knowledge of the blood-borne irritants of the bronchial centre is of recent origin, and my own interest in the subject was stimulated by a visit to America in the summer of 1919. Much important work on the subject has been carried out by Freeman,[1] of St. Mary's, and Walker,[2] of Harvard, work which has thrown light on the hitherto inexplicable individual variations in the ætiology of asthma.* The irritant is generally, but not always, a protein to which the individual is abnormally sensitive. The nature of these toxic idiopathies, as they have been called by Freeman, is obscure, but they present many analogies to experimental anaphylaxis, and it appears probable that they are really examples of anaphylaxis occurring in man owing to inherited or acquired sensitiveness to certain proteins. In guinea-pigs bronchial spasm is one of the characteristic phenomena of anaphylaxis. Whether a man who is sensitive to a certain protein will be unaffected

* Frank Coke's important investigations on the subject were published some weeks after the delivery of this lecture. Brit. Med. Jour., March 12th, 1921.

No. 5100.

by exposure to a moderate dose of it, or whether he will develop asthma, an urticarial or eczematous rash, or an acute gastro-intestinal attack, depends upon whether he has an irritable bronchial centre, an irritable skin, or an irritable digestive tract.

Walker found that in 52 per cent. of 400 cases of asthma the patient was specifically sensitive to one or more of his available proteins, as shown by the cutaneous tests, and that desensitisation generally prevented the development of asthma, whereas subcutaneous injection of the specific protein produced an attack of asthma. I believe that a still larger proportion of patients would give a positive reaction if they were tested whilst actually asthmatic, as the degree of sensibility varies with the state of the patient's general health, and he may fail to react to proteins during a period of freedom from attacks, although the same proteins may produce well-marked reactions during an asthmatic period.

The protein may gain access to the body by inhalation in the case of pollen, emanations from the hair and skin of animals, and the dust of cereal grains ; it is ingested in the case of a great variety of foods ; and, lastly, the protein may be derived from bacteria which have formed a focus of infection in the bronchi or less frequently the tonsils, nose, teeth, or intestines. The anaphylactic factor is most common in cases beginning in early life ; thus 80 per cent. of those beginning in the first 2 years of life, 65 per cent. from 2 to 15, 50 per cent. from 15 to 35, 25 per cent. from 35 to 50, and none beginning after 50 were of this type (Walker). The special liability in children is most marked with food proteins, and next with animal proteins ; the liability to bacterial proteins is equally distributed whatever is the age of onset up to 40.

Food.

Goodale[3] in 1916 showed that extracts of wheat foods gave positive skin reactions in asthmatics who had attacks of asthma when they ate bread. Walker has more recently investigated the question in connexion with a great variety of foods. In 68 out of his 400 cases the patient was sensitive to food protein. In more than half of them (35) the protein was derived from cereals, in most instances wheat (25), but occasionally maize (6), rice (3), rye (2), barley or oats, and sometimes from several sources in the same individual. Maize, oat, rye, and barley rarely caused symptoms before the war, as until the introduction of war bread few people ate enough of them to have any effect. Wodehouse has shown that different individuals are sensitive to different wheat proteins. In most cases the natural proteose of wheat is the most active and differs from the proteose produced artificially from the gluten of wheat. Heating, except to very high temperatures, does not affect the anaphylactogenic properties of wheat proteins.

Next to cereals come eggs among the foods which may cause asthma, and then potato, casein, and fish, especially lobster, oyster, salmon, mackerel, cod, and haddock. The proteins of beef, chicken, and other forms of meat, spinach and other vegetables, strawberries and other fruit are occasionally active, but generally in association with other food proteins. There are, indeed, few if any foods to which some individuals are not sensitive.

Only a small proportion of patients discover for themselves that the particular article of diet to which they are shown to be sensitive by the skin reaction gives them asthma, and in some cases eczema and urticaria as well. They have sometimes, however, a distaste for the food to which they are sensitive, especially in the case of eggs.

Pollen.

Freeman has found as the result of the long series of investigations on hay fever he has carried out during the last ten years that, although a patient suffering from hay fever or hay asthma may be

Y

shown experimentally to be sensitive to a variety of pollens, grass pollen is the only one of any importance in England. It is always present in the air during the grass-flowering season, from the middle of May to the beginning of August, except when recent rain has washed it away. It alone of English pollens is produced in sufficient amount, is sufficiently easily disseminated by light wind, and is capable of producing a strong reaction. Daisy pollen, for example, only flies a few yards in contrast to grass pollen which can fly many miles, and trees only pollinate for a few days instead of for several weeks. In America conditions are very different, and Walker has shown the need for investigating the sensitiveness of each patient to a large variety of pollens. The majority of cases of hay asthma are associated with hay fever, which occurs, of course, still more frequently as an independent condition.

Animal Emanations.

Hyde Salter[4] was the first to recognise that asthma may be caused by the emanation from animals. In 1859 he noted cases of asthma brought on by the presence of cats, horses, guinea-pigs, rabbits, hares, cattle, sheep, and deer. Cat and horse asthma are the most common, the others being comparatively rare. Many patients are at once aware of the presence of a cat in the room from the development of asthmatic symptoms, which are sometimes associated with nasal catarrh and even urticaria. Trousseau described a case of a woman who had an attack of asthma directly her feather-bed was shaken in her presence, and Salter had a patient who could not sleep upon a pillow stuffed with feathers. Freeman writes of a patient who said, "You must put your head on the pillow as upon a wasp's nest." Goodale in 1916 found that an alcoholic extract of the hair of cats produced a skin reaction in patients suffering from cat asthma, the reaction apparently indicating that the individual was anaphylactic to the proteins contained in the extract. Wodehouse[5] found that the substance in the hair of cats and other animals which gave rise to the reaction was not the keratin, which forms the main constituent of hair, nor the proteins of their blood, but various other proteins which he isolated from the dandruff of the animal's skin. Freeman has shown that a slighter reaction is also produced by the flesh, serum, fæces, and nasal mucus in individuals who are sensitive to the dandruff, and that sensitiveness to a horse is associated with a lesser degree of sensitiveness to other members of the horse-tribe, such as the zebra, but to a very slight extent, as a rule, to the donkey.

The quantity of specific protein required to cause an attack of asthma is, of course, exceedingly minute. The comparatively large quantity of foreign protein introduced into the circulation when horse serum is used therapeutically is sufficient to produce an attack in many asthmatics who are not otherwise liable to horse asthma. Anti-diphtheritic or other serum ought, therefore, never to be given to an asthmatic without preliminary desensitisation. In the absence of this precaution death from anaphylactic shock has occurred in a number of cases described by Collier, of Oxford, and others.

Bacterial Toxins.

It has long been recognised that asthma may be associated with infection of the bronchi, and less commonly of the teeth, nasal mucous membrane, tonsils, and intestines. The infection may give rise to the production of bacterial proteins to which the individual is abnormally sensitive, in which case the asthma is of anaphylactic origin, or the lesion produced may act as an irritant focus and give rise to reflex attacks of asthma. It is possible to distinguish between these two possibilities by testing the cutaneous reaction to the toxins of each organism isolated from the sputum or other infective material or to stock toxins obtained from various organisms;

a positive reaction is obtained in the anaphylactic but not in the reflex cases. Vaccination may lead to improvement in both classes, but this is likely to be more marked in the former. Dr. John Eyre tells me that the organism which most frequently has a specific relation with asthma is a bacillus of the Friedländer group; this is often found in the spirals coughed up during an attack.

Other Proteins.

Asthmatics are occasionally sensitive to other proteins as well as those already referred to. Thus in one of Walker's patients an attack was always produced in the presence of a flax-seed poultice, and in another the attacks were caused by tobacco smoke, as in a case described by Floyer in 1726. The patients were found by the skin reaction to be sensitive to a protein in flax-seed and tobacco respectively. In a third case a jewel polisher was found to be sensitive to protein obtained from the dust of the boxwood he used in his work. Sensitisation of this kind undoubtedly explains many of the remarkable idiosyncrasies shown by asthmatics.

Multiple Sensitisation.

Walker found that multiple sensitisation was uncommon in cases which begin later than the age of 10, but it is common if it begins in infancy. It is probable that sensitisation to one protein early in life tends to be followed by subsequent sensitisation to others. Skin reactions indicating multiple sensitisation do not necessarily indicate that the asthma is at the actual moment being produced by all the proteins, although each is a potential cause and requires separate consideration in determining what treatment should be undertaken.

REFLEX CAUSES.

The most important peripheral stimuli which may affect an irritable bronchial centre and produce asthma reflexly arise in the nose, bronchi, stomach, and bowel. There is a point on the mucous membrane of the nasal septum opposite the inferior turbinal which appears to be specially rich in afferent nerve fibres which may influence the bronchial centre. Touching this with a probe may cause an asthmatic patient to wheeze, and contact with a congested inferior turbinal may give rise to an attack of asthma. Congestion of the turbinal is most frequently caused by infection, but apart from this contact may occur in individuals with a narrow nose or deflected septum, especially when the turbinal swells as a result of gravity on assuming the horizontal position, this being one reason why sleep is much less likely to be interrupted by an attack of asthma if the patient sits in a chair instead of going to bed.

I have already pointed out that the association of bronchial infection with asthma is due to either or both of two factors—sensitiveness to the toxin of one or more of the infecting organisms, and a reflex caused by the irritation of the bronchial mucous membrane by the infection; the latter must be present alone when the cutaneous reactions are absent, but improvement results from vaccination. Distension of the stomach with food may cause asthma, especially in the evening, quite independently of the nature of the food. Similarly distension of the rectum with fæces produces reflex asthma in patients with an irritable bronchial centre immediate relief follows defæcation.

HYSTERICAL AND EMOTIONAL ASTHMA.

In an individual with an irritable bronchial centre, but never apart from this, asthma may be caused by an idea or an emotion. Thus if a patient has had an attack under certain conditions he will expect to have another if the conditions are repeated. When for any reason the conditions have altered, but without the patient's knowledge, he may yet be so convinced that an attack will occur that one

THE LANCET,]   DR. ARTHUR F. HURST: ASTHMA.   [MAY 28, 1921 1115

is produced. Asthma caused by auto-suggestion in this way is truly hysterical, though in the absence of an abnormal bronchial centre no amount of suggestion could cause bronchial spasm and hypersecretion. Trousseau describes the case of a lady, who always had asthma in the presence of roses and had an attack when she saw some artificial roses which she thought were real. On my first visit to Salisbury in 1908 I had a very severe attack, which was repeated the following year, but I had no further attacks on numerous occasions in 1918 and 1919 when I revisited the city, as I had meanwhile become firmly convinced that my second attack was brought on solely by expectation, whatever may have been the cause of the first. Many patients who learn to rely on certain remedies are sure to become asthmatic if they discover that they have forgotten to take their powder, inhalation, or injection with them. Some asthmatics have an attack with any little excitement, business worry, or annoyance, but a severe fright is more likely to stop an attack than to cause one.

THE SUPRARENALS IN ASTHMA.

The excitability of different nerve centres shows considerable individual variations. This is shown by the variability of the pupil reflexes, skin reflexes, and deep reflexes. I believe that asthma is due to a condition which is generally, or perhaps always, inborn, and often inherited, in which the broncho-motor part of the vagus nucleus is more active than in the average man. In some cases it is very slightly so; the individual may then never have an attack of asthma in his life or, as in several of my patients, only a few attacks under very special circumstances. In other cases it is very hypersensitive and the asthma is more severe and constant. The over-activity of the broncho-constrictor fibres of the vagus is kept in check by the broncho-dilator activity of the sympathetic nerve-supply to the bronchial muscles, which is largely dependent on the constant secretion of adrenalin.

Physical and mental fatigue is a very common cause of asthma. Many asthmatics are always ill when they over-work, but recover at once on a holiday. Asthma is always worse in the evening than in the morning, and many patients can eat a large breakfast without any unpleasant symptoms resulting; but the smallest dinner, consisting perhaps of no articles of diet which cannot be taken with impunity at breakfast, is followed at once by wheeziness. And even if no food is eaten at night asthma may develop, though less severely. If the patient sleeps in the afternoon he is often less asthmatic in the evening, or if he sleeps just before dinner he may be able to eat much more than would otherwise have been possible. As asthma is caused by over-activity of the bronchial muscles, it might have been expected that fatigue would result in their relaxation, and consequently in the relief of the asthma. But physical fatigue does not seem to influence involuntary muscles, and certainly it does not lead to the relaxation of the bronchial spasm. It is well known that extreme fatigue leads to marked exhaustion changes in the suprarenal gland. It is quite possible that the fatigue of each day is sufficient to cause a slighter degree of similar changes. The smallest diminution in the secretion of adrenalin would allow the over-activity of the vagal bronchomotor centre to have greater play and asthma would result. These considerations appear to afford an adequate explanation of the production of asthma by fatigue.

A toxic idiopathy or hypersensitiveness to a certain protein, according to certain French authors, depends in part upon the fact that the protein has the effect of depressing the activity of the suprarenals. This effect may manifest itself in depression of one or all of its normal activities, the chief being in connexion with the blood-vessels, the alimentary canal, and the bronchi. Acute and severe anaphylaxis produced by large doses of serum injected into an individual sensitised by a previous injection of serum affects all three. More commonly only those functions in which the adrenal control is specially important for the particular individual are affected. Thus an asthmatic will have an attack of asthma and a man with a sensitive vaso-motor system will develop urticaria or other vaso-motor disturbances in the skin. A man who tends to have gastro-intestinal attacks owing to the abnormal irritability of his digestive tract will vomit and have diarrhœa and abdominal cramp owing to exaggerated peristalsis and relaxation of the cardiac, pyloric, and ileo-cæcal sphincters; this explains idiosyncrasies to shell-fish, eggs, and other foods which are manifested by acute digestive disturbances. In some cases an attack of asthma will be accompanied by the vaso-motor changes, or alternate with them, or will be accompanied by the abdominal attack. In one of my patients an attack of diarrhœa is always preceded by a feeling of tightness in the chest, which may develop into definite asthma whilst the diarrhœa lasts, finally disappearing with it. Lastly, in some cases the idiopathy is manifested in an attack of hay fever.

It is a familiar fact that a severe fright may relieve an attack of asthma. A man in the middle of a severe attack was driving downhill when the brake refused to act; he was in immediate danger of dashing into a wall which faced him at the bottom of the hill, but at the very last moment he succeeded in regaining control of the car; when he drew up he found that he was breathing with perfect freedom. This was probably due to the stimulation of the sympathetic and of adrenalin secretion caused by the fright. The stimulation of suprarenal secretion by asphyxia, which is perhaps the cause of second wind in runners, explains also the spontaneous relief or "second wind" which an asthmatic may experience if he continues his exercise after walking has brought on a moderate degree of dyspnœa. Finally, the extraordinarily rapid effect of adrenalin injections in bringing relief to an acute attack of asthma in many individuals can best be explained by this theory. The dose required is less than that required to produce general symptoms, such as a rise of blood pressure and a rapid pulse, because adrenalin first acts upon any organ which is too much under vagal control at the moment. If any intestinal symptoms are present these are likely to be relieved at the same time.

INHERITANCE OF ASTHMA.

All writers have noted the frequency of a family history of the disease in asthmatics, a frequency which is much too great to be accidental. Thus in 39 per cent. of Salter's 217 cases there was a clear history of inheritance. The important question arises: What is it that is inherited? I think that there is sufficient evidence to prove that it is sometimes an irritable bronchial centre, sometimes a toxic idiopathy, and sometimes both. When an individual whose father or mother is asthmatic develops asthma in the absence of any evidence of a toxic idiopathy, or has his first attack of asthma as a sequel of an infection or after he has acquired in adult life a toxic idiopathy, he must have inherited an irritable bronchial centre. For there is no doubt that a toxic idiopathy may be acquired, especially as a result of prolonged exposure to emanations in the course of a man's occupation. In half of Walker's cases which began after the age of 50 the patient was sensitive to a protein with which he came in contact as a result of his work: thus several bakers were sensitive to wheat, an ostler to horse dandruff, and a coffee-sifter to the protein of green coffee husks. Trousseau described the case of a chemist who had a violent attack of asthma when linseed, scammony, and ipecacuanha were powdered in his laboratory, and four others who were sensitive to ipecacuanha only. If no toxic idiopathy is inherited or acquired in an individual who is a potential asthmatic as a result of having inherited a sensitive bronchial centre, he may transmit the tendency to his children without ever developing asthma himself. Thus the paternal grandfather and uncle and maternal grandmother and aunt but neither parent of one of my asthmatic patients suffered from asthma.

An individual may share with some of his relations an abnormal sensitiveness to a certain protein. Coke relates the cases of a woman who was sensitive to milk, and had severe asthma throughout her two pregnancies ; both children were fed on cow's milk ; the first had gastric symptoms for the first 6 weeks of its life, and the second died from asthma when 6 weeks old. More frequently a general tendency to toxic idiopathies is inherited ; Freeman has published numerous instances of this. This may manifest itself in different members of the family as asthma, hay fever, or digestive disturbances, depending upon the inheritance or acquisition of an irritable bronchial, nasal, or digestive system respectively.

Treatment.

Three things require consideration in discussing the treatment of asthma : (1) the irritable bronchial centre ; (2) the chemical, reflex, and psychical stimuli which may affect the centre ; and (3) the attack itself.

1. *The Irritable Bronchial Centre.*

Every asthmatic knows that the better his general health is the less liable he is to asthma. In other words, the irritability of his bronchial centre varies directly with the state of his health. For this reason he should avoid over-work and take adequate holidays. Nothing is likely to do him more good than a month in the Swiss mountains in the winter, where he will probably find that he can indulge in ski-ing, lugeing, and skating with a vigour and freedom from respiratory distress he has not known for months. He should try to take some exercise every day, and a great deal more during the week-end. Slight dyspnœa is no contra-indication, as it often disappears on persevering with the exercise. Most important of all, he should try his best to avoid all possible causes of asthma, as the longer he remains free from it the less irritable the centre will become, until finally after some years of inactivity it may cease to respond at all to stimuli which in the past invariably gave rise to attacks. The best cure of asthma is not to have it. It is almost always possible to find some place where the patient does not get asthma, and no asthmatic child should be allowed to go to a school where he is more or less constantly asthmatic.

I have found that the irritability of the bronchial centre can be to some extent reduced by giving between 3 and 5 grains of caffeine, with double the dose of phenazone, when the patient feels slightly asthmatic and fears that an attack will develop later, as, for instance, immediately after lunch and dinner or on going to bed.

2. *Chemical, Reflex, and Psychical Stimuli.*

(a) *Toxic idiopathies.*—When asthmatic attacks are caused by food proteins all that is generally necessary is to exclude from the diet the food to which the patient is found to be most sensitive by the cutaneous test. Long abstention probably results in desensitisation. If eczema or urticaria is present it often disappears at the same time. Desensitisation does not follow injection of the proteins or feeding in slowly increased quantities of the food. Desensitisation to pollen can almost invariably be brought about by the subcutaneous injections of progressively larger doses of the pollen extract during the weeks preceding each hay-fever and hay-asthma season.

A patient can often free himself from asthma by simply avoiding any animal to which he has been shown to be sensitive, or in the case of feathers by avoiding feather pillows, mattresses, and upholstery. When an asthmatic is sensitive to horse dandruff in a dilution of 1 in 10,000 or more desensitisation is necessary, as the dust of city streets contains sufficient of the protein to cause attacks. In such cases, and whenever avoidance of the animals is impossible or does not relieve the asthma, desensitisation should be undertaken with the specific proteins. Nothing but specific treatment is of any use ; thus an individual who is sensitive to horse serum can be desensitised with the serum if it is necessary to give him some antitoxin, but this has no effect on his asthma, even if he happens to be also sensitive to horse-dandruff proteins. A large proportion of cases are relieved ; at the same time the skin reaction disappears or is greatly reduced in intensity.

Idiopathy to bacterial toxins can generally be overcome by vaccination in the ordinary way with organisms isolated from the patient's bronchial secretion or material obtained from other infective foci. In determining which organisms are most important the cutaneous reactions give some help, but even if no reaction is obtained an autogenous vaccine may prove very useful in curing chronic bronchitis or rhinitis which has acted as a reflex cause of asthma. The reaction is generally negligible if the injection is made at night and the patient takes 10 or 15 grains of aspirin at the same time. Lastly, the daily life of each patient should be investigated in every detail in an attempt to find some special toxic idiopathy other than the familiar ones already described, which may be in part responsible for the asthma.

(b) *Reflex causes.*—Bronchitis should be treated by autogenous vaccines and small doses of iodide taken for long periods. A careful examination of the nose should be made and any obvious source of irritation should be removed, but no operation should be performed unless it is very clearly indicated, as I have seen several cases aggravated by such operations, and one of the worst cases I ever saw was a man of 50 who had his first attack of asthma immediately after a hypertrophied turbinal had been removed. I have seen several cases in which mere cauterisation of a sensitive point on the septum in an apparently normal nose, as advocated by Francis, has produced marked improvement, though rarely, if ever, complete disappearance of all attacks. In many cases an autogenous vaccine prepared from the nasal secretion will do away with the need for local treatment by relieving the congestion which is secondary to infection, and in any case it is a useful preliminary measure in order to diminish the severe reaction which occasionally follows an operation. Apart from the Friedländer bacillus, already referred to, Dr. Eyre finds that the *B. septus* isolated from the nasal secretion, and pneumococci, *M. catarrhalis* and streptococci from the nasal and bronchial secretion are the organisms most frequently found in the rhinitis and bronchitis associated with asthma.

Asthma caused by a gastro-bronchial reflex can be avoided by eating hardly anything for dinner, which should be as early as possible, and nothing at all on going to bed, as the reflex only comes into play as the day advances and the patient becomes more tired. I have already pointed out how much benefit he may derive by sleeping or resting for half an hour before his evening meal. Regulation of the quantity of food is of more importance than its quality, except for any toxic idiopathies which may be present, but the food, especially in the evening, should be as digestible as possible ; no better guide to a suitable diet could be found than that given in Dr. James Adam's little book on " Asthma."

The intestinal-bronchial reflex comes almost entirely from the pelvic colon and rectum, and regular habits and exercises to overcome dyschezia are generally sufficient to keep it in check. Aperients should be avoided as far as possible, but in some cases a small weekly dose of infusion of senna is needed to prevent a fæcal accumulation from forming.

(c) *Psychical causes.*—Psychotherapy is only useful in so far as explanation of the mechanism involved may lead an asthmatic to take a less hopeless view as to his chance of complete recovery. So long as he feels convinced that certain circumstances will inevitably cause an attack they will certainly do so. He should be persuaded to be optimistic about his condition, and hope and even expect that what has hitherto caused an attack will not necessarily do so in the future.

3. *The Attack.*

An attack of asthma can most readily be cut short by the subcutaneous injection of adrenalin. The most efficacious dose is very much smaller than that generally given. In many cases a single minim of 1 in 1000 adrenalin chloride is enough, more than two minims being rarely required. But the injection should be given at the beginning of an attack, directly a patient wakes in the night, for instance, and not half an hour or an hour later when it has reached its full development. The relief is so immediate that the patient often falls asleep within five minutes of waking in an attack. Such small doses give rise to no unpleasant sensations, such as frequently follow the injection of three or more minims, and the blood pressure does not rise at all. Consequently the treatment can be continued for long periods without any fear of ultimately causing arterio-sclerosis. It is the only form of injection which a patient should be allowed to use on himself; if he has to depend on someone else giving the injection he will rarely receive it at the right moment.

For slight attacks and for the feeling of slight dyspnœa, which may persist throughout the day when severe attacks occur at night, atropine and cocaine may be used with an atomiser.

No patient should be allowed to use any of the numerous powders which are used by inhaling the fumes produced when they are burnt, as they invariably aggravate any bronchitis which may be present, and actually give rise to bronchitis in patients who have hitherto been free from it. I have seen several patients who have only recovered from a prolonged attack of asthma, persisting for weeks or months, after they had been persuaded to spend their nights sleeping in an easy chair instead of lying down in bed. Lastly, I wish to emphasise the fact that these remarks on the treatment of the attack should not make us forget that our chief aim must be to devise such a course of action for the patient that he will eventually have no attacks to treat.

References.

1. J. Freeman : THE LANCET, 1920, ii., 229.

2. I. C. Walker: Journ. Med. Research, 1917, xxxv., 497 and 509 ; 1917, xxxvi., 231, 237, 243, 295, and 423 ; 1917, xxxvii., 51, 277, and 287 : Boston Med. Surg. Jour., 1918, clxxix., 288 ; Am. Jour. Med. Sciences, 1919, clvii., 409 ; and Arch. Int. Med., 1918, xxii., 466, and 1919, xxiii., 220.

3. J. L. Goodale : Boston Med. Surg. Jour., 1915, clxxv., No. 2, and 1916, No. 6.

4. Hyde Salter : Asthma, London, 1859.

5. R. P. Wodehouse: Jour. Immunology, 1917, iv., 227, 237, 243, and 417.

A NOTE ON THE INHALATION TREATMENT OF ASTHMA

By P. W. L. CAMPS, F.R.C.S., Surgeon to Teddington Cottage Hospital.

THE general practitioner sees few cases of asthma compared with the specialist consultant, but he probably sees them more often in their agony of distress and panic in the night hours, he realises how urgently relief is demanded and needed, he sees the home conditions and feels the fears and dreads of recurring incapacities, and perhaps experiences frequent loss of his own night's rest. The practitioner is expected to and would if he could exorcise the devils of every disturbance, and he eagerly searches not only in the main roads but in the byways for remedies by which to restore to efficiency and to preserve harmony and health, and so in asthma we often observe the effects of the vaunted cures in order to exclude them.

The most remarkable characteristics of asthma are the variability of the causes, the temporary nature of its apparent cure, and the multitude of remedies and their erratic benefits.

About three years ago I had three obstinate cases of asthma, who, tired of my efforts, sought relief by a treatment at that time advertised in the lay press, and having obtained it reported the good news to me in the right spirit. (Our failures seldom come back to us.) They had obtained relief by the use of inhalations of drugs vaporised by oxygen. I was interested and acquired an apparatus (and soon a second and later two more), and experimented with it and various drugs in both acute and chronic pulmonary cases as well as asthma. I convinced myself by some dramatic results in cases, in which other methods had failed, that this vaporising of drugs by means of oxygen administered to the patient through a mask had a field of usefulness which by means of scientific research would be considerably extended.

Applying the method to the treatment of asthma, I found that by inhalation of adrenalin in the solution known as apneugene, which I obtained from the suppliers of the apparatus, the attack of asthma was cut short or aborted, and then by

496

A note on the inhalation treatment of asthma. *Camps PWL*

INHALATION TREATMENT OF ASTHMA 497

administering at bedtime for three to five minutes at 7 litres of oxygen per minute, after a few nights the nocturnal attacks were prevented and the asthma habit was broken. Cessation of treatment was not followed by any return while the patient was living an ordinary life, until some gross error of living or other accident, such as the contagion of a cold or family anxiety, brought back attacks which yielded again at once to the treatment..

I have used adrenalin, glycerine, ephedrin, and chloretone, but I come back to the apneugene as the reliable preparation, and the Spiess–Drager or Hirth's as a good form of apparatus, by which to produce a very fine vapour or cloud of oxygen and atomised solution and to deliver conveniently to the patient in bed, in any position in which he is comfortable, through a lightly fitting mask which he may hold or which may be retained by elastic bands.

What is the physiological action or why relief comes about I know not, but there is no abdominal or other discomfort, such as occurs with an overdose of adrenalin injections, nor is there any rise of blood pressure; the patient is relieved and falls asleep.

Much work has been done in Germany on the physical aspect of the atomisation of the solution as regards the fineness of the particles under different pressures and as delivered from the mask, but much more is required, particularly on the action of drugs upon the nasal and bronchial mucous membrane, and the changes in absorption and the rate of absorption under varying conditions of the patient and under differing pressures of delivery.

The fact that oxygen is used must be stressed, as I am led to understand that compressed air fails to yield the same beneficial results in the treatment of asthma.

Though inhalation therapy dates back to over 2000 years ago, it is curious how little has been written about it, and though we all employ it in some form or other daily, but little scientific research has been carried out, and I commend it to those who have time and would advance our knowledge of a treatment which achieves good.

Research needs to be carried out along four paths: firstly, the physical, which is concerned with the preparation and state of the medicament and its conveyance to the patient; secondly, the physiological, which is concerned with the effects upon the mucous membrane, muscle and circulation of the respiratory tract and with the absorption of drugs; thirdly, the pathological, which is concerned with the effects of the treatment in

A note on the inhalation treatment of asthma. *Camps PWL*

498 INHALATION TREATMENT OF ASTHMA

various diseases, not only of the respiratory system; fourthly, the psychological, which is concerned in estimating the rôle of suggestion, as in my experience in general practice this is the most difficult element to eliminate in estimating the value of any treatment.

A note on the inhalation treatment of asthma. *Camps PWL*

862   NATURE. VOL. 219, AUGUST 24, 1968

New Class of Selective Stimulants of β-Adrenergic Receptors

THE duration of the bronchodilator action of isoprenaline (I, $R_1 = R_2 = OH$, $R_3 = Pr^i$) is limited by metabolism by catechol-O-methyl transferase (COMT) to the inactive ether (I, $R_1 = OH$, $R_2 = OMe$, $R_3 = Pr^i$) (ref. 1).

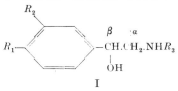

I

We have now prepared compounds where the *meta*-phenolic group of the catechol is replaced by related functions stable to COMT. When $R_2 = CH_2OH$ these are potent selective and long-lasting stimulants of β-adrenergic

Table 1. RELATIVE β-ADRENERGIC STIMULANT POTENCIES OF ARYLETHANOL-AMINES

Compound I	R_1	R_2	R_3	Bronchial muscle*	Cardiac muscle†
Isoprenaline	OH	OH	–CHMe₂	100	100
AH.3021	OH	–CH₂OH	–CHMe₂	40	0·1
AH.3365	OH	–CH₂OH	–CMe₃	100	0·05
AH.3923	OH	–CH₂OH	–CHMe.CH₂⟨⟩—OMe	150	0·075
AH.4553	OH	–CH₂OH	–CHMe.CH₂⟨⟩—OH	300	0·05
AH.3770	–CH₂OH	OH	–CHMe₃	0	0
AH.4045	OH	Me	–CMe₃	0	0·01
AH.4009	OMe	–CH₂OH	–CMe₃	0	0
AH.4665	OH	–CH₂OMe	–CMe₃	0	0

* Antagonism of the bronchoconstrictor action of acetylcholine in the anaesthetized guinea-pig[2]. Compounds are administered intravenously.
† Increase in contraction rate and isometric tension of isolated guinea-pig atria.

receptors in bronchial muscle and, in contrast to the catecholamines, show relatively little effect on cardiac muscle (Table 1). Their actions were antagonized by the β-adrenergic blocking drug propranolol. More detailed results of biological tests on a typical member of this series (AH.3365) are reported in the next communication.

The structural requirements of the ethanolamine side chain for potent β-stimulant activity broadly follow the pattern established for the catecholamines[3]. Thus the β-hydroxyl and the α-secondary amino functions are essential, the corresponding ethers and tertiary amines being inactive. Potency is enhanced in amines bearing branched alkyl chains containing additional aryl substituents and is reduced by alkylation at the α-carbon atom.

In the aromatic portion of the phenethanolamine the 4-hydroxyl group is vital and efficacy is destroyed by etherification. The proton is a key factor in the function of the hydroxymethyl group and both the methyl ether AH.4665 and the desoxy compound AH.4045 are lacking in β-stimulant effects. The loss of activity when the 3 and 4 substituents are reversed (AH.3770) parallels the observations of earlier workers[4] in compounds (for example, I, $R_1 = OH$, $R_2 = MeSO_2NH—$, $R_3 = Pr^i$) in which one of the phenolic groups of a catechol was replaced by the "bioisosteric" methanesulphonamide function. The explanation offered in the latter case—that the more acidic moiety (the sulphonamide) at the *para*-position induces an unfavourable fit on the receptor surface—clearly cannot apply in our examples where the pK_a of the phenol will be much lower than that of the hydroxymethyl group. Our results emphasize once more the differentiation between β-adrenergic receptors in smooth and cardiac muscle[5].

The capacity of the saligenin moiety to subserve as a

catechol is also demonstrated by the activity of our compounds at "metabolic" receptors[6] and at α-adrenergic receptors. Preliminary observations (personal communication from L. E. Martin) suggest that when 100 µg/kg is given to dogs intravenously the potent bronchodilators, for example AH.3365, are at least as effective as equal doses of isoprenaline in increasing serum concentrations of glucose and fatty acids. Further work is in progress to quantify these results and to assess their significance in the context of the concept of β-1 and β-2 receptors[7].

The racemic form of (I, $R_1 = OH$, $R_2 = —CH_2OH$, $R_3 = H$) is a directly acting α-adrenergic stimulant with a potency about one-fortieth of that of $R(-)$-noradrenaline when administered intravenously in the spinal cat.

Modern views on the function of the catechol portion of the catecholamines have modified Belleau's earlier postulate[8] that it fulfils a vital role in β-stimulant action by chelating with the magnesium atom of an ATP complex. Instead, it is now held[9] to potentiate an intrinsic effect of the remainder of the molecule by forming a localized water cluster that induces an ordering effect on a lipoprotein enzyme. It seems possible that the saligenin group in our compounds exerts a similar ordering function. The lower efficacy in promoting α-stimulation may be a consequence of the difficulty of inducing a conformational change of the type postulated by Belleau[9] for noradrenaline cocatalysis of phosphoryl group transfer which differs from that of the β-ordering process.

We thank Dr R. T. Brittain and his staff for providing the pharmacological results and Messrs D. T. Collin, J. C. Press and P. Toon for preparing some of the compounds.

D. HARTLEY
D. JACK
L. H. C. LUNTS
A. C. RITCHIE

Department of Chemistry,
Research Division,
Allen and Hanburys, Ltd,
Ware, Hertfordshire.

Received April 29; revised May 24, 1968.

[1] Iverson, L. L., *The Uptake and Storage of Noradrenaline in Sympathetic Nerves*, 70 (Cambridge University Press, 1967).
[2] Farmer, J. B., and Lehrer, D. N., *J. Pharm. Pharmacol.*, **18**, 649 (1966).
[3] Barlow, R. B., *Introduction to Chemical Pharmacology*, second ed., 294–318 (Methuen, London, 1964).
[4] Larsen, A. A., Gould, W. A., Roth, H. R., Comer, W. T., Uloth, R. H., Dungan, K. W., and Lish, P. M., *J. Med. Chem.*, **10**, 462 (1967).
[5] Lands, A. M., and Brown, jun., T. G., *Proc. Soc. Exp. Biol. and Med.*, **116**, 331 (1964).
[6] Ellis, S., Kennedy, B. L., Eusebi, A. J., and Vincent, N. H., *Ann. NY Acad. Sci.*, **139**, 826 (1967).
[7] Lands, A. M., Arnold, A., McAulift, J. P., Luduena, F. P., and Brown, jun., T. G., *Nature*, **214**, 597 (1967).
[8] Belleau, B., *Ciba Foundation Symposium on Adrenergic Mechanisms* (edit. by Vane, J. R., Wolstenholme, G. E. W., and O'Connor, M.), 233 (Churchill, London, 1960).
[9] Belleau, B., *Ann. NY Acad. Sci.*, **139**, 580 (1967).

α-[(t-Butylamino)methyl]-4-hydroxy-*m*-xylene-α¹,α³-diol (AH.3365): a Selective β-Adrenergic Stimulant

α-[(*t*-Butylamino)methyl]-4-hydroxy-*m*-xylene-α^1,α^3-diol (AH.3365), one of a new series of β-adrenergic stimulants described in the preceding communication, when tested on animals has been found to have a considerably greater action on bronchial smooth muscle than on other smooth muscles affected by β-stimulants. Relative potencies found for AH.3365, isoprenaline and orciprenaline in preventing bronchospasm induced by acetylcholine in guinea-pigs are given in Table 1 together with their potencies in relaxing spontaneous tone of isolated tracheal chain preparations. In the Konzett–Rössler preparation, similar orders of potency were found when the spasmogen used was histamine, 5-hydroxytryptamine or bradykinin. At equi-effective doses AH.3365 and orciprenaline had a similar duration of action and both were longer acting than isoprenaline in the *in vivo* tests. The ratios found on the tracheal chain preparation are different from those obtained in any *in vivo* experiment designed to measure airflow or airways resistance in any species tested so far.

Table 1. COMPARATIVE β-ADRENERGIC STIMULANT POTENCIES OF AH.3365, ISOPRENALINE AND ORCIPRENALINE IN THE GUINEA-PIG

Test preparation and spasmogen	Route of drug administration	Relative β-stimulant potency		
		AH.3365	Isoprenaline	Orciprenaline
Anaesthetized guinea-pig intravenous acetylcholine (Konzett and Rössler preparation)[1]	Intravenous	1	1	0·025
Conscious guinea-pig; aerosolized acetylcholine*	Oral	1	Poorly active: effect not dose related	
	Aerosol	1	0·1	0·01
Isolated tracheal chain[2]	*In vitro*	1	10	2

* Unpublished work of J. B. Farmer, V. A. Cullum and G. P. Levy.

NATURE, VOL. 219, AUGUST 24, 1968

Thus *in vitro* tests may give a poor estimate of the real bronchodilator activity of β-stimulants.

The cardiovascular actions of AH.3365 are less than those of isoprenaline or orciprenaline. When tested on isolated guinea-pig atria the stimulant effect of AH.3365 was found to be 2,000 times less than that of isoprenaline and half that of orciprenaline. Unlike isoprenaline, AH.3365 could prevent bronchospasm due to efferent vagal stimulation in anaesthetized cats or dogs in doses (0·5–5 μg/kg intravenously depending on species) which did not affect the heart rate or blood pressure. The bronchodilating potencies of the two drugs were similar in this test, but the vasodilator action of AH.3365, assessed by perfusing dog hind limb or by measuring blood pressure, was only about one-tenth that of isoprenaline.

$$HOH_2C \diagdown \atop HO-\!\!\!\!\underset{}{\diagup}\!\!\!\!\underset{^3H}{\overset{OH}{\underset{|}{C}}}.CH_2.NH.C\!\!\!\underset{\diagdown}{\overset{\diagup CH_3}{-CH_3}}\diagup \atop CH_3} \qquad (I)$$

AH.3365 specifically tritiated on the β-carbon (I) was used for metabolic studies in dogs and rats. In dogs given 1, 5 or 12·5 mg/kg of tritiated AH.3365 orally 70–80 per cent of the dose was excreted unchanged in the urine, which also contained an unidentified glucuronide equivalent to about 10 per cent of the dose administered. A similar excretion pattern was obtained in dogs which had received daily doses of AH.3365 for 3 months, suggesting that specific processing enzymes for the drug had not developed during that time.

In rats given doses between 25 and 200 mg/kg of tritiated AH.3365 orally 50–80 per cent of the administered radioactivity appeared in the urine within 48 h but only 20–40 per cent of this represented unchanged drug; the remainder was a glucuronide. AH.3365 or its metabolites are excreted in quantity in the bile of rats. For example, the bile collected over a 4 h period from rats given 20 mg/kg of tritiated AH.3365 intraperitoneally contained 27 per cent of the radioactivity administered. This probably explains why 20–40 per cent of the drug given orally is excreted in the faeces; it is probably in the form of metabolites. It is known that isoprenaline is rapidly inactivated by catechol-*O*-methyl transferase[3]. The metabolic studies reported here clearly show that AH.3365 is not affected by this enzyme and should therefore be a longer acting drug.

These results suggest that AH.3365 would be an improved bronchodilator, being more selective, longer acting and safer than isoprenaline, and more potent and probably less likely to cause side effects than orciprenaline. The early results of quantitative clinical studies agree with these conclusions. AH.3365, in a dose of 100 μg given by aerosol, has been shown to be a highly effective, long acting bronchodilator without observable side effects. Indeed, at least ten times this dose given by aerosol is needed to induce detectable effects on the heart and blood pressure. When given orally about 5 mg of drug is effective in adults, again without detectable cardiovascular actions. Full results of all these investigations will be published later.

R. T. BRITTAIN
J. B. FARMER
D. JACK
L. E. MARTIN
W. T. SIMPSON

Research Division,
Allen and Hanburys, Ltd,
Ware, Hertfordshire.

Received April 29, 1968.

[1] Konzett, H., and Rössler, R., *Arch. Exp. Pathol. Pharmak.*, **195**, 71 (1940).
[2] Farmer, J. B., and Lehrer, D. N., *J. Pharm. Pharmac.*, **18**, 649 (1966).
[3] Ross, S. B., *Acta Pharmacol. Toxicol.*, **20**, 267 (1963).

α-[(t-butylamino) methyl]-4-hydroxy-m-xylene -αl, α3-diol (AH.3365):
a selective β-adrenergic stimulant. *Brittain RT, Farmer JB, Jack D et al*

3 May 1969   BRITISH
                                              MEDICAL JOURNAL   287

Controlled Comparison of the Bronchodilator Effects of Three β-Adrenergic Stimulant Drugs Administered by Inhalation to Patients with Asthma

Y. F. J. CHOO-KANG,* M.B., B.SC., M.R.C.P.ED. ; W. T. SIMPSON,† M.B., CH.B.
I. W. B. GRANT,‡ M.B., F.R.C.P.ED.

British Medical Journal, 1969, **2**, 287–289

Summary: In a double-blind trial of the effect of inhaling three different β-adrenergic stimulants (isoprenaline sulphate 1,000 μg., orciprenaline sulphate 1,500 μg., and salbutamol 200 μg.) and a placebo on ventilatory function in 24 patients with chronic asthma salbutamol was found to have a much longer action than isoprenaline, and it produced a slightly more intense and prolonged effect than orciprenaline. In a double-blind subjective assessment 13 of the 24 patients selected salbutamol as the most effective preparation, while only five preferred isoprenaline and three orciprenaline. Hence salbutamol, given by inhalation, may prove to be the most effective drug at present available for the short-term relief of asthmatic symptoms.

Introduction

The β-adrenergic stimulant isoprenaline is a useful bronchodilator when administered by inhalation, but it has certain disadvantages. These consist of, firstly, a rather short duration of action owing to rapid metabolism by catechol-O-methyl transferase to the inactive 3-methoxy derivative (Paterson *et al.*, 1968), and, secondly, a marked action on cardiovascular β-adrenergic receptors, leading to tachycardia and increased cardiac output (Goodman and Gilman, 1965). Orciprenaline, another specific β-adrenergic stimulant (Engelhardt *et al.*, 1961 ; Shanks *et al.*, 1967), is effective both by inhalation and by mouth. After inhalation it has a duration of action longer than that of isoprenaline, and is less apt to produce cardiovascular side-effects (Holmes, 1968). In an effort to find a more powerful bronchodilator drug combining prolonged action with a minimum of undesirable β-adrenergic stimulant effects many compounds with structural resemblances to isoprenaline have recently been screened in research laboratories. One of these compounds, salbutamol (AH 3365), has now been released for clinical study, and the purpose of this communication is to assess the bronchodilator activity of this drug compared with that of isoprenaline, orciprenaline, and a placebo, administered by inhalation in each instance. Salbutamol was described by Hartley *et al.* (1968) and by Brittain *et al.* (1968). It differs from isoprenaline in that (*a*) the meta-OH is replaced by a primary alcohol group—CH₂OH, and (*b*) the N-isopropyl group is replaced by N-tertiary butyl. The first of these renders the compound stable to catechol-O-methyl transferase, while the second makes inactivation by N-dealkylation unlikely. A compound with these properties should have a prolonged action when inhaled, and should also be effective when given by mouth. Results in animals and preliminary trials in man (Brittain *et al.*, 1968) suggest that salbutamol is indeed a long-acting bronchodilator, effective both by inhalation and by

mouth with little action on the heart. The structural formulae of isoprenaline, orciprenaline, and salbutamol are shown in Fig. 1.

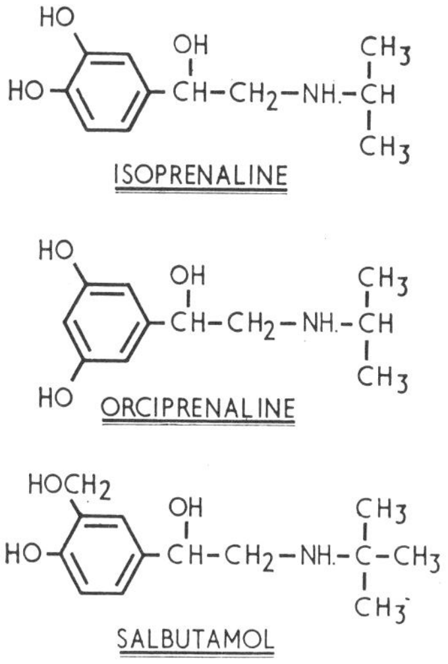

FIG. 1.—Structural formulae of isoprenaline, orciprenaline, and salbutamol.

Plan of Trial

The purpose of the trial was to compare the bronchodilator activity of isoprenaline, orciprenaline, salbutamol, and a placebo consisting simply of inert propellant. It was designed as a 4 × 4 "Latin square," in which the following were administered on consecutive days to each patient: isoprenaline sulphate 1,000 μg., orciprenaline sulphate 1,500 μg., salbutamol 200 μg., and propellant alone.

Each preparation was administered as two "puffs" of a pressurized aerosol, the isoprenaline and orciprenaline being the commercially available products Medihaler-IsoForte and Alupent respectively. (Alupent was repacked at a suitably adjusted concentration in a container to match the others.) The Latin square was repeated six times, the coding of the preparations being changed after each square. In this way all permutations of the four preparations were covered, and since the containers and applicators were identical in appearance it was virtually impossible for bias on the part of either observer or subjects to influence the results.

Forced vital capacity (F.V.C.) and forced expiratory volume in one second (F.E.V.₁) were measured on three occasions at 10-minute intervals before the drugs were administered, except in two instances where by oversight one recording was omitted. The measurements were repeated at 1 minute, 6 minutes, 20 minutes, 50 minutes, 80 minutes, 110 minutes, 140 minutes,

* Medical Registrar.
‡ Consultant Physician.
Respiratory Diseases Unit, Northern General Hospital, Edinburgh, and the Department of Respiratory Diseases, University of Edinburgh.
† Head of Medical Services, Allen & Hanburys Ltd.

E

Controlled comparison of the bronchodilator effects of three
β-adrenergic stimulant drugs administered by inhalation to
patients with asthma. *Choo-Kang YFJ, Simpson WT, Grant IWB*

170 minutes, 230 minutes, and 290 minutes after administration. Three readings were taken on each occasion. In the analysis of results the mean of the highest figures achieved on each of the pretreatment occasions was taken as a "mean best pretreatment figure"; this was the standard with which the best in each group of three post-treatment figures was compared.

A measure of subjective preference was obtained by asking each patient on completion of the trial which treatment had given most relief. Side-effects and other comments were noted if they were mentioned spontaneously. Patients' pulse rates were counted on two or three occasions before treatment and at 1, 6, and 20 minutes after treatment.

The entire procedure was carried out on each occasion by the same technician.

Patient Selection

The patients consisted of 7 men and 17 women, ranging in age from 28 to 71 years (mean 56·3 years). All had severe chronic asthma but had been stabilized for at least six months on treatment with a corticosteroid drug, in most instances prednisolone. They were selected on the basis of having shown a good response to inhaled isoprenaline at previous outpatient attendances, and, in order to ensure that this response would be reproduced in the trial itself, they were accepted for study only if the F.E.V.₁ was between 50 and 75% of the previous highest recording. Those patients who had been receiving prednisolone intermittently were given the drug daily throughout the period of the trial in order to minimize variations in the severity of the asthma. Corticosteroid dosage in terms of prednisolone ranged from 5 to 20 mg. per day.

The mean control value for F.E.V.₁ at the start of the trial was 1,189 ml. (range 390–3,450 ml.), and for F.V.C. was 2,253 ml. (range 880–5,500 ml.).

Results

The increases which occurred in F.E.V.₁ and in F.V.C. after treatment were calculated as percentages of the mean highest pretreatment values, and also in terms of mean total "area under the curve" obtained by integrating the changes in individual values throughout the period of the experiment. The mean highest pretreatment values for isoprenaline, orciprenaline, salbutamol, and placebo were as follows:

			F.E.V.₁	F.V.C.
Isoprenaline	..	..	1,190	2,250
Orciprenaline	..	..	1,250	2,330
Salbutamol..	..	..	1,230	2,300
Placebo ..	..	..	1,250	2,250

The mean percentage changes in F.E.V.₁ and in F.V.C. are shown graphically in Figs. 2 and 3. The mean changes in F.E.V.₁/F.V.C. (×100) are shown in Fig. 4. The integrated values for "area under the curve" in respect of F.E.V.₁ and F.V.C. are given in Tables I and II. The patients' preferences at the end of the trial are shown in Table III, and the percentage changes in heart rate from the lowest pretreatment values in Table IV.

TABLE I.—*"Area Under the Curve"—Integrated F.E.V.₁ Change*

Isoprenaline	..	..	64,600	Salbutamol	..	..	110,800
Orciprenaline	..	..	93,900	Placebo	..	..	20,600

A difference of 24,000 or more is significant at the 5% level.

TABLE II.—*"Area Under the Curve"—Integrated F.V.C. Change*

Isoprenaline	..	..	96,300	Salbutamol	..	..	160,000
Orciprenaline	..	..	126,200	Placebo	..	..	46,600

A difference of 40,500 or more is significant at the 5% level.

TABLE III.—*Patients' Preferences for Various Treatments*

Isoprenaline	..	..	..	5	Placebo	..	..	..	0
Orciprenaline	..	..	..	3	No preference	..	..	..	3
Salbutamol	..	..	..	13					

TABLE IV.—*Mean Percentage Change in Heart Rate*

Minutes After Administration	Isoprenaline	Orciprenaline	Salbutamol	Placebo
1	13·0*	1·6	3·5	2·9
6	10·8*	−0·6	4·1	2·7
20	3·3	1·1	0·5	0·8

* Significantly different from placebo values (P < 0·05).

Placebo

There was a slight and sustained rise in F.V.C. and F.E.V.₁ after the inhalation of placebo, but this change was negligible in comparison with that produced by all three active preparations. The response to placebo was, however, not significantly different from that of isoprenaline at 140, 170, and 190 minutes after inhalation, presumably because by then the pharmacological action of isoprenaline had come to an end.

Isoprenaline 1,000 µg.

The response to isoprenaline was significantly greater at one minute than that observed with either of the other two drugs. The effect reached a maximum at six minutes, was clearly on the wane after less than an hour, and had virtually disappeared at 140 minutes. In terms of F.E.V.₁/F.V.C. ratio patients were at this time no better than after placebo. Isoprenaline produced a significant increase in pulse rate one minute and six minutes after administration.

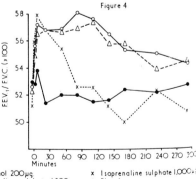

FIG. 2.—Percentage changes in F.E.V.₁ after the inhalation of salbutamol, orciprenaline, isoprenaline, and placebo. FIG. 3.—Percentage changes in F.V.C. after the inhalation of salbutamol, orciprenaline, isoprenaline, and placebo. FIG. 4.—Changes in F.E.V.₁/F.V.C. (×100) after the inhalation of salbutamol, orciprenaline, isoprenaline, and placebo.

Controlled comparison of the bronchodilator effects of three β-adrenergic stimulant drugs administered by inhalation to patients with asthma. *Choo-Kang YFJ, Simpson WT, Grant IWB*

3 May 1969   Asthma—*Choo-Kang et al.*   BRITISH MEDICAL JOURNAL   289

Orciprenaline 1,500 μg.

Orciprenaline was longer acting than isoprenaline, its effect on F.E.V.$_1$ reaching a plateau at between 20 and 120 minutes. The response to this drug was, however, less intense than that observed with either isoprenaline or salbutamol, the maximum mean increase in F.E.V.$_1$ being 38·7%, as compared with 47·9% for isoprenaline and 47·7% for salbutamol. The effect of orciprenaline on the heart rate did not differ significantly from that of the placebo.

Salbutamol 200 μg.

Although the response to salbutamol at one minute was not as great as that to isoprenaline 1,000 μg., there was a subsequent slow increase in effect over the next 60 minutes, in contrast with the rapid decline observed with isoprenaline. In terms of maximum improvement salbutamol equalled isoprenaline on F.E.V.$_1$ (47·7% v, 47·9%) and slightly exceeded it on F.V.C. (35·8% v. 30·7%). The bronchodilatation produced by salbutamol was much more prolonged than that produced by isoprenaline, and was well sustained for three hours. Even at five hours after salbutamol the mean F.E.V.$_1$ was still 26% above the control value, as compared with figures of 8% for isoprenaline, 19% for orciprenaline, and 6% for placebo. The effect of salbutamol on F.E.V.$_1$ and F.V.C. exceeded that of isoprenaline at 50 minutes and at all subsequent observations.

Compared with orciprenaline, salbutamol produced consistently greater improvement both in F.E.V.$_1$ and in F.V.C., but the difference was significant (P<0·05) only at 50 minutes in the case of F.E.V.$_1$ and at 50 and 170 minutes in the case of F.V.C. At most of the other times the value for P lay between 0·1 and 0·05, but support is given to the clinical, if not to the statistical, significance of this difference by the fact that 13 patients selected salbutamol as the best treatment, while only three preferred orciprenaline and five isoprenaline. The effect of salbutamol on heart rate did not differ significantly from that of placebo.

Discussion

The study described in this paper showed that the inhalation of salbutamol in a dose of 200 μg. provided effective bronchodilatation for a period of at least three hours without producing detectable cardiac stimulation. The bronchodilator activity of this dose of salbutamol was slightly more intense and prolonged than that of 1,500 μg. of orciprenaline, and equal in peak effect to that of 1,000 μg. of isoprenaline. Side-effects did not occur with either salbutamol or orciprenaline in the doses specified, but palpitations and tremor have been reported by Holmes (1968) with a higher dose of orciprenaline. Isoprenaline 1,000 μg. compared unfavourably with both salbutamol and orciprenaline, as the bronchodilator response, though initially more intense, remained effective for less than one hour and was accompanied by tachycardia.

From the data available in this study it is difficult to reach a firm conclusion on the relative therapeutic merits of salbutamol and orciprenaline, because the differences in the effects of these two drugs only rarely achieved statistical significance, and also because the dose of the one or the other may have been suboptimal. A more conclusive result might have been obtained by observing the bronchodilator response to graduated doses, but this would have been difficult to incorporate into a strictly controlled trial design and probably impracticable, since few patients will tolerate more than four days of this exacting type of investigation. The doses selected for study were those recommended by the manufacturers and normally prescribed in the treatment of asthma. As such, they were considered to provide a fair basis for comparison of the therapeutic value of the two drugs in clinical practice.

Under these circumstances the bronchodilator effect of salbutamol 200 μg. was slightly superior to that of orciprenaline 1,500 μg., and in the double-blind subjective assessment it was rated as the best of the four treatments by 13 patients, while only three preferred orciprenaline. These findings suggest that salbutamol, given by inhalation, may prove to be the most effective drug at present available for the short-term relief of asthmatic symptoms.

As a single dose of salbutamol administered by inhalation can provide effective bronchodilatation for three hours, it might be assumed that regular three-hourly inhalation would afford continuous relief of symptoms in chronic asthmatics. Preliminary studies of this kind of therapeutic regimen have, however, shown that the bronchodilator effect of salbutamol, like that of ephedrine when administered regularly by mouth (Laurence, 1966), gradually wanes after a period of one to three weeks. Until more information is available about the frequency with which tolerance can be induced by regular administration, it would be advisable to reserve salbutamol, like other β-stimulants, for the relief of acute asthmatic symptoms, and not to use it in an attempt to maintain continuous bronchodilatation.

Our thanks are due to Mr. A. J. Davey for the statistical analysis, and to Miss L. Tully for technical assistance.

REFERENCES

Brittain, R. T., Farmer, J. B., Jack, D., and Simpson, W. T. (1968). *Nature*, **219**, 862.
Engelhardt, A., Hoefke, W., and Wick, H. (1961). *Arzneimittel-Forschung*, **11**, 521.
Goodman, L. S., and Gilman, A. (1965). *The Pharmacological Basis of Therapeutics*, 3rd ed., p. 498. New York, Macmillan.
Hartley. D., Jack, D., Lunts, L. H. S., and Ritchie, A. C. (1968). *Nature*, **219**, 861.
Holmes, T. H. (1968). *Clinical Pharmacology and Therapeutics*, **9**, 615.
Laurence, D. R. (1966). *Clinical Pharmacology*, 3rd ed., p. 371. London, Churchill.
Paterson, J. W., Conolly, M. E., Davies, D. S., and Dollery, C. T. (1968). *Lancet*, **2**, 426.
Shanks, R. G., Brick, I., Hutchison, K., and Roddie, I. C. (1967). *British Medical Journal*, **1**, 610.

Controlled comparison of the bronchodilator effects of three β-adrenergic stimulant drugs administered by inhalation to patients with asthma. *Choo-Kang YFJ, Simpson WT, Grant IWB*

THE USE OF SUPRARENAL CORTEX EXTRACT IN THE TREATMENT OF BRONCHIAL ASTHMA*

A. H. FINEMAN, M.D.

NEW YORK

HARTMAN, Mac Arthur and Hartman[1] and Rogoff and Stewart,[2] working independently and at the same time, were the first investigators to isolate the cortical hormone of the suprarenal gland; but it remained for Swingle and Pfiffner,[3] in 1930, to prepare an extract which indefinitely maintained life, in normal condition, of suprarenalectomized animals. This contribution gave impetus to the clinical application of the extract in human beings suffering from Addison's disease, and many reports[4, 5, 6] of its beneficial effect have recently appeared in the literature.

The influence of the suprarenal cortex extract in conditions other than Addison's disease has been little studied. No work has been published of its use in the treatment of bronchial asthma. Patients suffering with severe and protracted asthma frequently complain of weakness, loss of appetite, loss of weight and exhaustion. The blood pressure is invariably low. There is, as a rule, a hypochlorhydria with a relatively low blood sugar. These findings are also present in Addison's disease except in a more marked degree. It seems plausible that some degree of cortical insufficiency may exist in patients with chronic asthma and that administration of the cortical hormone may prove of value in this condition.

For this investigation a study of four patients, three white and one colored, suffering with severe asthma was made. The youngest patient was twenty-two years and the oldest forty-three years. The age of onset was over twenty years in three cases and under this age in one. In three cases the onset was gradual. The duration of asthma before admission to the clinic was eighteen years in one, eight years in another, and six months in each of the other two cases. One patient was treated for more than two years before the suprarenal cortex extract was tried; the remaining three were under care for less than six months each and were selected because of the severity of the asthma.

A thorough history, a complete physical examination and roentgen-ray examination of the chest and nasal sinuses as well as electrocardiographic studies were made. A complete series of protein skin tests was performed. Three patients were found to be protein sensitive and one was non-sensitive.

Treatment with suprarenal cortex extract was begun in each case during the winter months, when asthma is usually aggravated. No other

*From the Allergy Clinic and Department of Medicine, Sydenham Hospital.

The use of suprarenal cortex extract in the treatment of bronchial asthma. *Fineman EH*

treatment was given while the cortical hormone was employed. Detailed records were kept of the effect of the extract on the asthmatic condition, appetite, strength, blood pressure, pulse and weight. The results of these observations are discussed under separate headings.

MATERIAL USED AND METHOD OF ADMINISTRATION EMPLOYED

The material used in this investigation was an aqueous extract* of fresh beef suprarenal cortex, prepared according to the method of Swingle and Pfiffner. Each cubic centimeter represented the hormone obtained from 30 grams of suprarenal cortex. In the present study quantitative figures of dosage are given in cubic centimeters of the extract or the equivalent amount of glandular tissue. This was found necessary for the time being because no uniform unit of dosage has been adopted.

The patients were first tested intradermally with the extract, and negative reactions were obtained. Treatment was begun with a dose of 0.5 c.c. which was gradually increased to 3.0 c.c. In one patient a maximum dose of 4.0 c.c. was given over a period of one month. Injections were given subcutaneously for the first few weeks and subsequently intramuscularly. Three to four injections were given weekly during the first month and one to two injections weekly thereafter. No soreness or redness appeared at the sites of injection, and no untoward systemic effects were encountered. The intravenous route was avoided because of the fear of general reactions.

Two patients were treated with the cortical extract for four months each; one patient for three months and one for six weeks.

EFFECT OF THE EXTRACT ON ASTHMA

Of the four patients treated with the suprarenal cortex extract, one showed marked improvement, one moderate, one slight and one no improvement. Detailed reports of the cases studied are as follows:

REPORT OF CASES

CASE 1.—P. H., colored, single, aged twenty-two years, was first seen at the allergy clinic on September 28, 1931. She gave a history of asthma of six months' duration. The onset was gradual with wheezing and cough, and subsequent attacks developed. There were at first free intervals of three to four weeks' duration; then the attacks became more

---

*The extract is marketed under the commercial name of Eschatin by the Parke, Davis & Company. The solution is clear, colorless and sterile. It contains minute quantities of epinephrine, less than one part in three million, but for clinical purposes the amount is considered negligible. The extract is comparatively stable, and its activity is maintained at refrigerator temperature for a long time. Since the early part of 1932 it has been assayed and standardized according to the dog unit suggested by Harrop et al. (Proc. Soc. Exper. Biol. & Med. **29**: 449, 1932). A dog unit of the extract is the minimum daily dose of cortical hormone per kilogram of body weight necessary to maintain normal physiologic conditions (appetite, body weight and the blood level of nonprotein nitrogen) in an adrenalectomized dog that has been previously held on a maintenance dose for a period of ten days. No definite standard of biologic assay of potency of the cortical extract has been uniformly accepted.

The use of suprarenal cortex extract in the treatment of bronchial asthma. *Fineman EH*

184 THE JOURNAL OF ALLERGY

frequent and more severe especially in the two months prior to admission to the clinic. No history of any other manifestations of allergy in the patient was obtained.

Protein skin tests with the scratch method elicited only the following positive reactions; ragweed (short), one plus; elm, three plus; coconut, two plus; and squirrel and goat hair plus-minus. Intradermal tests with many food extracts were negative. A moderately positive reaction to house dust was elicited.

May 20, 1932, roentgen-ray examination of the chest revealed an increase in size and density of the hilum shadows. The nasal sinuses were roentgenographically negative. The electrocardiogram was within normal limits. The blood count and urinalysis were normal.

The patient was observed for three and a half months and during this time had about two attacks of asthma weekly. She wheezed continually, and ephedrine hydrochloride was taken for relief. A tonsillectomy was performed with no beneficial effect.

On January 9, 1932, treatment with suprarenal cortex extract was begun. She weighed 104.5 pounds (47.5 kg.), and blood pressure was 104 mm. systolic and 86 mm. diastolic.

During the first month she received eleven injections of the extract subcutaneously, beginning with 0.5 c.c. which was increased to 3.0 c.c.; the last seven doses being 3.0 c.c. each. At the end of the second week wheezing disappeared and the patient felt better. Members of her family noticed she was lively and more active. At the end of the first month she was considerably improved, and repeated physical examination of the lungs revealed no sibilant râles. Her appetite was excellent and she gained three pounds (1.3 kg.). During the second month she received eight injections of the extract subcutaneously; each dose contained 3.0 c.c. She had no attacks of asthma and wheezed only occasionally. During the third month she received only one treatment weekly, 3.0 c.c. each; the last injection being given intramuscularly. She had no attacks and felt better than at any time in the previous year. During the fourth month of treatment she also received one injection weekly, but because of an insufficient quantity of extract on hand one injection contained 1.0 c.c., another 2.0 c.c. and the remainder 3.0 c.c. each. Improvement continued. She felt as though she were "cured of asthma." The extract was discontinued on May 9, 1932. She had received twenty-seven injections containing in all 72.5 c.c. (representing 2,175 grams of suprarenal cortex).

The result in this case was considered one of marked improvement. Attacks of asthma disappeared. The patient was able to work, had little or no difficulty in breathing and wheezed only occasionally. She felt much stronger and looked decidedly improved. July 11, 1932, she was doing well, had only one mild attack and weighed 110 pounds (50.0 kg.).

CASE 2.—J. P., aged twenty-six years was first seen at the clinic on November 30, 1931. He gave a history of asthma of six months' duration.

The onset was sudden. He was perfectly well until May, 1931, when his trouble began with an attack of wheezing, shortness of breath, cough and sneezing. Attacks recurred daily and required injections of epinephrine hydrochloride (1:1000). The condition became aggravated so that he had practically continuous asthma and could not work.

Physical examination revealed a robust young Italian, well developed and well nourished, dyspneic, wheezing and coughing. Sibilant and sonorous râles were heard throughout both lungs. The electrocardiogram revealed tachycardia with tendency toward right axis deviation. The blood count was normal.

Roentgen-ray examination of the chest showed moderate hilum enlargement, and the nasal sinuses were negative except for slight clouding of the antra. Protein skin tests with the scratch and intradermal methods were negative. The patient was observed for one month and was having constant asthma.

On December 28, 1931, treatment with suprarenal cortex extract was begun. The patient's blood pressure was 104 mm. systolic and 74 mm. diastolic, and his weight was 180.5 pounds (82.0 kg.).

During the first month he received thirteen injections of the extract subcutaneously, beginning with a dose of 0.5 c.c., which was gradually increased to 3.0 c.c.; the last eight injections being 3.0 c.c. each. He seemed to be improved for eight to ten hours after treatment and sometimes for one to two days. He wheezed less, his appetite was improved and he gained five pounds (2.2 kg.). During the second month he received eleven injections of 3.0 c.c. each. The first three injections were given subcutaneously and the remainder intramuscularly. The patient showed definite improvement and felt better than at any time in the previous eight months. In the third month of treatment he received eight injections of the extract intramuscularly; the first five doses contained 3.0 c.c. each and the subsequent three doses 4.0 c.c. each. He was not so well as he had been the month before. Attacks returned and were severe. During the fourth month he received ten injections; seven doses contained 4.0 c.c. each, two 3.0 c.c. each, and one only 1.0 c.c. He was generally improved and had only two or three attacks but none severe. The last injection was given on April 22, 1932. He had received forty-two injections, a total of 126.5 c.c. (representing 3,795 grams of suprarenal cortex).

The result in this case was considered one of moderate improvement. About three or four weeks after discontinuance of the extract asthma became aggravated and wheezing more constant.

CASE 3.—S. P., female, unmarried, aged twenty-nine years, was first seen in the allergy clinic on November 22, 1929. She gave a history of asthma of eighteen years' duration. In childhood attacks occurred every few months and lasted a day or two. Gradually her condition grew worse, and wheezing spells became more frequent and more severe. In the six months before admission to the clinic attacks occurred practically daily

The use of suprarenal cortex extract in the treatment of bronchial asthma. *Fineman EH*

and asthma was constant.   No other form of allergy was present in the patient.   The family history revealed asthma in a maternal cousin and a brother.

Physical examination revealed a thin, frail, sallow, markedly underweight and undernourished female, appearing chronically ill with dyspnea and wheezing.   There was moderate anteroposterior enlargement of the chest with hyperresonance on percussion.   Throughout both lungs there were numerous sibilant and sonorous râles.   The heart was normal and the electrocardiogram showed a right axis deviation.   The blood pressure was 100 mm. systolic and 70 mm. diastolic.   Her weight was 84.5 pounds (38.4 kg.).

Skin tests were performed with the scratch method, and plus-minus reactions were obtained to cat hair, dog hair, lettuce and beet.   An ophthalmic test with dry pollen was negative.

April 29, 1930, roentgen-ray examination of the chest showed general parenchymatous changes in the middle thirds of both lungs.   The hilum shadows were markedly increased in size and density.   Roentgen-ray examination of the nasal accessory sinuses revealed the left antrum cloudly as compared to the right.

The patient received injections of nonspecific therapy and autohemotherapy in addition to various dietary regimens.   Asthma was somewhat relieved, but generalized weakness became more apparent.   She complained of vague pains in the arms and legs and was easily fatigued.

On February 15, 1932, treatment with suprarenal cortex extract was begun.   At this time the patient was wheezing nearly constantly and complained of difficulty in breathing.   Her blood pressure was 96 mm. systolic and 70 mm. diastolic, and her weight was 85 pounds (38.6 kg.).

During the first month she received ten injections of the extract, beginning with a dose of 0.5 c.c. which was gradually increased to 4.0 c.c.   All injections but one were given subcutaneously; one dose of 4.0 c.c. was administered intramuscularly.   During this time she showed definite improvement.   There was less wheezing and less heaviness in the chest. She felt stronger and was more active.   Before the use of the cortical extract she had no desire for food, but after two weeks of treatment her appetite improved markedly and she gained four pounds (1.8 kg.).   During the second month ten injections of 3.0 c.c each were given; four subcutaneously and six intramuscularly.   She claimed that she felt better than at any time in the previous six months or year.   During the third month she received seven injections of the extract intramuscularly; four doses contained 3.0 c.c. each, one 2.0 c.c. and two doses 1.0 c.c. each. Asthma returned.   The last injection was given May 9, 1932.   She had received twenty-seven injections, a total of 70.5 c.c. of the extract (representing 2,115 grams of suprarenal cortex).   During the following months attacks of asthma recurred but were not severe.

The result in this case was considered one of slight improvement.   The striking change noted was the increase in appetite and strength while under treatment with the cortical hormone.

CASE 4.—J. C., aged forty-three years, male, was first seen at the clinic on May 11, 1931. He gave a history of asthma of eight years' duration. Wheezing and heaviness in the chest followed a "head cold." Attacks became severe and frequent and later occurred three and four times daily. He soon learned the use of the hypodermic syringe and would inject himself with 0.5 c.c. of epinephrine hydrochloride (1:1000) five to ten times daily. He was practically in continuous asthma and had been unable to work for a few years.

Physical examination revealed a thin, pale-faced man appearing chronically ill with dyspnea and wheezing. The chest was emphysematous, and sibilant and sonorous râles were heard throughout both lungs. No abnormalities of the heart were noted. The blood pressure was 112 mm. systolic and 70 mm. diastolic.

June 23, 1931, roentgen-ray examination revealed some parenchymatous changes in both apices and an increase in size and density of the hilum shadows. Roentgen-ray examination of the nasal accessory sinuses showed small and large cells somewhat cloudy.

Protein skin tests with the scratch method elicited positive reactions with the following: timothy, three plus; June grass, and sweet vernal grass, four plus; orchard grass and plantain, one plus. Intradermal tests with a solution of ragweed short (1:50 dilution) gave a two plus reaction and ragweed giant a plus-minus.

He received pollen treatment and other forms of therapy with no apparent relief from asthma.

On November 23, 1931, treatment with suprarenal cortex extract was begun. At this time his blood pressure was 110 mm. systolic and 78 mm. diastolic, and his weight was 150 pounds (68.1 kg.).

During the first week he received six injections subcutaneously of 0.5 c.c. each of the extract. At first he seemed somewhat improved for a few hours after treatment but then attacks of asthma recurred. During the second week three injections of 1.0 c.c. each were given. Wheezing was somewhat diminished and his chest felt clearer. In the third week he received one injection of 2.0 c.c. Asthma was severe. The following week he received two injections of 3.0 c.c. each, but no signs of improvement were noted. His weight at the end of the month was 152 pounds (69.0 kg.), a gain of two pounds (0.9 kg.).

Treatment was discontinued for seven weeks and when resumed injections were given intramuscularly. Five injections were given within two weeks without beneficial effect, and the last treatment was administered on March 2, 1932.

Seventeen injections were given in all, a total dosage of 26.0 c.c. This patient received much less of the extract than any of the other three cases and when seen again on April 1, 1932, he was having severe asthma.

The use of suprarenal cortex extract in the treatment of bronchial asthma. *Fineman EH*

188 THE JOURNAL OF ALLERGY

EFFECT OF THE EXTRACT ON OTHER SYMPTOMS

Strength.—In three of the four cases a decided increase in strength was noted. One patient felt much stronger after one month of treatment and was able to work. Another showed increased vitality and was able to walk for long distances. The generalized fatigue and vague pains in the extremities disappeared. The patient who showed no improvement in asthma exhibited no increase in strength as a result of treatment.

Appetite.—Three of the four patients showed definite increase in appetite. In one case this was very striking.

Weight.—Gain in weight was observed in three patients. During the interval of relief from asthma there was an average gain in weight of four and one-half pounds (2.0 kg.). One patient showed a gain of nine pounds (4.0 kg.) after two months' treatment. With the return of symptoms of asthma the weight curve declined. The unimproved patient showed slight increase in weight temporarily.

EFFECT OF THE EXTRACT ON BLOOD PRESSURE AND PULSE RATE

Blood pressure estimations were taken frequently during the course of treatment. Both arms were used in each case and at each sitting. No significant change in blood pressure was noted during or at the end of treatment in any case. In three patients readings were also taken twenty minutes and a half hour after injections of 2.0 c.c. and 3.0 c.c. of the extract. No immediate rise in blood pressure was noted.

The pulse rate was taken frequently in each case during the course of treatment, but no appreciable change was observed.

COMMENT

The susceptibility of the suprarenal glands to acute and chronic diseases elsewhere in the body has been emphasized in recent years.[7] Degenerative changes in the cortex with replacement by fibrous tissue and atrophy have been described. Such changes are presumed to be toxic in nature and secondary to an underlying systemic cause. In the more recent reports[8, 9, 10] on the pathology of asthma, including autopsied material of patients dying from this condition, no mention is made of the microscopic anatomy of the suprarenal glands. It seems likely that close study of these structures may reveal secondary pathologic changes in the cortex or medulla similar to those noted in other chronic diseases. Particularly in cases of severe and chronic asthma are such changes to be looked for.

That some degree of cortical insufficiency exists in patients suffering with chronic asthma was deemed probable, and based upon this assumption the suprarenal cortex extract was administered as a replacement therapy in the four cases studied in this series. It was also believed possible that the cortical hormone may stimulate the production of epinephrine in the body and thus produce a favorable influence on bronchial asthma. According to Goldzieher[11] "destruction of one part of the suprarenal gland (cortex or medulla) will obviously involve the other, first by impairing its function and finally by producing morphological changes, such as atrophy." There is some experimental work which lends support to the view of a synergistic action between these two hormones. In the four cases of asthma included in this report suprarenal cortex extract was used to the exclusion of epinephrine in order to determine the influence of the cortical hormone on asthma and associated symptoms. Epinephrine was used only as an emergency measure, and therefore no data on the possible synergistic action of these two preparations can be submitted. At no time was any evidence obtained to suggest antagonistic action between them. In no case was an attack of asthma induced following the use of the suprarenal cortex extract, and in a total of 113 injections no untoward local or systemic reactions were encountered.

It is also possible that the cortical hormone may act on the liver and help regulate the carbohydrate metabolism. It has been suggested[12] that this is the prepotent function of the suprarenal cortex as determined by the rise in blood sugar following the use of the cortical hormone in Addison's disease. Chemical studies of the blood in cases of asthma must be carried out before any statement can be made concerning its influence on metabolism in allergy.

It is interesting to note that Perla and Marmorston-Gottesman[13] demonstrated increased resistance to infection, toxins and histamine poisoning in suprarenalectomized animals treated with cortical hormone. This suggests the possible clinical use of the extract in human beings manifesting evidence of cortical insufficiency as a result of chronic infectious diseases or in cases of allergic nature.

CONCLUSIONS

1. Four patients, ranging in age from twenty-two to forty-three years, and suffering with severe asthma (three protein-sensitive and one non-sensitive) were treated for a period of from one to twenty-seven months with little or no improvement. Suprarenal cortex extract was then used; and the effect of the hormone on asthma, strength, appetite, weight, pulse and blood pressure was carefully noted.

2. Treatment with the extract was begun with dosage of 0.5 c.c. and increased up to 4.0 c.c., the maximum dose. Injections were given three to four times weekly during the first month and once or twice weekly thereafter. Subcutaneous and intramuscular injections were administered in each case. Two patients received treatment for four months, one for three months and one for six weeks.

3. One patient showed marked improvement in asthma, one moderate, one slight and one no improvement.

4. In three of the four patients a decided increase in strength and appetite was noted, with an average gain in weight of four and one-half

The use of suprarenal cortex extract in the treatment of bronchial asthma. *Fineman EH*

pounds (2.0 kg.). The general condition of the patient was definitely improved in these three cases.

5. No appreciable change in blood pressure was noted during or at the end of the course of treatment. No influence on the pulse rate was observed.

6. The results obtained with the suprarenal cortex extract in the four cases studied and reported in this paper warrant its further trial in a larger series of cases, employing larger dosage and utilizing, if necessary, the intravenous route.

REFERENCES

1. Hartman, F. A., Mac Arthur, C. G., and Hartman, W. E.: A Substance Which Prolongs the Life of Adrenalectomized Cats, Proc. Soc. Exper. Biol. & Med. **25**: 69, 1927.
2. Rogoff, J. M., and Stewart, G. N.: The Influence of Adrenal Extracts on the Survival Period of Adrenalectomized Dogs, Science **66**: 327, 1927.
3. Swingle, W. W., and Pfiffner, J. J.: An Aqueous Extract of the Suprarenal Cortex Which Maintains the Life of Bilaterally Adrenalectomized Cats, Science **71**: 321, 1930.
4. Rowntree, L. G., Greene, C. H., Swingle, W. W., and Pfiffner, J. J.: Addison's Disease, Experiences in Treatment With Various Suprarenal Preparations, J. A. M. A. **96**: 231, 1931.
5. Rowntree, L. G., Greene, C. H., Ball, R. G., Swingle, W. W., and Pfiffner, J. J.: Treatment of Addison's Disease With the Cortical Hormone of the Suprarenal Gland, J. A. M. A. **97**: 1446, 1931.
6. Harrop, G. A., and Weinstein, A.: Addison's Disease Treated With Suprarenal Cortical Hormone (Swingle-Pfiffner), J. A. M. A. **98**: 1525, 1932.
7. Guttman, P. H.: Addison's Disease—A Statistical Analysis of Five Hundred and Sixty-Six Cases and a Study of the Pathology, Arch. Path. **10**: 742, 1930.
8. Kountz, W. B., and Alexander, H. L.: Death From Bronchial Asthma, Report of Three Cases, Arch. Path. **5**: 1003, 1928.
9. Steinberg, B., and Figley, K. D.: Pathology of Asthma; Nonbacterial Allergic and Bacterial Types Based on Autopsy Material, Jour. Lab. & Clin. Med. **13**: 921, 1928.
10. Harkavy, J.: Observations on Fatal Bronchial Asthma, Report of Two Cases, J. Allergy **1**: 136, 1930.
11. Goldzieher, M. A.: The Adrenals, New York, 1929, p. 273, the Macmillan Co.
12. Britton, S. W., and Silvette, H.: The Apparent Prepotent Function of the Adrenal Glands, Am. J. Physiology **100**: 701, 1932. Ed. J. A. M. A. **99**: 657, 1932.
13. Perla, D., and Marmorston-Gottesman, J.: Injections of Cortin on Resistance of Suprarenalectomized Rats—Biological Assay of Extracts of Suprarenal Cortex, Proc. Soc. Exper. Biol. & Med. **28**: 475, 1931. Effect of Injections of Cortin on Resistance of Suprarenalectomized Rats to Histamine Poisoning, Proc. Soc. Exper. Biol. & Med. **28**: 650, 1931.

PRELIMINARY OBSERVATIONS ON THE EFFECT OF ADRENOCORTICOTROPIC HORMONE (ACTH) IN ALLERGIC DISEASES

JOHN E. BORDLEY, RICHARD A. CAREY, A. McGEHEE HARVEY, JOHN E. HOWARD, ALBERT A. KATTUS, ELLIOT V. NEWMAN AND WALTER L. WINKENWERDER

From the Departments of Medicine and Otolaryngology of the Johns Hopkins Medical School and Hospital

Received for publication September 26, 1949

In April, 1949 Hench and his collaborators (1) described the dramatic effect of cortisone and adrenocorticotropic hormone (ACTH) in patients with rheumatoid arthritis. In a subsequent report (2) suggestive results were obtained with cortisone in acute rheumatic fever. In one case ACTH was administered in small doses for a period of seven days. Fever subsided within forty-eight hours and articular symptoms within four days.

The experimental studies of Rich and Gregory (3, 4) suggested a relationship between the hypersensitive state and the rheumatic diseases. The possible usefulness of ACTH in the control of the hypersensitivity state was first explored in a patient with severe exfoliative dermatitis due to iodine. The unique rapidity of recovery in this critically ill patient stimulated the trial of ACTH in other allergic states.

In the second patient extensive giant urticaria, joint pains and fever associated with a "serum disease type" sensitivity to penicillin were abolished within twenty-four hours after ACTH was begun.

The prompt control of the chronic asthmatic state and the striking alterations in the tissues of the upper respiratory tract in five asthmatic patients form the basis of this preliminary report.

In two patients the asthma was thought due to combined external and intrinsic factors. In the other three it was of the intrinsic type. The age of the patients ranged from 26 to 63 years, and the duration of the asthma from 5 to 23 years. The sputum in all contained many eosinophils. In several of the patients no more than partial and very temporary relief was obtained by the administration of adrenalin, aminophyllin, and ether by rectum.

396

The initial daily dose of ACTH varied between 30 and 100 mgm. given intramuscularly, divided in equal portions at six hour intervals. Unequivocal benefit was noted in from four to forty-eight hours. Complete freedom from all asthmatic symptoms occurred within one to eight days. In four of the patients there was total disappearance of sputum, and abnormal physical signs in the chest. In the fifth patient, who was six months pregnant, rhonchi persisted although she was free of asthmatic symptoms. Coincident with symptomatic relief, tracings of the expiratory phase of respiration showed improvement with removal of the relative obstruction to outflow.

Treatment was maintained for eleven to twenty-one days. The daily dose was gradually reduced after clinical recovery; the total amount administered ranging from 360 to 775 mgm. One patient has remained asymptomatic for one month after therapy was stopped.

Detailed examinations of the upper respiratory tract, including nasopharyngoscopy, were made on four of the patients. Three patients had a pale, edematous, polypoid nasal mucous membrane which was bathed with a thick mucopurulent discharge. During therapy the membrane became bluish pink in color, was covered with clear mucus, and the edematous, polypoid appearance was no longer present. The breathing space was greatly enlarged. The lymphoid tissue in the nasopharynx, which was covered with a thick discharge, was pale and edematous. During treatment the edema subsided, an orange pink color developed, the crypts became more prominent, and it was easily outlined from the surrounding mucous membrane. There was no gross change in the volume of the lymphoid tissue present. In two patients there was complete obstruction of the nose by polyps. These began to shrink on the third day of treatment and by the end of therapy had completely vanished in one and almost completely in the other. The three cases with mucous membrane abnormalities had antral clouding on roentgenological examination which cleared during the administration of ACTH. Several small polyps had reappeared in one patient on the twenty-third day after cessation of therapy.

The intradermal reactions to inhalant and bacterial antigens were followed in three patients. Two showed marked skin sensitivity to pollens and other extrinsic antigens. In one the sensitivity was greatly diminished during treatment but returned to its original level three weeks after cessation of ACTH. In the other patient no alteration was

Preliminary observations of the effect of adrenocorticotropic hormone (ACTH) in allergic diseases. *Bordley JE, Carey RA, Harvey et al*

398 BORDLEY ET AL.

observed. In both patients serum reagin titration revealed no change. The intradermal reaction to bacterial antigens decreased significantly in two patients and did not change in another. In one the sensitivity has returned to the pretreatment level three weeks after discontinuance of ACTH.

The previously described (1, 2) metabolic effects of ACTH in no instance were a serious complicating factor in these cases.

These clinical studies suggest that ACTH may have an important action in blocking various hypersensitivity reactions. Further observations are necessary to establish its efficacy in allergic states, and the effects of ACTH in other types of hypersensitivity are under study.

The ACTH used in these studies was supplied by Armour and Company through the courtesy of Dr. John R. Mote.

We wish to thank Dr. Walter Baetjer, and Dr. Milton Sherry for permission to treat patients under their care.

BIBLIOGRAPHY

1. HENCH, P. S., KENDALL, E. C., SLOCUMB, C. H. AND POLLEY, H. F.: The Effect of a Hormone of the Adrenal Cortex (17-hydroxy-11-dehydrocorticosterone: Compound E) and of Pituitary Adrenocorticotrophic Hormone on Rheumatoid Arthritis; Preliminary Report. Proc. Staff Meeting Mayo Clin., 1949, **24**, 181.
2. HENCH, P. S., SLOCUMB, C. H., BARNES, A. R., SMITH, H. L., POLLEY, H. F. and Kendall, E. C.: The Effects of the Adrenal Cortical Hormone 17-hydroxy-11-dehydrocorticosterone (Compound E) on the Acute Phase of Rheumatic Fever: Preliminary Report. Proc. Staff Meeting Mayo Clin., 1949, **24**, 277.
3. RICH, A. R. AND GREGORY, J. E.: Experimental Evidence that Lesions with the Basic Characteristics of Rheumatic Carditis Can Result from Anaphylactic Hypersensitivity. Bull. Johns Hopkins Hosp., 1943, **73**, 239.
4. RICH, A. R.: Hypersensitivity to Iodine as a Cause of Periarteritis Nodosa. Bull. Johns Hopkins Hosp., 1945, **77**, 43.

THE EFFECT OF ADRENOCORTICOTROPIC HORMONE (ACTH) AND CORTISONE ON THE COURSE OF CHRONIC BRONCHIAL ASTHMA

RICHARD A. CAREY, A. McGEHEE HARVEY, JOHN E. HOWARD
AND WALTER L. WINKENWERDER

Department of Medicine, Johns Hopkins University School of Medicine

Received for publication August 7, 1950

INTRODUCTION

In an earlier report the dramatic relief of chronic intractable bronchial asthma during the administration of ACTH was described (1). During the past ten months further observations have been made concerning the immediate response to the administration of ACTH and cortisone, the most effective dosage schedules, the duration of the remissions, and the response to subsequent administration of these hormones after relapse. In addition, a control study designed by Dr. Margaret Merrell of the Department of Biostatistics has been carried out in order to evaluate the influence of psychogenic and environmental factors on these observations. The present communication describes the effect of ACTH in 23 patients with chronic intractable asthma in the majority of whom there occurred complete remission of all signs and symptoms of the disease for periods up to ten months. Cortisone has been given to five similar patients with less improvement noted from exhibition of this hormone in the doses used.

MATERIAL AND METHODS

In order to mimimize the influence of psychogenic and environmental factors only patients who had had constant asthma for at least two months were included in the study. All patients had a severe chronic form of the disease and had received no satisfactory relief from any other type of treatment, including symptomatic measures and desensitization. It can be seen from the tables that the series was about evenly divided between males and females. The ages ranged from 26 to 75 years and the duration of the asthma from 6 months to 45 years. All patients were considered to have intrinsic asthma and in four one or more extrinsic factors were thought to play a rôle.

387

388   RICHARD A. CAREY ET AL.

Each day that the patients were under observation an assessment of their clinical status was made using both subjective and objective criteria. The most useful subjective manifestations were degree of dyspnoea, feeling of tightness or weight on the chest, effort in breathing, and capacity for exertion. Among the objective data recorded were ability to lie flat in bed, respiratory rate at rest and after exertion when possible, use of accessory muscles of respiration, character and distribution of auscultatory signs, amount and character of the sputum, vital capacity, and spirometric tracings.

In evaluating benefit which resulted from the ACTH or cortisone, subjective relief was considered complete when, without adjuvant treatment, the patient no longer experienced any sense of respiratory discomfort, even to the feeling of weight on the chest. The latter symptom, occurring in the early morning on waking, was usually the last to disappear. Remission from asthma was considered objectively complete when musical and other rales had been inaudible by stethoscopic examination for 48 hours, even after mild exertion. In those patients who were tested spirometrically, the return of the expiratory phase of respiration to the normal pattern coincided with the patients' statement of subjective relief.

In the special control group only those patients were used who had had asthma for at least five years, with no freedom from symptoms for at least two months despite vigorous symptomatic therapy. Any obvious infection in the lower respiratory tract was cause for exclusion from the group, as was the possibility that any of the symptoms might be of cardiac origin. Each patient had to express complete willingness to be hospitalized for at least a month and to cooperate in any procedures indicated in the study. The patients agreed to stop all adjuvant drugs but one (usually they chose a spray or aminophylline suppositories) during the experimental period, and even this one was to be used only with concurrence of the doctor. In an emergency the physician conducting the study, and who was the only person knowing whether placebos or ACTH was being given, was to decide the need of any additional treatment.

The drug being tested (ACTH or cortisone) and the placebo were indistinguishable, the ACTH control being a standard solution of pitressin in saline made up in old ACTH bottles; the cortisone control

The effect of adrenocorticotropic hormone (ACTH) and cortisone on the course of chronic bronchial asthma. *Carey RA, Harvey AM, Howard JE et al*

was a suspension of cholesterol, kindly furnished by Merck and Company. The patients were all told they were to receive ACTH or cortisone, and together with the nurses and attendants were all unaware that a control study was being carried out. Each day independent observations were made by two physicians who did not know the identity of the material being used; and these observers did not have access to the patient's weight chart, eosinophil chart or results of other collateral studies. Standard courses of treatment were arbitrarily decided upon. In the case of ACTH, 100 mgm., 75 mgm., 50 mgm., 40 mgm. and 20 mgm. per day were given for two day periods, a total period of ten days' administration of the drug. Cortisone was given 200 mgm. the first day and 100 mgm. daily for the next seven days. The ACTH and cortisone were both administered intramuscularly, one-fourth the daily dose being given every six hours.

The patients were assigned to two groups in random fashion. A list giving an order of assignment was prepared by Dr. Merrell, and was available only to the one physician who knew the identity of the drug being given to the patient. The placebo was administered for five or eight days, either before or after the course of the active agents. Thus, a given patient might receive placebos for five days, followed by ten days of ACTH, ten days of ACTH followed by placebo, placebo for five days followed by cortisone or vice versa.

The assessment of clinical status was made after five, eight and fifteen days in each instance.

Before administration of either ACTH or cortisone to any patient the following studies were carried out: 1) eosinophil counts (blood and sputum), 2) measurement of daily sputum volume, 3) determination of vital capacity during the maximal relief obtained by the most effective symptomatic therapy (epinephrine or aminophylline), 4) hematocrit, sedimentation rate, white cell and differential counts, 5) blood non-protein nitrogen and sugar, serum chloride and bicarbonate concentrations, 6) daily blood pressure recording, 7) morning weight with empty bladder, 8) electrocardiogram and determination of venous pressure.

After treatment was begun, blood pressure, vital capacity and sputum volume were recorded daily. Eosinophil counts were taken each morning, four hours after the morning injection, until they reached

The effect of adrenocorticotropic hormone (ACTH) and cortisone on the course of chronic bronchial asthma. *Carey RA, Harvey AM, Howard JE et al*

390   RICHARD A. CAREY ET AL.

TABLE 1

Age, Sex and Duration of Asthma in the Patients Treated for the First Time with ACTH

CASE	HISTORY NO.	SEX	AGE	ASTHMA Years	ASTHMA Type	ACTH Total mgm.	ACTH Starting dose per day	ACTH Days	EOSINOPHILES Before RX	EOSINOPHILES Minimum after RX	EOSINOPHILES Fall %	EOSINOPHILES Fall On day	COMPLETE REMISSION On day	COMPLETE REMISSION Duration days	REMISSION %
1 R. M.	511025	F	40	18	E & I	440	50	12	1100	22	98	5	4	86	100
2 H. N.	231977	M	63	18	I	578	50	16	1050	66	94	5	7	105	100
3 E. M.	512303	M	34	2	E & I	732	20	21	484	11	97	5	7	263+	100
4 W. S.	170250	M	38	12	I	338	50	11	821	66	92	2	2	25	100
5 F. L.	434666	F	54	27	I	527	100	12	360	66	72	5	7	60	100
6 J. B.	170223	F	44	8	I	477	80	10	462	11	98	2	3	70	100
7 D. H.	336367	M	41	5	I	798	140	10	300	33	89	7	4	40	100
8 B. M.	200493	F	75	12	I	570	100	10	286	0	100	2	3	116	100
9 O. Z.	358563	M	57	2	I	193	25	11	1056	88	92	4	5	7	100
10 M. G.	528824	M	57	½	I	600	100	10	1496	0	100	2	8	75+	100
11 J. F.	528483	M	28	6	I	1248	100	18	899	6	99	3	11	15	100
12 M. H.	527856	F	46	9	I	570	100	10	550	0	100	7	4	100+	100
13 H. W.	532987	M	55	12	I	240	50	6	528	286	46	3	5	51+	100
14 B. de S.	530526	M	53	1	I	285	85	4	858	77	91	4	3	3	100
15 M. S.	435221	F	26	4	I	786	80	14	605	154	75	5	4	14+	100
16 N. B.	100080	F	26	23	I	826	100	16	524	67	87	5	None		95
17 H. S.	512338	M	44	1½	I	232	50	9	921	715	23	3	None		40
18 L. I.		F	65	45	E & I	190	25	8	2800	160	94	6	None		50
19 J. G.	535594	F	56	26	E & I	695	100	13	572	11	98	2	None		50

In type of asthma, I signifies intrinsic, E that extrinsic factors—such as inhalants—were thought to play a role. Maximal and minimal blood eosinophile counts are given and the day on which the fall was greatest. The day after ACTH administration on which all symptoms and signs of asthma were first absent is listed as day of complete remission. Duration of remission in most instances was determined from the patients' own evaluation, usually the time when spray or suppository therapy became necessary again for comfort.

The effect of adrenocorticotropic hormone (ACTH) and cortisone on the course of chronic bronchial asthma. *Carey RA, Harvey AM, Howard JE et al*

minimal levels; thereafter counts were made at 2-day intervals until discharge. Other blood counts and chemical determinations were carried out twice weekly. Most of the patients kept a daily biographical record of their course while in the hospital.

The ACTH used was ACTH Armour, the doses listed are in milligrams of Armour Standard, and the daily dose was always divided into four equal parts given intramuscularly at six hour intervals. The daily dose of cortisone acetate (Merck) is also expressed in milligrams and this hormone was administered in a similar manner. In those patients not in the control series the dosage schedules of ACTH and cortisone varied widely. In several instances dosage was higher or lower than intended, owing to error in assay of the ACTH. In most patients the starting dose was 50 to 100 mgm. per day, and after one to three days on this schedule the dose was gradually lowered. To one patient, critically ill in status asthmaticus, it was deemed wise to give a larger initial dose (100 mgm. in first six hours) to be certain of obtaining the earliest possible maximal effect. In another instance 20 mgm. per day was given at the start in an effort to determine minimal effective dosage.

The total amount of ACTH given in the initial course of treatment in these patients varied from 190 to 1248 mgm., with an average of 423 mgm. The duration of therapy varied from four to twenty-one days with an average of 11.6 days. The patient receiving the largest total dosage (Case 11, Table 1) was sensitive to acetyl salicylic acid and after his asthma had cleared ACTH was continued at a high dosage for greater safety while he was being challenged with aspirin. The patient receiving the longest period of treatment (21 days in Case 3, Table 1) started at a low daily dose which was gradually raised in an effort to determine the minimal level at which response occurred. The treatment schedules for cortisone are presented in Table 3.

RESULTS

Fifteen of the nineteen patients (Table 1) achieved subjective and objective remissions of their asthma while taking ACTH. The four who did not obtain complete freedom from asthma (the last four in Table 1) experienced 50 per cent or more reduction in severity, as judged by themselves and the observers.

The effect of adrenocorticotropic hormone (ACTH) and cortisone on the course of chronic bronchial asthma. *Carey RA, Harvey AM, Howard JE et al*

There was noticeable symptomatic improvement, both to patient and physicians, often within four hours, always within thirty-six. The rapidity with which complete relief was attained varied; in some instances adjuvant therapy, which served as an excellent guide to the subjective status, was no longer necessary after a few hours; in others, such medication could not be comfortably abandoned for nearly a week. In this group, early improvement did not necessarily indicate eventual freedom from asthma, though other factors may have played a rôle in those who did not achieve complete remission, as will be mentioned later.

In attempting to evaluate the effect of the dosage level on the completeness of the freedom from asthma, the variability of the disease from patient to patient must be considered despite the fact that all but two of these individuals had severe constant asthma and were free of complicating pulmonary infection. In reviewing those patients (the last four in Table 1) who failed to obtain complete remission, it is noted that patients #17 and #18 received very small doses. This was unintentional and due to an error in assay of the ACTH not discovered until later However, patient #9, who because of the error in assay, received no greater dose, obtained complete relief on the fifth day; and patient #3, who was purposely begun on 20 mgm. per day and the dose increased to 30 mgm. on the sixth day, experienced a total remission of asthma on the seventh day. In order to observe the effects on nasal polyps, the dose was increased further and later was gradually reduced. The total period of treatment was 21 days. He has had no asthma during the succeeding ten months, despite severe upper respiratory infections, although the polypi have recurred. Furthermore, cases #16 and 19 were begun on 100 mgm. ACTH per day and received total doses considerably in excess of that given to many patients who achieved complete and lasting remissions. Patient #16 was in her sixth and seventh months of pregnancy while the ACTH was given. She experienced prompt relief and was free of all subjective manifestations by the fifth day, but the auscultatory signs never entirely disappeared. Two days after ACTH was stopped, coincident with an upper respiratory infection, the asthma recurred in sufficient severity to require epinephrine. She continued to have asthma with approximately 50 per cent of its previous severity until delivery. Since then asthma has been very mild. Similar postpartum alleviation followed two of her four

The effect of adrenocorticotropic hormone (ACTH) and cortisone on the course of chronic bronchial asthma. *Carey RA, Harvey AM, Howard JE et al*

EFFECT OF ACTH AND CORTISONE ON BRONCHIAL ASTHMA   393

previous pregnancies, though after two other deliveries her asthma became greatly exaggerated.

Patient # 19 had had asthma for more than 25 years and had always noted a marked exaggeration in damp and humid weather. During most of the time she was receiving ACTH, the weather was extremely hot and humid, and the patient herself stated that previous experience made her certain that she would have required almost constant injections and sprays had it not been for the beneficial action of ACTH.

The duration of the complete remissions from asthma has varied from three days up to ten months. The average length of the freedom from any difficulty has been 68 days. The patients with the longest remissions after ACTH were # 1, 2, 3 and 8 in Table 1, the duration of complete freedom being 86, 105, 263 and 116 days, respectively. The patients whose remissions were shortest were # 4, 9, 11 and 14, with freedom for only 25, 7, 15 and 3 days, respectively. Comparison of these two groups discloses that a patient in the short remission group received the largest total dose and was treated for the longest period, that two of the group with short remissions began on 100 mgm. per day, whereas only one patient with a long remission began on so high a dose. However, the patient with the shortest remission of all was treated with the smallest dose over the fewest days. It is worthy of note that in no instance thus far has the severity of asthma in the relapse been as great as prior to administration of ACTH.

It seems likely that in two of the failures, larger doses of ACTH would have effected complete asthmatic remissions. However, one patient refused to submit to another trial with ACTH, owing to unpleasant side effects experienced in the first course even with the small dose, and the other patient has moved to a distant part of the country so that the effects of a second course of ACTH could not be observed.

The response to second and third courses of ACTH

Seven of the patients have received more than one course of ACTH. All of these had responded to their first course with complete remissions. Each likewise responded to the subsequent courses with disappearance of all symptoms and signs of asthma. Table 2 depicts the dosage schedule, promptness and duration of remissions with *each* of their courses of ACTH.

The first patient's second course of ACTH was much briefer than

The effect of adrenocorticotropic hormone (ACTH) and cortisone on the course of chronic bronchial asthma. *Carey RA, Harvey AM, Howard JE et al*

394   RICHARD A. CAREY ET AL.

TABLE 2
Dosage and Results After the First and Subsequent Courses of ACTH

CASE	HISTORY NO.	COURSE NO.	ACTH Total (mg.)	ACTH Starting dose/day (mg.)	ACTH Days	REMISSION %	REMISSION On day	REMISSION Duration	INTERVAL BETWEEN COURSES (days)	EOSINOPHILES Before RX	EOSINOPHILES Min. after	EOSINOPHILES Fall %	EOSINOPHILES On day
1 O. Z.	358563	1	193	25	11	100	5	7	...	1056	88	92	4
		2	200	50	4	100	3	80	133	363	0	100	3
2 J. B.	170223	1	477	80	10	100	3	70	...	462	11	98	2
		2	200	50	4	100	2	14	105	561	0	100	4
		3	288		5¼	100	3	30*	48	517	0	100	3
3 H. N.	UMH 14912	1	578	50	16	100	7	105	...	1050	66	94	5
	231977	2	570	100	10	100	9	55	172	275	55	80	5
		3	950	50	17	100	16	21+	44	2079	33	99	4
4 D. H.	336367	1	798	140	10	100	4	40	...	300	33	89	7
		2	225	50	5	100	5	55	55	132	220	0	—
5 R. M.	511025	1	440	50	12	100	4	86	...	1100	22	98	5
		2	200	40	5	100	4	11	224	1056	0	100	3
6 J. F.	528483	1	1248	100	18	100	11	15	...	899	6	99	3
		2	1641	100	26	100	15	14+	63	781	0	100	15
7 B. de S.	530526	1	285	85	4	100	3	3	...	858	77	91	4
		2	210	40	5¼	100	3	3	6	1331	163	88	3

* This patient continued to receive ACTH twice weekly (see text).

The effect of adrenocorticotropic hormone (ACTH) and cortisone on the course of chronic bronchial asthma. *Carey RA, Harvey AM, Howard JE et al*

the previous one, the daily initial dose having been doubled. Thus, he received in four days (50 mgm. per day) as much ACTH as he had received in 11 days previously. The response was more rapid, complete remission occurred within three days, and the duration of the second remission was 80 days as compared with 7 days following the first course. The interval between the two courses was 133 days; so that the patient had had asthma for 126 days prior to his second administration of ACTH. It should be noted, however, that the asthma was only 75 per cent as severe as when the first course was begun.

In the second case the second course of ACTH was begun 105 days after termination of the first, when mild asthma had been present (estimated at 50%) for 33 days. In the second period of treatment the patient received 50 mgm. ACTH per day (as opposed to 80 mgm. initial dose in the first course), but with a *total* dose only two-fifths of the first and for four days total treatment rather than ten. Remission was equally prompt but lasted only two weeks. Then, after asthma of only mild severity had been present for six weeks, a third course of ACTH was given, identical with the second except that 50 mgm. was given daily for six days instead of four. Prompt remission again resulted, and the patient was then given 80 mgm. per day in *two* doses on two days out of each week for two weeks, then 40 mgm. per day in two doses twice each week. Asthma recurred on the twenty-ninth day.

Patient #3 had three courses of ACTH. His first two courses were of approximately the same *total* dosage, but initial dosage was smaller with the first course and injections were given over 16 days as compared with ten. The former resulted in a complete remission lasting 105 days, the latter only 35 days. His third course of ACTH was complicated by the development of pneumococcal pneumonia on the third day. Penicillin promptly overcame this infection and treatment with ACTH was not interrupted. However, he continued to have slight oppression in breathing and a few expiratory wheezes were heard until the seventeenth day of treatment. By the time the pneumonia developed, his asthma had cleared sufficiently so that antiasthmatic drugs were no longer necessary, and none was required during the remainder of his hospital stay. This patient is now being given 50 mgm. ACTH in two divided doses, two days out of each week, to see the effect of this procedure on the duration of freedom from asthma.

The effect of adrenocorticotropic hormone (ACTH) and cortisone on the course of chronic bronchial asthma. *Carey RA, Harvey AM, Howard JE et al*

396   RICHARD A. CAREY ET AL.

The fourth patient had a higher than average initial dosage, 140 mgm. per day (because of error in assay) in his first course which lasted ten days. The second course consisted of five days with 50 mgm. ACTH given each day and was begun 15 days after mild recurrence in which adjuvant therapy was required only at night. Remission from this second course lasted slightly longer than after the first.

In patient #5, both first and second courses were given with the same initial dose, duration of course one being twelve days as opposed to five days for the second. Remission in the second instance was but 11 days as compared with 86 for the first, although the asthma was much less severe.

In the sixth and seventh patients, the first and second courses were very similar and the duration of remissions, brief in both, was almost identical after the two courses.

In summary of the effects of subsequent courses of ACTH given 6 to 224 days after asthmatic relapse had occurred, it may be said that beneficial response was in every instance just as prompt and just as complete as with the first course. When the same starting dose was used but the length of administration and total dose decreased, the duration of the remission induced was greatly shortened in three (cases 2, 3 and 5); on the other hand, patient #4 achieved an equally long remission from one-third the initial dose and one-third the total dose. In one patient doubling the initial dose (25 up to 50 mgm. per day) resulted in a faster remission and a ten-fold increase in the duration of freedom from asthma, despite the fact that his total dosage in the two courses was the same. It should perhaps be re-emphasized that in no instance had the severity of the asthma reached the same degree as it was before the initial course of ACTH was given.

Treatment with Cortisone

Cortisone has been given to five patients with asthma. With one exception their asthma was similar in type and severity to that of the group who received ACTH. To patients 1, 2, 3 and 4 (first course) the dose of cortisone given was 200 mgm. on the first day and 100 mgm. thereafter for seven days (Table 3). A second course with double this dosage was given to patient #4, 45 days after the first course at a time when the asthma was of approximately equal severity. To the fifth patient cortisone was given 300 mgm. the first two days, and 200 mgm. thereafter for nine days. The daily dose was divided into four equal parts and administered intramuscularly at intervals of six hours.

The only patient in this group to achieve complete subjective and objective freedom from asthma was patient ♯5, who not only received the largest doses of cortisone, but whose asthma was very mild as compared with any other member of this series. The medication was given to him primarily to note its effect on a large accumulation of nasal polypi. His remission from asthma lasted 51 days, the symptoms recurring with approximately their former severity coincident with an

TABLE 3

Dosage of Cortisone Given to Four Patients and to One Patient Twice and Resulting Remission and Effect on Eosinophile Count

CASE		HISTORY NO.	SEX	AGE	ASTHMA		CORTISONE			EOSINOPHILES				REMISSION	
					Yrs.	Type	Total	In-itial dose	Days	Be-fore RX	Low-er after RX	% fall	Day	%	Day
							mg.	mg.							
1	H. S.	230494	M	63	27	I	900	200	8	440	319	27	9	40	7
2	H. P.	523671	M	50	20	E & I	900	200	8	1221	77	94	6	25	7
3	F. L.	434666	F	54	27	I	900	200	8	1342	22	98	8	50	8
4	S. S.	118083	F	57	7	I	900	200	8	605	66	89	2	30	6
							1800	400	8	1892	11	99	9	25	6
5	J. S.	530174	M	40	4	E & I	2300	300	11	231	66	72	6	100	5

upper respiratory infection. The other patients failed to improve more than moderately in their own opinion or as judged by the various criteria described above. None of these patients showed further improvement after cortisone was stopped.

Four of the patients treated originally with cortisone were later given ACTH (Table 4). Patients 1, 2 and 4 received ACTH eight days after completion of their courses of cortisone. The dose of ACTH was larger than usual, due to an error in assay, yet in two of the three symptoms were no more improved than they had been with cortisone. It was felt that perhaps the capacity of the adrenal to respond to ACTH had been impeded by the previous cortisone, yet the eosinophil response, edema formation and rise in urinary 17-ketosteroids (of the two whose urine

The effect of adrenocorticotropic hormone (ACTH) and cortisone on the course of chronic bronchial asthma. *Carey RA, Harvey AM, Howard JE et al*

398   RICHARD A. CAREY ET AL.

was studied) revealed as vigorous response to ACTH as in the other patients to whom ACTH was given. In addition, patient #3 received a third course of ACTH after an interval of five months. The initial dose on this occasion was 75 mgm. as compared to 140 with the first course of ACTH and the total amount 785 mgm. over thirteen days as compared to 798 mgm. over ten days. With the third course there was complete suppression of the asthma. Patient #2 achieved a complete remission when ACTH was given eight days after completion of the cortisone course.

TABLE 4

Results of ACTH Given 8 Days after a Previous Course of Cortisone, and After Further Intervals Following the Cortisone

CASE	HISTORY NO.	ACTH				DAYS SINCE CORTI-SONE	REMISSION			EOSINOPHILES			
		COURSE	Total	Initial dose/ day	Days		%	Day	Dura-tion	Max.	Min.	% fall	On day
			mg.	*mg.*									
1 H. P.	523671	1	798	140	10	8	50	7	—	440	11	97	5
2 S. S.	118083	1	798	140	10	8	100	8	14	187	0	100	2
		2	650	50	13	54	100	13	14	671	0	100	13
3 H. S.	230494	1	798	140	10	8	50	6	—	418	0	100	3
		2	1150	50	22	75	100	21	?	484	0	100	3
4 F. L.	434666	2	570	100	10	60	80	10	—	1034	0	100	10

A comparison of the results in this small group treated with cortisone with the results of the larger group treated with ACTH indicates that, in the dosages of the two drugs employed, cortisone compares unfavorably with ACTH in alleviating the signs and symptoms of bronchial asthma. Clinical improvement was, furthermore, noted earlier in every instance after ACTH than after cortisone. From the small number of observations it cannot be decided whether a previous course of cortisone, ending eight days before ACTH was used, reduced the likelihood of optimal clinical response to ACTH.

Results of the control studies

The procedure outlined was carried out in eleven instances, using ACTH with seven patients, cortisone with four. In the group receiving

The effect of adrenocorticotropic hormone (ACTH) and cortisone on the course of chronic bronchial asthma. *Carey RA, Harvey AM, Howard JE et al*

ACTH (Table 5), four of the seven received placebo first, and during the five or eight days there was no evidence of clinical improvement. By the fifth day of ACTH administration, there was uniform agreement of improvement in all; in four, all symptoms and signs of asthma had disappeared, in the remaining three improvement was estimated to be better than 75 per cent.

Results in the four patients in the cortisone group were more difficult to evaluate, since none of these patients achieved more than 50 per cent amelioration of their symptoms even at the end of cortisone

TABLE 5

Results in Control Series Treated with ACTH and Placebos

CASE	PLACEBO FIRST	PLACEBO AFTER ACTH	CLINICAL EVALUATION AT DAY 5	CLINICAL EVALUATION AT DAY 15
1 B. M.	X		No change	Complete remission
2 J. B.		X	Complete remission	Complete remission
3 D. H.		X	Complete remission	Complete remission
4 M. H.	X		No change	Complete remission
5 H. N.	X		No change	Complete remission
6 J. F.		X	80% improvement	Complete remission
7 F. L.	X		No change	80% improvement

For details see text.

administration. However, at the fifth day there was a uniformity of opinion that no improvement was present in the two patients who had received placebo, whereas slight or doubtful improvement was the interpretation after five days of cortisone.

Clinical evaluation at the 15th day disclosed that six of the seven patients in the ACTH group were entirely free of asthma; the seventh was adjudged 80 per cent improved. In the group receiving cortisone, it was judged at the 15th day that the patients were all better, but the improvement was variously estimated between 25 and 50 per cent. It was obvious in the group treated with ACTH that the results were clear cut in their indication that the clinical improvement following ACTH is due to the effects of the hormone and cannot be attributed to environmental or psychogenic factors.

The effect of adrenocorticotropic hormone (ACTH) and cortisone on the course of chronic bronchial asthma. *Carey RA, Harvey AM, Howard JE et al*

400   RICHARD A. CAREY ET AL.

COLLATERAL STUDIES

Eosinophils

Eosinophil counts were obtained on all the patients four hours after the first medication and each morning thereafter until the lowest level was reached. In the patients given ACTH (Tables 1 and 2), maximum fall in eosinophils occurred between the second and seventh days with one exception (second course of patient 6 in Table 2). In those patients who achieved complete remissions from their asthma, the fall in eosinophils was 72 per cent or greater, with the single exception of patient 13, who despite entire freedom from asthma within five days never manifested reduction in eosinophils to more than 50 per cent of his starting level. In the four patients whose asthma was not completely relieved, there was an equally great and prompt fall in eosinophils in three (patients 16, 18 and 19 in Table 1), though only a 23 per cent fall in patient 17. Reduction in the blood eosinophil count has been considered the most sensitive test of adrenal cortical activity (2). From this experience with asthmatic patients one might conclude that maximal relief from asthma may not occur unless the eosinophil count falls 75 per cent by the fifth day of administration, but a 90 per cent or better fall in eosinophils need not indicate that good clinical response will occur. In those patients treated with cortisone or with cortisone and ACTH at different times (Tables 3 and 4), the eosinophil fall with ACTH is seen to be usually more prompt. Some patients showed 100 per cent reduction of eosinophils during cortisone therapy without complete alleviation of asthma.

Throughout the entire group of patients who achieved complete remissions under ACTH, there is a striking correlation between the day on which freedom from asthma became total and the day on which maximum eosinophil fall was reached. Exceptions were always on the side of maximal eosinophil fall preceding complete symptomatic remission, as exemplified by patients 10 and 11 in Table 1.

Toward the end of each course of ACTH, usually when the dose fell below 30 mgm. per day, the eosinophil count rose (though rarely to the initial height), while the asthma remained completely in abeyance. Thus, the rise in eosinophils, after previous fall under the influence of ACTH, offered no clue as to the duration of the remission or the in-

The effect of adrenocorticotropic hormone (ACTH) and cortisone on the course of chronic bronchial asthma. *Carey RA, Harvey AM, Howard JE et al*

cipiency of symptomatic relapse. Chart I depicts a typical pattern of the eosinophil count in relation to asthmatic symptoms during and after administration of ACTH.

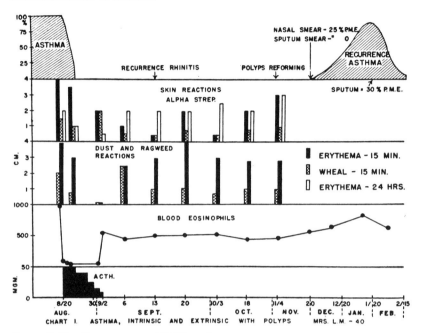

CHART I. THE RESPONSE TO ACTH OF SYMPTOMS AND THE BLOOD EOSINOPHILES IN A PATIENT WITH ASTHMA.

Skin reactions to various antigens

Skin tests to several inhalent and bacterial antigens were made prior to, during and after ACTH and cortisone administration. The majority of the tests carried out during drug administration were done on or between the third to the fifth day of therapy. Injections were made intradermally on the forearm or upper arm using a 25 gauge needle. As a rule, skin tests were carried out only once during drug administration for fear that repeated injections of antigens might modify not only the local skin response but also the antibody titer. In three patients giving typical skin reactions to ragweed pollen, the serum reagin titer using the serum dilution method, was determined. One recipient only was used for the several sera obtained from each individual patient.

The effect of adrenocorticotropic hormone (ACTH) and cortisone on the course of chronic bronchial asthma. *Carey RA, Harvey AM, Howard JE et al*

In the majority of patients the immediate skin reactions to pollens, dust and to bacterial antigens, and also the 24-hour reactions to the latter were partially or completely suppressed. In several patients, after ACTH administration was stopped the skin reactions were larger and more intense than those observed prior to drug administration. In several the erythema observed during the treatment period, though as large in extent as noted prior to injections of ACTH, was less intense, and the immediate whealing response was also reduced.

No constant relationship between the size of skin reactions as modified by ACTH and the response of asthmatic symptoms to this drug was noted. Skin reactions were reduced on the third day of ACTH, at a time when the asthma had greatly improved in patients 1 and 7 (Table 1) and symptoms disappeared entirely the following day. However, in patient 1 of Table 4, the skin reactions to inhalant antigens were reduced on the fifth day, but maximal relief from asthma did not obtain until the seventh day of ACTH, and the patient was never entirely relieved of symptoms. There was no correlation between gain in weight which occurred in 50 per cent of the cases studied with the changes in skin reactions.

There was variability in the time of reappearance of skin reactions when suppression was noted during drug administration. In several patients who were tested within three to five days after treatment was terminated, the reactions had reappeared, a few exceeding the pre-treatment size. In others, suppression of the reactions was noted up to two weeks beyond the period of hormone administration. In Case 1, Table 1, the skin reactions as recorded were still suppressed on the second day after ACTH was stopped. When the tests were repeated on the sixth post-treatment day reactions to four antigens had reappeared but the partial suppression of the dust reaction remained about the same.

Five patients in the series gave typical immediate reactions to inhalant antigens, three to ragweed pollens and two to dust. Two of the former were clinically sensitive to ragweed pollen and asthmatic symptoms were worse during the ragweed season. Significant reduction in skin reactions was noted in four of the five patients while receiving ACTH, and essentially no change was observed in the fifth.

The serum reagin titer determined in the three pollen sensitive cases,

The effect of adrenocorticotropic hormone (ACTH) and cortisone on the course of chronic bronchial asthma. *Carey RA, Harvey AM, Howard JE et al*

TABLE 6
Intrinsic Asthma

EFFECT OF ACTH AND CORTISONE ON BRONCHIAL ASTHMA   403

	DEC. 10	11	12	13	14	15	16	17	18	19	20	21	22	23	24	25	26	27	28	29	30
Staph. Aureus	1.0 / 0	1.0	+ / −				+ / −	0.5				0								0.6 / 1.2	1.0
Pneumococcus	1.0 / 2.5	2.5	+ / −				+ / −	0.5				0								0.5 / 1.0	1.0
H. Influenzae	1.0 / 3.75	2.5	+ / −				+ / −	1.0				0								0.8 / 2.0	+ / −
Staph. Toxin	1.0 / 2.5	3.0 / 2.5	2.5				0.7 / 2.5	1.5				0.9 / 2.5	2.0 / *							0.9 / 2.5	3.5
Tuberculin 1-100,000	0	0.5 / 0.5	0.5				0	0.7				0	0	0						0	2.0
Tuberculin 1-10,000	0	1.75 / 1.75	1.75				0	1.0				0	0.05 / ±	0						0	1.5
Dust	1.0 / 2.5	−	−				+ / −					0								+ / −	−
Eosinophiles	286		300	99	55	55				33		44		264					429		
Weight	136½		136	134½	135	136½	138¾	138	140	141	141½	142½	143	140½	140¼	139½	137	136½	136½	136½	137¾
ACTH mgm.				140	140	105	105	70	70	56	56	28	28	0	0	0	0	0	0	0	0

Effect of ACTH (Case 7, Table 1), on skin reactions to bacterial and inhalant antigens (dust). First column of figures of each series of tests represent immediate reactions; second column, the 24-hour reactions; and third column the 48-hour reactions. With one exception, definite reduction in all reactions on the 4th day of ACTH, and complete suppression on 9th day. When retested on 7th post-treatment day, reactions reappeared.

Upper numerals ÷ diameter of wheals.

Lower numerals ÷ diameter of erythema.

Where only one row of figures is recorded, values represent diameter of erythema.

* Mild reaction, erythema very faint.

I very faint reaction, erythema only.

The effect of adrenocorticotropic hormone (ACTH) and cortisone on the course of chronic bronchial asthma. *Carey RA, Harvey AM, Howard JE et al*

in two of which the skin reactions were suppressed (Patient 1, Table 1, Patient 1, Table 4), was not significantly altered. In Patient 1 of Table 1 passive transfer studies were done on the third and fifth days of drugs administration, and on the sixth day after withdrawal of ACTH. It is fully realized that these observations on skin reaction to inhalant antigens and serum reagin titers are very limited and that no definite conclusions can be drawn.

Immediate and delayed (24 hour) reactions to bacterial antigens were significantly reduced during ACTH administration. The antigens used were bacterial vaccines prepared in the usual manner and included strains of Staphylococcus albus and aureus, several strains of strep-tococci, one Pneumococcus, Staphylococcus Toxin, and Tuberculin (Old Tuberculin). Positive immediate wheal-erythema reactions were obtained in ten patients, and in seven the reactions were significantly reduced during ACTH administration. The 24-hour reactions were reduced in eight of eleven patients. *Table* 6 (Case 7, Table 1) illus-strates a typical experiment in this group, and includes the reactions to Tuberculin which were likewise suppressed. Of the three patients exhibiting positive Tuberculin reactions prior to ACTH, significant suppression of the reaction was noted in all three instances.

The comparative effect of cortisone and ACTH administration on skin reactions to both inhalant and bacterial antigens was observed in four patients. Cortisone preceded ACTH administration in each case. In the dosage used cortisone was definitely less effective than ACTH in reducing skin reactions. In two patients (No. 1, 4, Table 4) exhibiting positive reactions to pollens and/or dust, the reactions were definitely reduced in one, and slightly in the other. When ACTH was given further reduction in size of the reactions was noted.

Of the immediate and delayed (24 hour) bacterial reactions obtained in the four patients prior to cortisone, the only change was in the delayed reactions (24 hour) in one patient. However, when ACTH was administered, marked reduction of both immediate and delayed re-actions were observed in three, but no further reduction in size of the delayed reactions already suppressed by cortisone was noted.

Metabolic effects

The metabolic effects of ACTH and cortisone in the asthmatic patients followed in general those reported for the entire group of disease states so far treated in this clinic (3). Weight gain of more than five pounds occurred in approximately two-thirds of the patients; manifest edema developed in one-half. There was prompt return to pretreatment status within a few days of discontinuation of the drugs; often in the patients given ACTH weight loss began when the dose was reduced below 30 mgm. per day. Rises in blood pressure of more than 25 mm. systolic or 15 mm. diastolic occurred in five of the twenty-three patients. Fasting blood sugar rose more than 20 mgm. per 100 cc. in 50 per cent, but in no instance did glycosuria occur. No patient developed hirsutism, amenorrhea or striae. Acne appeared in six of the group and was quite severe in one. One patient developed asymptomatic hypokalemia; she was elderly and the most undernourished in the group. Serum CO_2 rose between 3 and 8 meq. in 50 per cent of the group. The hematocrit fell in all patients, the average being 7 mm. (Wintrobe); the degree of blood dilution manifested by the hematocrit was, however, not correlated with the amount of weight gain or the presence or absence of edema.

DISCUSSION

It has been conclusively demonstrated that stimulation of the adrenal glands by ACTH and administration of cortisone result in alleviation of the clinical manifestations of chronic bronchial asthma in the majority of cases treated. Coincidentally with the studies outlined in this report, Randolph and Rollins (4) and Rose (5) observed improvement in asthmatic patients following exhibition of ACTH. The site of operation and mechanism of the beneficial actions are as yet unknown.

The various factors which determine the length of freedom from symptoms have not been elucidated, but it is quite clear that an equally satisfactory response can be obtained following a second and third course of treatment without the necessity for more intense or prolonged administration. The experiences of the past year which are reported here indicate, when one reviews the duration of the remissions obtained, that this form of therapy represents an important advance in the management of patients with severe asthma who cannot be satisfactorily controlled by the other means available. In one instance of severe status asthmaticus described the administration of ACTH was a life-saving measure. Much more is to be learned concerning the ideal

The effect of adrenocorticotropic hormone (ACTH) and cortisone on the course of chronic bronchial asthma. *Carey RA, Harvey AM, Howard JE et al*

form of treatment with ACTH and cortisone and this may prove variable from patient to patient. The evidence thus far suggests that there may be a reasonably predictable period of remission for each patient of such duration that intermittent short courses of ACTH can keep the intractable type of asthma under continual control. However, there is little known at present about the effects of long-term administration of ACTH and further experience is needed before the value and safety of this type of therapy can be fully assessed.

Adrenal cortical extracts have previously been given to patients with bronchial asthma. Fineman (6) administered small doses of eschatin at one to three day intervals because the weakness, anorexia, weight loss, low blood pressure and hypochlorhydria, frequently seen in sufferers from chronic asthma, suggested the presence of adrenal insufficiency. Two of the four patients so treated showed improvement. Cohen and Rudolph (7) used Interrenalin (Rogoff), but their patients manifested no evidence of any change in the severity of the asthma.

Evidence that the adrenal glands are in some way related to the phenomena of hypersensitivity is not new. Dale suggested that histamine released from the tissues might be the causative agent in anaphylactic shock. Though many discrepancies have fallen in the way of this theory, there is still a certain body of evidence indicating that histamine or a related substance is one of the factors in the anaphylactic type of allergy. Dale (8) found that the blood pressure lowering effect of histamine is ten-fold greater in the adrenalectomized than in normal cats and Banting and Gairns (9) observed histamine to be thirty times more toxic in dogs whose adrenal glands had been removed. Kellaway and Cowell (10) showed that it was loss of the adrenal cortex rather than the medulla which was responsible for the increased toxicity of histamine. In all of the cases of asthma studied by Rose there was an increased excretion of histamine in the urine before treatment and in five patients marked reduction in output of histamine after ACTH therapy was begun. Preliminary observations on certain of our patients by Dr. David B. Grob has shown similar results, but in many instances as the dose of ACTH was reduced excretion of histamine again rose at times exceeding the pretreatment amounts. Grob also administered histamine intracutaneously both before treatment and when the asthma was in remission under ACTH therapy. At each time the cutaneous

The effect of adrenocorticotropic hormone (ACTH) and cortisone on the course of chronic bronchial asthma. *Carey RA, Harvey AM, Howard JE et al*

response was identical. Furthermore, curare injected intracutaneously (11) produced the same response whether ACTH was being administered or not. Thus, ACTH in doses sufficient to induce a clinical remission in asthmatic patients does not inhibit the capacity of the epidermal tissues to release histamine or respond to its intracutaneous injection. Curry and his coworkers (12) have studied the effect of ACTH on the evanescent attack of asthma induced by the injection of histamine in which there is a reduction in vital capacity and maximum minute ventillation. Significant protection against the action of histamine could not be obtained by the administration of ACTH suggesting that benefit obtained in patients with asthma with the hormone is not through an antihistaminic action.

Asthma is a disease generally recognized as resulting from sensitivity to an antigen-antibody combination. Mirick (13) has shown that, in patients in whom either ACTH or cortisone is being administered, antibodies to pneumococcus polysaccharide are produced quantitatively and qualitatively just as well as in normal controls. Chow finds that the titer of complement in the plasma rises when ACTH is administered; in contrast to the inactivation of complement by nitrogen mustard (14), which also suppresses local tissue sensitivity (15). In the few patients in this series which were studied serum reagin titers did not change during ACTH therapy. There is no evidence thus far that the beneficial action of ACTH in asthma is mediated by a reduction of either circulating antibody or complement.

The impression is gained that the "resistance" to the hypersensitivity which is conferred by the adrenal activation is a relative one, capable of being broken through if the challenging stimulus is large enough. The degree and duration of the resistance to the asthma seems highly variable, and dependent on factors as yet undetermined. Thus far, however, no patients have been met in whom there has not been conferred considerable clinical benefit from exhibition of ACTH.

A much larger experience with the use of ACTH and cortisone in asthmatic subjects, together with a greater knowledge of their mode of action, is required before a proper evaluation of the therapeutic implications of these agents can be made. On the present evidence it seems that they may be used profitably as therapeutic adjuvants for brief periods in severe asthmatic states, provided they are not given

The effect of adrenocorticotropic hormone (ACTH) and cortisone on the course of chronic bronchial asthma. *Carey RA, Harvey AM, Howard JE et al*

408 RICHARD A. CAREY ET AL.

to patients to whom the other physiologic effects of these hormones might prove dangerous.

SUMMARY

1. It has been conclusively demonstrated that stimulation of the adrenal glands by ACTH and administration of cortisone in sufficient doses have a beneficial effect on the clinical manifestations of chronic bronchial asthma. Complete remissions lasting from four days to over ten months have been obtained.

2. The various factors which determine the length of freedom from symptoms have not been determined, but an equally satisfactory response can be obtained following a second and third course of treatment with ACTH.

3. A much longer experience is necessary before a proper evaluation of the therapeutic implications of these agents can be made. At present it seems that they may be used profitably for brief periods of time in severe asthmatic states, provided they are not given to patients to whom other physiological effects of these hormones might prove dangerous.

ACKNOWLEDGEMENTS

Part of the ACTH used in these studies was supplied by Armour and Company through the courtesy of Dr. John R. Mote. The cortisone and part of the ACTH was purchased through a grant-in-aid from the U. S. Public Health Service. The metabolic studies, to be reported later in detail, were supported in part by a contract between the Johns Hopkins University and the Office of Naval Research.

BIBLIOGRAPHY

1. BORDLEY, J. E., CAREY, R. A., HARVEY, A. M., HOWARD, J. E., KATTUS, A. A., NEWMAN, E. V. AND WINKENWERDER, W. L.: Preliminary observations on the effect of adrenocorticotropic hormone (ACTH) in allergic diseases. Bull. Johns Hopkins Hosp., **85:** 396, 1949.
2. THORN, G. W.: Proc. of First Clinical ACTH Conference, John R. Mote, Editor. Philadelphia, The Blakiston Co., p. 7, 1950.
3. To be published.
4. RANDOLPH, T. G. AND ROLLINS, J. P.: Relief of allergic diseases by ACTH therapy. Proc. of First Clinical ACTH Conference, John R. Mote, Editor, The Blakiston Co., Philadelphia, 1950, p. 479.
5. ROSE, B., Pare, J. A. P., Pump, K. AND STAFFORD, R. L.: Preliminary report on adrenocorticotropic hormone (ACTH) in asthma. Canad. Med. Assn. J., **62:** 6, 1950.

The effect of adrenocorticotropic hormone (ACTH) and cortisone on the course of chronic bronchial asthma. *Carey RA, Harvey AM, Howard JE et al*

EFFECT OF ACTH AND CORTISONE ON BRONCHIAL ASTHMA   409

6. FINEMAN, A. H.: The use of suprarenal cortex extract in the treatment of bronchial asthma. Jour. Allergy, **4**: 182, 1932–33.
7. COHEN, M. B. AND RUDOLPH, J. A.: Studies on the relation of the adrenal glands to allergic phenomena. III. On the specific therapeutic effects of cortical adrenal extracts in asthma. Jour. Allergy, **6**: 279, 1934–35.
8. DALE, H. H.: The Nature and Cause of Wound Shock. The Harvey Lectures, 1919–1920.
9. BANTING, F. G. AND GAIRNS, S.: Suprarenal insufficiency. Amer. J. Physiol., **77**: 100, 1926.
10. KELLAWAY, C. H. AND COWELL, S. J.: On the concentration of the blood and the effects of histamine in adrenal insufficiency. J. Physiol., **57**: 82, 1923–24.
11. GROB, D., LILIENTHAL, J. L., JR. AND HARVEY, A. M.: On certain vascular effects of curare in man: the "histamine" reaction. Bull. Johns Hopkins Hosp., **80**: 299, 1947.
12. CURRY, JOHN S., ROCHE, R. J., DOOLIN, P. D. AND KYLE, L. H.: An experimental study of ACTH in induced asthma. 1950 Proc. South. Soc. for Clin. Res., 4th Annual Meeting, p. 6, New Orleans, March 18, 1950.
13. MIRICK, G. S.: To be published.
14. WATKINS, W. M. AND WORMALL, A.: Inactivation of complement by nitrogen mustard. Nature, **162**: 535, 1948.
15. BECKER, R. M.: Suppression of local tissue reactivity by nitrogen mustard, benzol and x-ray irradiation. Proc. Soc. Exper. Biol. & Med., **69**: 247, 1950.

APPENDIX

Three case reports will be given, representative of the entire group and showing some special feature of interest for discussion.

Case 1

    M. G. (JHH 528824).

A 52-year-old white male butcher, who had no family history of allergic disease. In 1941, during treatment for a parotid abscess with a sulfonamide, hives appeared and the drug was stopped. In July, 1947 he suddenly developed bouts of sneezing and rhinorrhea. Nasal polypi were removed without alteration of the symptoms which continued summer and winter but were readily relieved by antihistaminic drugs.

On September 22, 1949 the patient wakened feeling weak and dyspneic. His doctor made the diagnosis of asthma and gave aminophyllin both intramuscularly and intravenously. Respiration became progressively more difficult and the following day the patient was admitted to a hospital where, for two weeks, he was treated in an oxygen tent with various antiasthmatic drugs. Improvement was only transitory, and in the succeeding four months he was hospitalized on five occasions. In two especially grave episodes, the patient became unconscious and developed circulatory collapse. At no time since onset of the asthma, even in

The effect of adrenocorticotropic hormone (ACTH) and cortisone on the course of chronic bronchial asthma. *Carey RA, Harvey AM, Howard JE et al*

410   RICHARD A. CAREY ET AL.

hospitals and with the use of every adjuvant measure, had he even temporarily experienced comfortable breathing.

He was admitted on February 13, 1950, having lost approximately 30 lbs. in weight since the onset of his illness. Height was 64 inches, weight 129 lbs. Temperature normal, pulse 100, respirations 28, blood pressure 150/90. Oral hygiene was poor. He was in obvious distress, using the accessory muscles of respiration. Nail beds and lips were cyanotic. There was stridor, and asthmatic wheezes were audible all over the lungs. The chest was emphysematous. No abnormalities were made out in examination of the heart, abdomen, genitalia or nervous system. Urine was normal as was the erythron. Eosinophiles were 15 to 30% of the total white count which varied between 8 and 13 thousand. Serologic tests for syphilis were negative. Roentgenogram of the chest revealed only emphysema and old pleural adhesions at the right base. The laryngologist found small polyps in the ethmoid regions, and there appeared to be polyps or cysts in the antra radiologically. Vital capacity was 1.8 litres, after epinephrine 2.4 litres. Electrocardiogram was interpreted as showing left axis deviation and minor non-specific S-T changes. Serum CO_2 was 30 and chloride 97 meq. per litre; blood non-protein nitrogen and sugar were normal.

The patient's condition changed but little in the following month, during which time he was never free of respiratory distress. Sputum consisted of 1 to 2 ounces of thick whitish material, culture of which grew no pathogens. One or more times daily his steady asthmatic state would become suddenly worse, and for these exacerbations intravenous aminophyllin gave the best, but only partial, relief. He was given at varying times oxygen, helium, subcutaneous epinephrine in aqueous solution and in oil, aminophyllin, rectal ether, epinephrine spray, Isoprel, iodides and penicillin. His attending physicians, having exhausted their therapeutic armamentarium, suggested that ACTH be tried. At this time the physical and laboratory examinations were essentially as recorded above. A muscle biopsy disclosed no evidence of periarteritis nodosa.

ACTH was begun at noon on March 9th. 50 mg. was given as the initial dose and thereafter 25 mg. was given every six hours for 48 hours. From the 11th to the 13th he received 80 mg. ACTH per day; from the 13th to the 15th of March 50 mg. per day; from the 15th to the 17th 40 mg. per day, and 20 mg. per day until the 19th when the drug was discontinued.

On the afternoon of March 10th, 24 hours after ACTH was begun, improvement became apparent. During the previous 24 hours, the patient had constant severe respiratory difficulty, despite sitting bolt upright, and despite administration of helium and oxygen, together with the following drugs: 2 cc. epinephrine aqueous, 3 cc. epinephrine in oil, 2.5 gms. aminophyllin intravenously and 45 cc. paraldehyde. He had been unable to take any food and was fed parenterally. By supper time on the 10th he was able to eat and at 8 p.m. was reading a newspaper. Oxygen and helium were not necessary thereafter. On the 11th of March he was able to walk about and perform his own toilet with little discomfort. Both objectively and subjectively he improved steadily, and from the 11th to the 13th required but three

The effect of adrenocorticotropic hormone (ACTH) and cortisone on the course of chronic bronchial asthma. *Carey RA, Harvey AM, Howard JE et al*

injections of epinephrine and no further adjuvant medication was given. He had lost all subjective asthma by March 16th, but the chest was not clear to stethoscopic examination until March 25th. On the 28th the patient was discharged entirely comfortable, though on this day the examiner heard again a few transient wheezes after coughing.

Other features of interest during his course include the following: When ACTH was started, the eosinophile count was 1496 per c.mm.; eight hours later it was 242; the following morning 55 and 30 hours after beginning the drug, the count was zero. Thereafter the daily count fluctuated between 100 and zero (average 30) until March 20th when there was a sudden rise to 700 eosinophiles per c.mm. This was the morning after ACTH had been discontinued, and sterile saline injections were being given. From this time until discharge, the eosinophile count ranged between 300 and 500 per c.m 1.

The blood pressure *fell* progressively during ACTH administration, coincident with improvement in the asthmatic status, and likewise coincident with reduction in the enormous quantity of drugs he had been receiving, including epinephrine. By the third day the patient was eating well and soon developed a ravenous appetite. There was a 4 lb. gain in weight over the first three days of ACTH; thereafter the weight remained essentially stationary until discharge. His diet, while on ACTH, was as desired except that there was restriction of sodium chloride to 4 grams daily.

Serum CO_2 began at 30 meq. per litre and chloride at 96.8. After one week of ACTH, CO_2 was 34.3, chloride 100 and the serum sodium had risen from 136.8 to 146 mg/e. At this time serum potassium was 3 meq.

Four days after ACTH was discontinued, when the patient was continuing to gratify a very large appetite, he experienced postprandially one evening substernal discomfort lasting for half an hour. The symptoms disappeared spontaneously and did not recur; there were no cardiovascular changes noted and the electrocardiogram showed no alteration.

After discharge the patient remained free of asthma for more than two months. At the end of three months he is still active and suffers only minor asthmatic discomfort easily relieved by sprays.

Case 2

M. S. (JHH 435221).

A 26-year-old white married female had for seven years suffered with repeated upper respiratory infections. A maternal aunt has asthma. Wheezing respiration began three years ago during a cold; the first severe attack of asthma occurred two years ago during an attack of bronchitis. It was known that she had a chronic infection of the right lower lobe, thought to be bronchiectasis or congenital cystic disease. She did not react to inhalants by skin tests. Acute febrile respiratory episodes responded to penicillin, but the patient was never free of a productive cough

The effect of adrenocorticotropic hormone (ACTH) and cortisone on the course of chronic bronchial asthma. *Carey RA, Harvey AM, Howard JE et al*

412   RICHARD A. CAREY ET AL.

or asthmatic wheezing and was incapacitated so that she had to be waited upon at home.

The patient was admitted on March 8, 1950 with an exacerbation of her asthma. She was emaciated (weight 85 lbs.), anxious, moderately cyanotic, severely orthopneic. There were wheezes and sticky rales throughout both lungs. There were no signs of cardiac insufficiency; blood pressure was normal; abdominal, pelvic and neurologic examinations revealed no abnormalities. There was no fever, and the recovered sputum was small in amount, though it was believed that she swallowed large quantities. Cultures of the sputum disclosed normal flora, and no tubercle bacilli were found. Routine studies of the blood revealed 6 to 8% eosinophiles; urine and stool examinations were normal.

Penicillin and aureomycin brought about little improvement in the patient's symptoms which were mainly those of constant asthma with episodes of severe exacerbation in which she became cyanotic and often vomited. Oxygen, epinephrine, aminophyllin and antihistaminic drugs gave only transient and partial relief. Bronchoscopy and pulmonary visualization with lipiodol could not be carried out satisfactorily. For more than a month, every effort was made to cope with asthma in order to evaluate the pulmonary infection and prepare her for possible surgical therapy. These measures were unavailing, and the patient's status was unimproved six weeks after her admission.

It was decided to use ACTH therapeutically in order to overcome the asthma, and make bronchoscopic and lipiodol studies possible. At noon on April 25th, ACTH was begun, 80 mg. Armour standard being given daily until May 2nd, 50 mg. per day until May 5th, 37.5 mg. per day to May 7th and 25 mg. per day until discontinuance on May 9th.

Within 12 hours the patient felt more comfortable, and she required but one injection of epinephrine during the night. By the next morning, breathing was easier than at any time since admission and the patient ate breakfast without difficulty and was laughing and talking. The patient continued to improve steadily and by May 2nd there were neither subjective nor objective evidences of asthma. Sputum virtually disappeared, and the patient was able to be up and about the ward freely. Appetite was excellent.

On May 4th bronchoscopy and bronchography were carried out successfully with little discomfort to the patient. Bronchograms of the other lung were made on May 9th with no difficulty. Since these studies revealed saccular bronchiectasis of the right middle lobe and the other lobes were not involved, on May 17th right middle lobectomy was carried out. Sections revealed saccular bronchiectasis and areas of partial atelectasis. Postoperative course was uneventful, and there has been no recurrence of asthma to this date (two months).

Collateral studies carried out coincident with ACTH administration disclosed the following: Eosinophiles, prior to ACTH, varied between 5 and 600 per c.mm., fell to 250 eighteen hours after the first dose, to 130 at 42 hours, but never below this point. The counts ranged between 165 and 275 until May 9th, one day after

The effect of adrenocorticotropic hormone (ACTH) and cortisone on the course of chronic bronchial asthma. *Carey RA, Harvey AM, Howard JE et al*

EFFECT OF ACTH AND CORTISONE ON BRONCHIAL ASTHMA   413

ACTH was discontinued, when they rose to 935 and remained in this area thereafter. The eosinophiles fell to zero during the first 48 hours after operation.

On a routine ward diet, the patient gained 4 lbs. in the first four treatment days; weight was stable thereafter until operation. No edema was apparent. Hematocrit fell from 41 mm. (Wintrobe) to 34 mm. on May 5th, but had returned to 40 mm. by May 15th. There was no significant change in blood pressure, or in the concentration of chloride, CO_2 or total protein in the serum.

Case 3

R. M. (JHH 511025).

A registered nurse, aged 40, who first entered the hospital in November, 1932 with a febrile pneumonitis. For two months she remained ill with fever, cough, dyspnea and extensive infiltrative lesions of the lungs. White blood count ranged between 10 and 15 thousand per c.mm. with eosinophils always between 20 and 30 per cent. No tubercle bacilli or other pathogens were ever recovered from the sputum. Recovery set in spontaneously and was amazingly rapid with considerable clearing of the roentgenogram. She was sent to a tuberculosis sanitorium in March 1933 for bed rest. In April 1933, at the sanitorium, the former symptoms recurred and for six weeks she again suffered from a severe febrile respiratory illness. Roentgenograms again revealed extensive infiltration in both lung fields extending out from the hilar areas. Again there was complete recovery.

During the winter of 1933–1934 she developed constant nasal congestion which has persisted. The sense of taste and smell gradually disappeared.

In 1946, during a short febrile illness thought to be bronchitis, wheezing first appeared. During the next three years asthmatic symptoms steadily increased, the nose remained constantly obstructed and nasal polypi began to develop.

In May, 1949 all symptoms became worse. Dyspnea prevented walking except at the slowest pace, and orthopnea was so severe as to require the upright position for sleep. Pyribenzamine relieved the nasal symptoms slightly but did not alleviate the asthma. For two weeks prior to admission to the hospital on August 17, 1949 asthma had been constant and severe with no relief from sedatives, antihistamines and sympathomimetic drugs.

Examination revealed oral temperature of 99.4 F., pulse 128, respirations 36, B.P. 124/76. She appeared tired and ill with noisy labored breathing. The chest was emphysematous. Percussion note was hyperresonant and sibilant and sonorous rales were everywhere audible over the lungs. The nose was completely obstructed by large nasal polypi readily visible. Cardiac, abdominal and neurological examination revealed no abnormalities.

Serologic tests for syphilis negative. Hemoglobin 16 gms., hematocrit 49, sedimentation rate 0. White blood count 8 thousand, eosinophils 8.5 %. The urine and stool were normal as were the blood sugar and NPN. Roentgenogram disclosed fibroid infiltration of the right apex without evidence of activity, thickened pleura at both apices, normal heart and aorta.

The effect of adrenocorticotropic hormone (ACTH) and cortisone on the course of chronic bronchial asthma. *Carey RA, Harvey AM, Howard JE et al*

414 RICHARD A. CAREY ET AL.

During the first three hospital days the patient experienced constant respiratory difficulty despite all the simpler antiasthmatic remedies. Each night rectal ether was required to afford rest. Coughing was very frequent and severe when awake, productive of about a cupful of mucoid sputum per day; normal flora were grown on culture.

It had been planned to remove the nasal polypi and perform radical antral operations when the asthmatic state had been sufficiently controlled. Since no improvement had been manifest within the three days of hospitalization it was decided to see the possible effect of ACTH administration. This was begun at 6 a.m. August 20 in doses of 12.5 mgm. (Armour Standard) given every 6 hours. The clinical course is graphically represented in Chart I.

Within three hours after the first injection the patient became aware of extraordinary subjective relief. At five hours respirations had fallen to 20 per minute, pulse rate was 92, and only a few inspiratory and expiratory wheezes were heard on auscultation. By midafternoon the patient could inspire fully, which she rarely had been able to do for three years. That night she slept without sedation and the following day she performed her own toilet, walked in the corridor without respiratory embarrassment and could lie flat on the bed. No adjuvant therapy was required after ACTH was begun. On the third day of ACTH the patient suddenly noticed that she could taste and smell. It was discovered that the nasal polypi had shrunk and breathing space was plentiful. One of the earliest evidences of improvement noted by this patient had been diminution in both the nasal and bronchial secretions which had practically disappeared after 48 hours on ACTH. On the fourth day of administration of the hormone all signs and symptoms of asthma had disappeared. Asthmatic symptoms did not recur for 86 days after discharge from the hospital. Total ACTH given was 440 mgm. over a period of 12 days.

224 days after ending of the first course of ACTH the patient returned to the hospital for a second course of the drug. At this time the asthma was not nearly so severe as when the first course was given. 40 mgm. ACTH was administered per day for five days. Improvement was again manifest within 4 hours of the first dose. All signs and symptoms of asthma had disappeared by the fourth day. However, 11 days after ACTH was stopped the patient began to notice wheezing and mild respiratory embarrassment.

The effect of adrenocorticotropic hormone (ACTH) and cortisone on the course of chronic bronchial asthma. *Carey RA, Harvey AM, Howard JE et al*

G

The Journal of Allergy

VOL. 22   JANUARY, 1951   No. 1

Original Articles

ORAL CORTISONE IN INTRACTABLE BRONCHIAL ASTHMA*

PRELIMINARY REPORT

EMANUEL SCHWARTZ, M.D., BROOKLYN, N. Y.

REPORTS by Randolf and Rollins,[1] and Carryer and associates[2] have shown that cortisone given intramuscularly produced a marked symptomatic improvement in intractable asthma. Careful search of the literature to date has not revealed any report on the use of cortisone acetate tablets orally in the treatment of intractable bronchial asthma.

A study has been undertaken to determine whether oral cortisone† will influence intractable bronchial asthma. The patients in this study were observed daily. This report deals with the results with the first 3 patients and it is contemplated to summarize at a future date the results in a larger series of cases treated with oral cortisone acetate.

CASE REPORT

CASE 1.—F. N., a 10-year-old girl, had perennial bronchial asthma for the past 8 years and atopic eczema since she was 3 months old. A severe incapacitating bronchial asthma had been present for 3 months prior to the onset of oral cortisone therapy. Oxygen inhalation and repeated injections of intramuscular epinephrine and intravenous aminophyllin were required several times during the day and at night and produced slight and temporary relief. Intracutaneous tests to the common allergens showed positive reactions to lamb, chicken, chocolate, almond, walnut, peanut, house dust, timothy, and ragweed. Complete avoidance of all foods that showed positive skin reactions and hyposensitization to house dust, ragweed, and timothy did not alter the course of her asthma. In 1948 she lived in Tucson, Arizona, for 1 year without any change in her condition.

When cortisone was first given, the patient had severe asthmatic symptoms. On Sept. 29, 1950, an initial dose of a 25 mg. tablet of cortisone acetate was given orally and followed by 25 mg. every 4 hours for 4 doses for the first 24 hours. The daily dose for the second day was also 100 mg. in 4 divided doses of 25 mg. each. For the next 4 days 50 mg. were given daily in divided doses of 25 mg. every 12 hours. One hour after the second dose of 25 mg. of oral cortisone a remarkable and dramatic improvement set in. Her symptoms of asthma were completely relieved and the chest was clear of wheezes and râles on examination. She had a sense of well-being, her appetite and strength improved, and she was so completely relieved of her asthmatic symptoms that she returned to school on the fourth day of therapy. A maintenance dose of 25 mg. of cortisone before bedtime was established with complete relief of symptoms. With omission of this single dose her asthmatic symptoms returned. Her weight remained constant; there was no evidence of fluid retention, nor glycosuria, and there were no hormonal or other side effects.

*From the Division of Allergy of the Department of Medicine, The Long Island College Hospital, and The State University of New York Medical Center at New York City, College of Medicine.

†Cortisone Acetate tablets were furnished through the courtesy of Merck & Company, Inc., Rahway, N. J.

1

CASE 2.—C. W., a 31-year-old man, had bronchial asthma during childhood. There was no history of a recurrence of asthma until the spring of 1949. From then on his symptoms were perennial and were exaggerated in the late summer and early fall of 1949, and again in the spring and late summer and early fall of 1950. Hyposensitization to timothy produced slight improvement. At the beginning of August, 1950, his asthmatic symptoms increased in severity and were continuous. Hyposensitization to ragweed and house dust did not alter the course of his asthma.

Previous to oral cortisone therapy the patient had an incapacitating intractable asthma for 2 months. He used Isuprel by inhalation 4 or 5 times every night and 2 or 3 times each day. On Oct. 1, 1950, an initial dose of 50 mg. of cortisone was given orally and the total dose for the first day was 200 mg. in 4 divided doses of 50 mg. each. The daily dose for the second day was also 200 mg. in divided doses, and for the next 5 days 100 mg. daily was administered in 4 divided doses of 25 mg. each. On the first day of oral cortisone therapy, 1 hour after the third dose of 50 mg., or 9 hours after the onset of cortisone therapy, his difficulty in breathing disappeared. The wheezing of the chest and the cough were considerably less severe. The first night after cortisone was started, Isuprel was used on 1 occasion. On the second day he was completely free of all symptoms and the chest was clear on examination. On the third day of therapy a mild attack of asthma was promptly relieved by the inhalation of Isuprel. At the end of 1 week the daily dose was gradually decreased and a maintenance dose of 25 mg. before bedtime was established. At times it was necessary to step up the daily dose to 50 mg. Except for an occasional slight wheezing of the chest the patient had no other complaints. If the cortisone were discontinued for 1 day the symptoms would return.

The weight remained constant, and the urinary output was adequate; there was no other evidence of fluid retention and there were no other side effects.

CASE 3.—C. M., a 35-year-old housewife, had chronic asthma and vasomotor rhinitis for 11 years. Since December, 1949, her attacks increased in number, severity, and duration. A severe, continuous asthma was present for 6 months previous to oral cortisone therapy. Vaponephrine, Isuprel, and Adrenalin 1-100 by inhalation were required several times each day and at night. During this period it was impossible for her to attend to her household duties.

She was clinically sensitive to horse dander and house dust. Complete avoidance of horse dander, hyposensitization to house dust, catarrhal vaccine therapy, and a course of treatments with large doses of Pregnenolone did not alter her asthma.

When cortisone was first given the patient had severe asthmatic symptoms. An initial dose of a 50 mg. tablet of cortisone acetate was given orally and followed by 50 mg. every 4 hours for the first 24 hours. During the first 24 hours she showed improvement and Isuprel by inhalation was used on 1 occasion that night, whereas the night before the use of cortisone, aerosol Isuprel was required every 15 minutes. The daily dose for the second day was also 200 mg. in 4 divided doses of 50 mg. each, and for the next 5 days 100 mg. were given daily in 4 divided doses of 25 mg. each. From the third night on she slept well and had no asthmatic symptoms. On arising every morning she had mild asthma which was promptly relieved by inhalation of Isuprel. A maintenance dose of 25 mg. in the morning and 25 mg. before bedtime controlled her asthma. On the second day of therapy she was able to resume all of her household duties without discomfort. Examination of the chest previous to cortisone therapy always showed a marked wheezing type of respiration and many sibilant and sonorous râles. Although cortisone produced a remarkable improvement clinically, the chest still revealed wheezing respiration and râles, but to a lesser extent than previously.

During the first 3 days of oral cortisone therapy, the patient gained 3 pounds and the urinary output was approximately one-half the fluid intake. From the fourth day on the urinary output was adequate, with a subsequent loss of the weight gained previously. There was no glycosuria and there were no hormonal or other side effects.

DISCUSSION

The relief with oral cortisone tablets was attained during administration and immediately following. It seemed that the relief compared favorably with that produced by intramuscular cortisone. Relief occurred within hours after the onset of therapy. However, it should be emphasized that it was confined to the period during its administration. On inadequate dosage, or after the cortisone was discontinued, the asthmatic symptoms returned. After therapy was stopped the symptoms had a tendency to return more quickly than after intramuscular cortisone. The relief was much greater than that previously obtained with hyposensitization or with any other medication.

SUMMARY

1. Three patients received cortisone acetate tablets orally for severe, chronic, intractable bronchial asthma.

2. Each patient experienced prompt relief from symptoms of bronchial asthma which had been continuously present, in the first patient for three months; in the second, for two months; and in the third, for six months.

3. With proper dosage, symptomatic relief was confined to the period during which oral cortisone was administered.

4. Except for an initial gain in weight and also an initial decrease in urinary output in one patient, there were no hormonal or other side effects.

REFERENCES

1. Randolf, T. G., and Rollins, J. P.: Effect of Cortisone on Bronchial Asthma, J. ALLERGY 21: 288, 1950.
2. Carryer, H. M., Koelsche, G. A., Prickman, L. E., Maytum, C. K., Lake, C. F., and Williams, H. L.: The Effect of Cortisone on Bronchial Asthma and Hay Fever Occurring in Subjects Sensitive to Ragweed Pollen, J. ALLERGY 21: 282, 1950.

798 THE LANCET] ORIGINAL ARTICLES [OCT. 20, 1956

CONTROLLED TRIAL OF EFFECTS OF
CORTISONE ACETATE IN CHRONIC ASTHMA

REPORT TO THE MEDICAL RESEARCH COUNCIL BY THE SUBCOMMITTEE ON CLINICAL TRIALS IN ASTHMA *

THE asthma subcommittee was appointed specifically to investigate the value of cortisone in patients with asthma. Cortisone was chosen because of the ease of its administration compared with corticotrophin. It was decided that controlled trials in two phases of the disease would be necessary. The trial in patients with status asthmaticus is the subject of a separate report (Medical Research Council 1956). The present report concerns

---

* The members of the subcommittee are : Prof. R. V. Christie, F.R.C.P., Dr. J. G. Scadding, F.R.C.P., Dr. J. T. Boyd, Dr. W. Brockbank, T.D., F.R.C.P., Dr. E. T. Conybeare, O.B.E., F.R.C.P., Dr. J. J. R. Duthie, F.R.C.P.E., Dr. A. W. Frankland, Dr. R. Kauntze, M.B.E., F.R.C.P., Dr. M. C. S. Kennedy, Dr. H. Nicholson, F.R.C.P., Prof. G. W. Pickering, F.R.C.P., Prof. F. T. G. Prunty, F.R.C.P., Dr. R. S. Bruce Pearson, F.R.C.P., Sir John Taylor, C.I.E., D.S.O.

The subcommittee was appointed by the Collagen Diseases and Hypersensitivity Panel of the Medical Research Council whose members are : Prof. G. W. Pickering, F.R.C.P., Dr. E. G. L. Bywaters, F.R.C.P., Prof. R. V. Christie, F.R.C.P., Dr. J. J. R. Duthie, F.R.C.P.E., Prof. J. F. Danielli, Dr. P. G. H. Gell, Prof. J. H. Kellgren, F.R.C.P., F.R.C.S., Dr. D. A. Long, Prof. A. Neuberger, F.R.S., Dr. H. Nicholson, F.R.C.P., Prof. F. T. G. Prunty, F.R.C.P., Dr. A. H. T. Robb-Smith, F.R.C.P., Prof. G. Payling Wright, F.R.C.P.

THE LANCET]   ORIGINAL ARTICLES   [OCT. 20, 1956   799

a trial carried out at six centres † in the United Kingdom, in which patients with chronic asthma received either cortisone or placebo tablets. Previous reports suggesting very favourable results with cortisone in chronic asthma have already appeared (Lowell et al. 1953, Savidge and Brockbank 1954, Davies and Williams 1955).

An underlying difficulty of therapeutic trials in asthma is the incompleteness of our knowledge of its causes. Many authorities agree that in many younger patients asthma is due to extrinsic causes, such as sensitivity to plant and other antigens (see Pickering 1952). On the other hand, clinical experience shows that, particularly in older patients, inflammatory and other changes ("chronic bronchitis") play an increasingly important rôle in maintaining disability.

It was intended that this study should be on the effects of cortisone on " chronic bronchial asthma " and not on chronic pulmonary infection. For this reason it was stipulated that the patients selected should not have evidence of severe broncho-pulmonary infection. It was hoped that the patients could be admitted to the trial at a uniform rate throughout the year to minimise the effect of seasonal factors.

A further consideration was the importance of the psychogenic factor. It was essential that patients should be completely ignorant of which of the alternative treatments they were receiving. Apart from the usual measures to ensure this, special precautions were taken to make the placebo tablets, as far as possible, identical with the cortisone tablets. The general plan of the trial involved administration of the tablets in each group for a continuous period of six months, supplemented by the usual antispasmodic therapy. This was to be succeeded by a follow-up period of three months. It was desired to determine the possibility of withdrawing cortisone treatment during this period and the relative condition of the patients who had received the two types of treatment.

Material and Methods

Type of Patient

The trial was carried out among patients with chronic asthma attending hospital outpatient departments. It was agreed that patients to be included in the trial must (a) be between 14 and 60 years of age ; (b) have an asthma history of not less than three months' duration ; and (c) have had no complete remission of more than two weeks during the preceding 3 months. An additional criterion was that the dyspnœa present should, in the opinion of the physician, be due in large part to bronchial asthma ; patients with severe broncho-pulmonary infection were excluded. Those with any signs or history of cardiac failure or tuberculosis were excluded because of the possibility of untoward effects of cortisone.

Allocation to Treatment

The two treatment groups were constituted by random allocation. Patients in one group received cortisone acetate and in the other group placebo tablets. The latter each contained quinine dihydrochloride 0·6 mg., lactose 138 mg., starch 22 mg., and a trace of magnesium stearate, and were indistinguishable, as regards size,

† The Centres taking part in the trial were : Manchester Royal Infirmary (Dr. W. Brockbank, Dr. R. S. Savidge, Dr. H. Brebner) ; Wright-Fleming Institute, St. Mary's Hospital, London (Dr. A. W. Frankland, Dr. S. Lewis) ; Guy's Hospital, London (Dr. R. Kauntze, Dr. J. R. Trounce) ; King's College Hospital, London (Dr. R. S. B. Pearson, Dr. F. I. Rackow) ; Brompton Hospital, London (Dr. J. G. Scadding, Dr. J. Pepys) ; University College Hospital (Dr. H. Nicholson, Mrs. M. E. Turner-Warwick). The subcommittee is indebted to Dr. J. T. Boyd, of the Medical Research Council's Statistical Research Unit, for his analysis of data in the trial.

shape, colour, and bitterness, from the cortisone tablets (25 mg.).

Supplies of tablets sufficient to treat each patient were made available to participating hospitals in bottles labelled and numbered 1, 2, 3, 4 . . . Within each centre the bottles were allocated to patients in the same order as that in which they were admitted to the trial. The contents of individual bottles were determined by a random-order list, which was held centrally ; they were not disclosed to either clinicians or patients until the end of the trial. Should the clinician decide on ethical grounds that the patient was doing so badly that, in the event of his receiving placebo tablets, cortisone or other treatment (such as corticotrophin) should be given, he could be quickly informed of the nature of the treatment and the patient withdrawn from the trial.

Treatment

A standard initial dosage was agreed on and was applicable to patients receiving both cortisone and placebo tablets. Each patient received 300 mg. of cortisone acetate, or the equivalent number of placebo tablets, on the first day of the trial ; 200 mg. on the second and third days ; and 100 mg. daily for the next 4 days. After the first week the physician was asked to adjust the dosage to suit requirements of individual patients. It was specified that, at all dosage levels, tablets should be given in divided doses as follows :

Dosage (mg.)	Number of tablets (25 mg.)		
	Morning	Midday	Evening
300·0	4	4	4
200·0	3	2	3
100·0	1 1/2	1	1 1/2
87·5	1	1	1 1/2
75·0	1	1	1
62·5	1	1/2	1
50·0	1/2	1/2	1
37·5	1/2	1/2	1/2
25·0	1/2	..	1/2

All the patients were to be treated for 24 weeks and followed up for 12 further weeks, during which an attempt was to be made to withdraw the drug, aiming at total withdrawal. In addition to the trial tablets all the patients received any antispasmodic therapy considered necessary by their physician.

Assessment

Clinical assessment of each patient was required on entry to the trial, and then once every fortnight during the treatment and follow-up periods. Each assessment included (a) physical examination ; (b) an evaluation of exercise tolerance using five arbitrarily defined grades ; (c) an arbitrary assessment of incapacity for work due to asthma during the previous fourteen days ; and (d) a measurement of vital capacity. Side-effects of the trial tablets and additional requirements of standard antispasmodic therapy were recorded.

Results

96 patients from six centres were admitted to the trial, 49 being allocated to treatment with cortisone and 47 to the control group. Details of the patients by sex, age, duration of asthma, number of previous attacks of status asthmaticus, and time of year in which they were admitted to the trial are given in table I. There was a slightly higher proportion of younger women in the control group, but in other respects the two groups were closely similar.

Withdrawals from Trial

The penultimate column in table II records the number of patients removed from the trial on account of either treatment changes or failure to attend for subsequent assessments. Altogether 9 cortisone and 10 control patients were removed from the trial during the treatment period, the reasons for their removal being as follows :

Cortisone :

1. Male, aged 28 years ; appendicectomy followed by acute psychoneurotic illness. Treatment stopped after 2 weeks.

800   THE LANCET]   ORIGINAL ARTICLES   [OCT. 20, 1956

TABLE I—COMPARISON OF PATIENTS IN CORTISONE AND CONTROL GROUPS AT START OF TRIAL

Age and sex distribution					Duration of asthma		
Age (yr.)	Cortisone		Control		Duration (yr.)	Cortisone	Control
	M	F	M	F			
Under 30	6	3	5	6	Less than 5	6	7
30–	2	6	4	10	5–	8	7
40–	7	10	5	9	10–	16	22
50–59	5	9	4	3	20 +	17	11
Not stated	0	1	1	0	Not stated	2	0
Total	20	29	19	28		49	47

No. of previous attacks of status asthmaticus			Seasonal distribution		
No. of attacks	Cortisone	Control	Month of admission to trial	Cortisone	Control
0	22	19	Jan.–March	15	13
1–3	16	17	April–June	8	6
4–6	4	6	July–Sept.	4	6
7 +	3	2	Oct.–Dec.	21	22
Not stated	4	3	Not stated	1	0
Total	49	47		49	47

2. Female, age not stated ; acute duodenal ulcer. Treatment discontinued after 2 weeks.

3. Male, aged 54 years ; little help from tablets, " sudden panics," very considerable psychological element present. Removal from trial after 2 weeks.

4. Female, aged 55 years ; admitted to hospital in status asthmaticus ; trial abandoned after 2 weeks.

5. Male, aged 48 years ; defaulted after 8 weeks.

6. Female, aged 40 years ; became pregnant. Obstetrician requested discontinuation of trial after 12 weeks.

7. Male, aged 17 years ; severe and persistent status asthmaticus at 20 weeks. Withdrawn from trial and put on known cortisone.

8. Female, aged 35 years ; defaulted after 20 weeks.

9. Female, aged 54 years ; removed from trial after 20 weeks' treatment, owing to incidental finding of a tuberculous kidney.

Control :

1. Male, aged 57 years ; defaulted after 2 weeks.

2. Male, aged 45 years ; admitted to hospital in status asthmaticus and removed from trial after 2 weeks.

3. Female, aged 57 years ; defaulted after 4 weeks.

4. Male, aged 41 years ; defaulted after 8 weeks.

5. Female, aged 21 years ; admitted to hospital in status asthmaticus and removed from trial after 8 weeks.

TABLE II—PHYSICAL EXAMINATION (NUMBER OF PATIENTS WITH GIVEN CLINICAL GRADES * AT DIFFERENT POINTS OF TREATMENT)

Time of assessment	Treatment group	Clinical grade			No. removed from trial	Total
		1	2	3		
Start of trial	Cortisone	3	14	31	..	48†
	Control	6	19	22	..	47
Week 2	Cortisone	18	16	14	..	48*
	Control	12	14	21	..	47
Week 4	Cortisone	17	15	13	4	49
	Control	11	18	16	2	47
Week 6	Cortisone	18	14	13	4	49
	Control	13	13	18	3	47
Week 8	Cortisone	20	11	14	4	49
	Control	13	12	19	3	47
Week 16	Cortisone	20	13	10	6	49
	Control	18	11	10	8	47
Week 24	Cortisone	15	12	13	9	49
	Control	19	9	9	10	47
Follow-up	Cortisone	11	7	17	14	49
	Control	16	7	12	12	47

* Clinical grades (based on auscultatory findings) :
Grade 1: no added sounds.
Grade 2: rhonchi present, but not constant and widespread.
Grade 3: constant and widespread rhonchi.
† No record was made for 1 patient in the cortisone group.

6. Female, aged 48 years ; admitted to hospital in status asthmaticus and removed from trial after 10 weeks.

7. Female, aged 33 years ; defaulted after 10 weeks. Later stated she had no asthma for 3 months after giving up tablets.

8. Female, aged 50 years ; admitted to hospital in status asthmaticus and removed from trial after 12 weeks.

9. Male, aged 55 years ; admitted to hospital in status asthmaticus and removed from trial after 18 weeks.

10. Male, aged 33 years ; defaulted after 18 weeks.

The most frequent causes of removal from the trial were therefore default of the patient and onset of status asthmaticus. Each of these causes was responsible for the removal of 5 patients from the control group (i.e., together they explained all removals from this group), and 2 from the cortisone-treated patients.

Clinical Assessment

Physical examination.—The results of physical examination on entry and at different points of treatment are presented in table II. At the start of the trial the cortisone group has, by chance, the less favourable pattern in this respect, 31 patients being assessed as having constant and widespread rhonchi (i.e., grade 3), compared with 22 patients similarly assessed in the control group. By

TABLE III—NUMBER OF PATIENTS WITH GIVEN GRADE OF EXERCISE TOLERANCE AT DIFFERENT POINTS OF TREATMENT *

Time of assessment	Treatment group	Exercise tolerance					No. removed from trial	Total
		1	2	3	4	5		
Start of trial	Cortisone	1	7	18	16	6	..	48†
	Control	2	7	17	11	10	..	47
Week 2	Cortisone	6	16	13	7	6	..	48†
	Control	2	11	13	11	10	..	47
Week 4	Cortisone	5	23	9	4	4	4	49
	Control	4	9	15	7	10	2	47
Week 6	Cortisone	5	21	11	3	5	4	94
	Control	2	13	12	10	7	3	47
Week 8	Cortisone	8	21	7	5	4	4	49
	Control	4	10	13	11	6	3	47
Week 16	Cortisone	11	17	11	2	2	6	49
	Control	9	9	11	3	7	8	47
Week 24	Cortisone	8	20	5	6	1	9	49
	Control	9	11	13	4	..	10	47
Follow-up	Cortisone	4	14	10	5	2	14	49
	Control	6	10	10	4	5	12	47

* Exercise-tolerance grades were :
Grade 1: as good as that of others of same age and build.
Grade 2: able to walk with others of same age and build on level, but cannot keep up on hills or stairs.
Grade 3: unable to keep up with normals on level, but can walk a mile or more at own speed.
Grade 4: unable to walk a mile, even at own speed, without occasional rests.
Grade 5: unable to leave house without transport because of breathlessness.

† No record was made for 1 patient in the cortisone group.

the end of the first 2 weeks of treatment the relative positions of the groups are reversed : 18 patients in the cortisone group are now free from added sounds (i.e., grade 1), compared with only 12 in the control group ; and the number of cortisone patients in grade 3 is reduced from 31 to 14, while the number of control patients placed in this grade remains virtually the same at 21. The improvement shown by the cortisone group during the first 2 weeks reaches levels of technical significance ($\chi^2 = 17\cdot28$, n = 2, P<0·001), and their advantage at this stage is the more noteworthy in view of the group's relatively unfavourable position at the start of the trial. In both groups, apart from minor fluctuations, there are no further changes up to week 8, but thereafter a more definite improvement is shown by the control group, with the result that by 16 weeks the initial advantage of the cortisone group has disappeared and the patterns displayed by the groups are closely similar. At the end of the treatment period (i.e., at 24 weeks) auscultation did not reveal any added sounds in 15 of the cortisone patients and 19 patients in the control group.

Controlled trial of effects of cortisone acetate in chronic asthma. *Medical Research Council*

TABLE IV—ABILITY TO WORK DURING PREVIOUS FORTNIGHT

Time of assessment	Treatment group	Able to work		Unable to work	No. removed from trial	Total
		Full time	Part time			
Start of trial	Cortisone	20	11	17	..	48*
	Control	16	14	17	..	47
Week 2	Cortisone	26	3	19	..	48*
	Control	18	13	16	..	47
Week 4	Cortisone	25	7	13	4	49
	Control	20	11	14	2	47
Week 6	Cortisone	26	8	11	4	49
	Control	18	11	15	3	47
Week 8	Cortisone	28	5	12	4	49
	Control	19	13	12	3	47
Week 16	Cortisone	28	8	7	6	49
	Control	23	8	8	8	47
Week 24	Cortisone	27	8	5	9	49
	Control	24	7	6	10	47
Follow-up	Cortisone	24	5	6	14	49
	Control	18	9	8	12	47

* No record was made for 1 patient in the cortisone group.

Exercise tolerance.—Table III presents the results of exercise-tolerance assessments of patients in the two groups. At the start of the trial there was a close similarity between cortisone and control patients in their distribution over the five arbitrary grades. At the end of the first fortnight, however, the cortisone group shows an advantage, in that a larger proportion of them are placed in the two highest grades, 1 and 2. Thus, at this stage, 22 cortisone patients were assessed as at least able to walk on the level as well as others of the same age and build, compared with 13 patients in the control group. Correspondingly at the other end of the scale there are 21 control patients who are unable to walk a mile, even at their own speed (i.e., grades 4 and 5), but only 13 cortisone patients. This advantage to the cortisone group is somewhat increased up to week 8 and, though subsequently diminished by a late improvement among the control patients, remains evident to the end of the treatment period, when 28 of the cortisone patients are placed in the two most favourable grades compared with 20 patients in the control series. These differences between the treatment groups as regards exercise tolerance reach levels of technical significance‡ for the assessments at weeks 4, 6, and 8.

Ability to work.—Data concerning the patients' working histories during different fortnightly periods are given in table IV. The histories of the two groups for the fortnight preceding the start of the trial were reasonably comparable. The numbers of patients totally unable to work were 17 in each group, and for both cortisone and control patients these numbers declined until, at the end of the treatment period, there were only 5 and 6 patients respectively remaining in this category. Again at the start of the trial there were 31 cortisone and 30 control patients who were at least able to do some work. Among these patients, however, there was a slightly higher proportion of the group allocated to cortisone who were able to work full time (20 of 31 compared with 16 of 30 control patients). This difference between the proportions of full-time workers among those able to work increased during the early stages of the trial until, by week 8, 28 of the 33 cortisone " workers " were doing full time compared with 19 of the corresponding 32 control patients. After week 8, however, the difference between

‡ The distributions of the cortisone and control groups were compared after combining grades 1 and 2 and grades 4 and 5. Application of the χ² test to these comparisons at weeks, 4, 6, and 8 gave the following values :
Week 4 χ² = 10·22   n = 2, P<0·01
Week 6 χ² = 6·19   n = 2, P<0·05
Week 8 χ² = 9·46   n = 2, P<0·01

the treatment groups diminished, and by week 24 the proportions of " workers " working full time were almost identical ; 27 of 35 cortisone patients and 24 of 31 control patients.

Vital capacity.—Recordings of vital capacity at both the start of the trial and the end of the treatment period were available for 37 cortisone and 36 control patients. From these paired recordings there was no evidence of any material difference between the vital-capacity changes in the two treatment groups (table V). In the cortisone group 19 patients showed an increase and 18 a decrease in vital capacity, while the corresponding numbers among the control series were 21 and 14 respectively. The average changes were positive and at a similar level in both groups.

Side-effects

Possible side-effects were recorded in 27 of the patients receiving cortisone. Most of these patients had more than one complication, the most frequent being weight gain, œdema, and hypertension. Details of the side-effects were as follows (the figures in parentheses indicating the number of control patients for whom similar findings were recorded) :

	No. of patients
Weight gain of more than 20 lb.	6 (2)
Weight gain of 10–20 lb.	17 (4)
Œdema	10 (2)
Hypertension (rise of diastolic pressure exceeding 20 mm. Hg with a minimal final diastolic pressure exceeding 90 mm. Hg)	11 (3)
Moon-face	3 (0)
Albuminuria	3 (0)
Glycosuria	1 (0)
Raised jugular venous pressure	1 (0)

Examination of changes in weight during the first 4 weeks of treatment revealed that 15 cortisone patients

TABLE V—CHANGES IN VITAL CAPACITY DURING TREATMENT PERIOD (BASED ON PAIRED RECORDINGS FOR 37 CORTISONE AND 36 CONTROL PATIENTS)

Change in vital capacity (c.cm.)		Treatment group	
		Cortisone	Control
+ve	1000 +	3	2
	500–	8	7
	1–499	8	12
	0	..	1
−ve	1–499	11	12
	500 –	6	2
	1000 +	1	..
Total		37	36
Average change (c.cm.)		+130	+140

had gained more than 5 lb. during this period. The weight gain for 4 of these patients was in the range of 10–15 lb., and for a single patient the gain exceeded 15 lb. During the same period only 3 patients in the control group gained 5 lb. in weight, and in each case the gain was less than 10 lb.

Use of other Antispasmodic Treatment

Nearly all the patients in both treatment groups received antispasmodic treatment throughout the trial. The use of antispasmodics in the two groups was very similar, and at no time during the trial were more than 5 of the cortisone-treated and 4 placebo-treated patients not receiving these drugs.

Follow-up

Though it was hoped, if possible, to withdraw the tablets during the 12-week follow-up, many patients in both treatment groups were still receiving tablets at the end of this period. The individual dosages of trial tablets being administered at the end of the follow-up are given in table VI, which also presents, for comparison, details of maintenance doses at the mid-point of the treatment period. At the end of the follow-up tablets had been

Q 2

802 THE LANCET] ORIGINAL ARTICLES [OCT. 20, 1956

TABLE VI—DAILY DOSES BEING ADMINISTERED AT MID-POINT OF TREATMENT PERIOD, AND END OF FOLLOW-UP PERIOD

Tablets daily (cortisone 25 mg. or placebo equivalent)	No. of patients on given dose			
	Mid-point of treatment period		End of follow-up period	
	Cortisone	Control	Cortisone	Control
8	..	1	..	..
6	1	1	..	..
5	1	2	1	..
4	8	14	1	1
3½	1	1	..	..
3	15	15	5	6
2½	4	3	2	1
2	8	2	4	5
1½	5	1	2	..
1	1	..	3	2
½	..	..	1	..
0	..	..	16	20
Patients removed from trial	5	7	14	12
Total	49	47	49	47

completely withdrawn from only 16 of the cortisone and 20 of the control patients remaining in the trial, and in both groups there were patients still receiving as many as four tablets daily.

Of the 77 patients remaining in the trial at the end of the treatment period 7 (5 cortisone and 2 control) failed to complete their 12-week follow-up :

Cortisone :

1. Male, aged 42 years ; status asthmaticus during 4th week of follow-up, admitted to another hospital and died about a fortnight later without cortisone or corticotrophin treatment (cortisone had been withdrawn before the onset of status asthmaticus).

2. Male, aged 26 years ; defaulted after 2 weeks' follow-up (receiving cortisone 25 mg. daily before default).

3. Male, aged 52 years ; defaulted after 4 weeks' follow-up (not receiving cortisone at time of default).

4. Male, aged 41 years ; transferred to different asthma clinic after 6 weeks' follow-up, was well on ephedrine, no further record (not receiving cortisone when transferred).

5. Male, aged 53 years ; removed from trial after 6 weeks' follow-up, " has had a very bad month and is very wheezy," transferred to known cortisone (at time of removal from trial patient was receiving cortisone 50 mg. daily).

Control :

1. Female, aged 52 years ; no detailed records available after end of treatment period, was reported to have been subsequently admitted to hospital without either cortisone or corticotrophin producing any effect on her symptoms.

2. Female, aged 24 years ; admitted to another hospital in status asthmaticus after 8 weeks' follow-up, no further records available (dosage of placebo tablets had been reduced from 2½ to ½ tablet daily at time of onset of status).

The results of follow-up physical examinations and assessments of exercise tolerance and ability to work are presented in the bottom rows of tables II, III, and IV respectively. In each of these respects both groups showed some deterioration from the assessments (week 24) at the end of the treatment period. There was, however, little difference between the two treatment groups in the follow-up evaluations of physical findings, exercise tolerance, and ability to work. These final assessments were made for 35 patients in each group, of whom 11 patients treated with cortisone and 16 in the control group had clear chests on auscultation ; 18 cortisone and 16 control patients were assessed as at least " able to walk on the level " with others of same age and build ; and 29 cortisone and 27 control patients were working during the previous fortnight, the numbers doing so full-time being 24 and 18 respectively.

Discussion

The sample of patients studied was regarded as satisfactory for the purpose of this trial. Although the attempt to admit patients to the trial evenly through the year was not successful, the seasonal distribution in the two groups was similar. 36 of the 49 patients given cortisone and 35 of the 47 receiving placebo were admitted between October and March inclusive.

There is unequivocal evidence of a slight but definite advantage for the cortisone-treated patients as regards improvement in physical signs and exercise tolerance from the 2nd to the 8th week of treatment. From then on to the 24th week of treatment in both respects the control patients gained ground, with the result that at the end of this period there was very little to differentiate between the two groups. As regards increased ability to work, the use of cortisone showed no advantage in enabling those to work who were initially unable to do so. Among those initially fit for part-time work return to full-time work was slightly facilitated by cortisone during the first 8 weeks ; but after this the control patients gained and were as well off as those treated with cortisone. Thus the patient was at first better off from the point of view of exercise tolerance when treated with cortisone, but this improvement was not so great as to make a really significant gain in work capacity, and there was no diminution of the need for antispasmodic therapy. There was a slightly higher proportion of young patients in the control group, but separate analysis of the groups under and over the age of 40 years revealed that the older patients responded, if anything, better to cortisone. The changes in vital capacity showed wide and similar variations in the cortisone and control groups. The personal impressions of the clinicians were that 23 of the cortisone patients were improved during the trial, compared with 12 of those receiving placebo. These impressions may in a few cases have been influenced by a feeling of well-being by the patients or possibly by the coexistence of side-effects, such as œdema.

The reasons leading to patients being withdrawn from the trial are of interest. There were 9 of these in the cortisone group. Two who defaulted may be presumed to have little help from cortisone. Two actually developed status asthmaticus in spite of the benefit of cortisone in this condition (see Medical Research Council 1956), one while receiving cortisone 100 mg. daily and the other 75 mg. Of the patients on placebo treatment only 10 were withdrawn ; 5 defaulted presumably because of inadequate benefit, and the other 5 developed status asthmaticus. These differences give support to the previous findings of early advantages for the cortisone patients.

In view of the findings during the follow-up period of 3 months it is noteworthy that difficulties were encountered in withdrawing tablets from both groups of patients, 19 remaining on cortisone and 15 on placebo tablets. Since physicians had been asked to withdraw tablets if possible during this period, it is clear that patients receiving either type of tablet thought they were deriving benefit from them. The numbers of tablets of each kind given during the follow-up period were similar. These facts confirm the conclusion, based on assessment at the end of the 6 months' treatment period, that at this stage cortisone was causing no specific benefit. The reasons given for the removal of patients from the trial during the follow-up period are similar to those given for removal during the course of the trial. One patient was removed from the trial and given cortisone, although it later became apparent that at the time of withdrawal from the trial he had in fact been receiving cortisone 50 mg. daily.

Further observations of interest were made over an interval of from 6 to 22 months after the follow-up period. Data were available from 36 patients who received cortisone in the trial. 22 were still receiving it, and 12 of these were reported to be doing well ; 14 were

THE LANCET]   ORIGINAL ARTICLES   [OCT. 20, 1956 803

not receiving it, and 7 of these were reported to be well. At one of the hospitals there was a tendency to avoid the further use of cortisone, whereas, by contrast, at four others the tendency was to continue it. The reasons for these tendencies were not clear. Information was available about 27 patients who had received the placebo in the trial. Treatment without cortisone was continued in 10 patients, of whom 6 were reported to be well. Seventeen received cortisone or corticotrophin after the end of the trial, and 6 of these were reported to be well. The proportion of patients whose asthma was controlled is strikingly similar in the various groups, but some patients who had not received cortisone in the trial appeared to benefit later from the administration of either cortisone or corticotrophin.

The side-effects of cortisone during this trial were not particularly troublesome and, with one or two doubtful exceptions, did not necessitate interruption of treatment. The psychoneurosis which developed in one patient and the duodenal ulcer in another after 2 weeks' treatment may have been caused in part by cortisone, but may have been of old standing and exacerbated by it. It is possible that in the patient in whom tuberculosis of the kidney was discovered after 20 weeks' treatment the progress of this condition may have been accelerated.

The patient dying in status asthmaticus after the withdrawal of cortisone might be cited as a warning about possible dangers of this procedure. The unequivocal side-effects are, of course, those usually associated with cortisone, headed by significant weight gain in 50% and oedema in 20%. There seemed to be no evidence that the onset of oedema was associated with any important degree of cardiac failure. A much smaller, but noticeable, proportion of patients receiving the placebo were recorded as having gained weight and developed oedema. The remaining side-effects of cortisone were mild. A few patients developed hypertension of mild degree and insufficient to be a practical problem. None of the cortisone-treated patients had to be withdrawn from the trial on account of side-effects, but this may be due to careful selection of the patients admitted to exclude those with cardiac failure and other contra-indications.

Conclusion

The general conclusion to be drawn from the trial is that the patients receiving cortisone were subjectively and objectively improved during the first 2 months of treatment to a greater extent than those receiving the placebo, both groups simultaneously receiving antispasmodics. The early improvement with cortisone treatment was hardly sufficient to make a significant contribution to improved capacity for work, and cannot by any standard be regarded as dramatic or as great as that shown in patients with status asthmaticus (see Medical Research Council 1956). This early improvement was not maintained, and by the end of the trial the cortisone-treated group showed no significant advantage over the control group.

Summary

The effect of cortisone-acetate tablets was compared with that of placebo tablets in outpatients with chronic asthma, simultaneously receiving routine antispasmodic treatment.

96 patients were studied: 49 in the cortisone group and 47 in the control group. Treatment continued for 6 months.

Particularly as regards diminution of rhonchi and exercise tolerance, there was a partial, but significant, advantage to the cortisone-treated group during the first 8 weeks. From then to the end of the 6 months and during 3 months' follow-up this advantage gradually disappeared.

Difficulty was encountered in withdrawing both cortisone and placebo tablets in the follow-up period.

In the selected patients studied side-effects of cortisone in the doses used were not severe enough to cause practical difficulties.

We wish to thank the physicians who referred cases for inclusion in the trial, and Messrs. Roussel Laboratories Limited, who very generously provided the large number of placebo tablets.

REFERENCES

Davies, B. M., Williams, D. A. (1955) *Brit. med. J.* ii, 293.
Lowell, F. C., Schiller, I. W., Leard, S. E., Franklin, W. (1953) *J. Allergy,* **24**, 112.
Medical Research Council (1956) *Lancet,* ii, p. 803.
Pickering, G. W. (1952) *Brit. med. J.* i, 1207.
Savidge, R. S., Brockbank, W. (1954) *Lancet,* ii, 889.

Controlled trial of effects of cortisone acetate in chronic asthma. *Medical Research Council*

CONTROLLED TRIAL OF EFFECTS OF
CORTISONE ACETATE IN STATUS ASTHMATICUS
REPORT TO THE MEDICAL RESEARCH COUNCIL BY THE SUBCOMMITTEE ON CLINICAL TRIALS IN ASTHMA *

SINCE the early reports of the use of cortisone in asthma (e.g., Carryer et al. 1950) there has been a good deal of agreement about its value in the treatment of patients in status asthmaticus. Recent papers (Ball 1954, Pearson 1955) have reported satisfactory results from the treatment of small groups of patients suffering from this condition. It is known, however, that the treatment of status asthmaticus with antispasmodic drugs is successful in a high proportion of patients, and it seemed advisable to compare, with proper precautions, the effectiveness of cortisone with that of antispasmodic drugs. Cortisone was selected for the trial because it was known to be likely to become freely available and also because of the ease of its effective administration by mouth compared with corticotrophin, which must be given by intramuscular injection. Thirteen centres participated in the trial.†

Material and Methods

Type of Patient

It was agreed that the patients in status asthmaticus to be included in the trial must (a) be more than 14 years of age ; (b) have had at least one previous severe attack of asthma ; and (c) not have received any previous cortisone therapy. All patients admitted to hospital who met these requirements received " standard " treatment during the first 24 hours. The " standard " treatment received was determined by the normal practice of the clinician in charge of the patient, and might include (a) adrenaline 1 in 1000 solution subcutaneously, (b) aminophylline intravenously, (c) isoprenaline 1% inhaled,

---

* The members of the subcommittee are given on p. 798.

† Centres taking part in the trial :. Chase Farm Hospital (Dr. T. Simpson) ; Crumpsall Hospital, Manchester (Dr. R. W. Luxton) ; Guy's Hospital, London (Dr. R. Kauntze, Dr. J. R. Trounce) ; King's College Hospital, London (Dr. R. S. B. Pearson, Dr. F. I. Rackow) ; Manchester Royal Infirmary (Dr. W. Brockbank, Dr. R. S. Savidge, Dr. Hugh Brebner) ; Northern General Hospital, Edinburgh (Dr. I. W. B. Grant, Dr. A. R. Somner) ; Queen Elizabeth Hospital, Birmingham (Prof. W. M. Arnott, Dr. John Butler) ; Royal Hospital, Sheffield (Prof. C. H. Stuart-Harris) ; St. Bartholomew's Hospital, London (Dr. N. Oswald) ; St. David's Hospital, Cardiff (Dr. D. A. Williams) ; St. Thomas's Hospital, London (Dr. H. J. Anderson, Dr. D. S. Cadman) ; University College Hospital, London (Dr. H. Nicholson, Mrs. M. E. Turner-Warwick) ; Wright-Fleming Institute, St. Mary's Hospital, London (Dr. A. W. Frankland). The subcommittee is indebted to Dr. J. T. Boyd, of the Medical Research Council's Statistical Research Unit, for his analysis of data in the trial.

804 THE LANCET] ORIGINAL ARTICLES [OCT. 20, 1956

(d) oxygen, (e) antibiotics, and (f) sedatives. During the first 12 hours an attempt was made to establish the dosage of antispasmodic required, and, whenever possible, the dosage established was not increased, nor were any additions made to therapy, during the second 12 hours. At the end of this initial treatment period patients who remained in status asthmaticus were admitted to the trial, which was thus concerned only with those in whom " standard " methods of treatment had failed over a period of 24 hours.

Allocation of Treatment

In a trial of this nature it was obviously impossible that the control group should receive placebo treatment alone, and on ethical grounds it was desirable that the cortisone group also should continue to receive the benefit of normal standard treatment for status asthmaticus. The contrast made, therefore, was between standard methods plus cortisone and standard treatment alone. The two treatment groups were formed by random allocation at the time of admission to the trial. Cortisone acetate was given in the form of 25 mg. tablets, and patients not receiving cortisone were given placebo tablets prepared so as to be as nearly as possible indistinguishable in size, shape, colour, and taste from the cortisone tablets (see Medical Research Council 1956).

Supplies of tablets were made available to centres in labelled bottles each containing sufficient to treat one patient and numbered 1, 2, 3, 4 . . . Within each centre numbers were allotted to patients in the order in which they were admitted to the trial. The contents of individual bottles were determined by a random-order list, which was held centrally ; they remained unknown to clinicians and patients in the participating centres during the whole course of the trial.

Treatment

A standard dosage schedule was agreed on and was applicable to patients receiving both cortisone and placebo tablets. The specified course, given in divided doses, was as follows :

Day 1.—350 mg. : 2 tablets immediately, 1 tablet every hour for 8 hours, 1 tablet every 4 hours.
Day 2.—200 mg. : 2 tablets every 6 hours.
Days 3–9.—Dosage reduced by 25 mg. daily.
Day 3.—175 mg. : 2 tablets, followed by 2 tablets 6 hours later, then $1\frac{1}{2}$ tablets every 6 hours.
Day 4.—150 mg. : $1\frac{1}{2}$ tablets every 6 hours.
Day 5.—125 mg. : 2 tablets, then 1 tablet every 6 hours.
Day 6.—100 mg. : 1 tablet every 6 hours.
Day 7.—75 mg. : 2 tablets, then 1 tablet after 12 hours.
Day 8.—50 mg. : 1 tablet 12-hourly.
Day 9.—25 mg. : $\frac{1}{2}$ tablet 12-hourly.
Days 10–14.—No cortisone or placebo tablets given.

The total amount of cortisone given to patients in the " treated " group was thus 1·25 g., while the control patients received, in total, an exactly equal number of placebo tablets (50). All the patients continued to receive whatever standard treatment was considered necessary by their physicians, and the proviso was made that, in the event of any patient's condition causing serious concern, the tablets might be discontinued and the patient receive any treatment, including known cortisone, preferred by the clinician.

Assessment of Patients

Clinical assessment of each patient was required twice on the day immediately before the start of treatment with cortisone or placebo tablets, twice on the first day of the trial, and then once daily for 14 days, or until the patient was discharged from hospital. Each assessment included (a) an evaluation of the degree of bronchial obstruction present, using five arbitrarily defined clinical grades ; and (b) temperature, respiration-rate, and pulse-rate, for each of which recorded maxima and minima were requested. In addition, details were required of the

TABLE I—COMPARISON OF PATIENTS IN CORTISONE AND CONTROL GROUPS AT START OF TRIAL

Age and sex distribution					Seasonal distribution		
Age (yr.)	Cortisone		Control		Month of admission	Cortisone	Control
	M	F	M	F			
Under 20	0	1	1	0	Jan.–March	6	4
20–	1	3	2	2	April–June	4	5
40–	2	6	5	5	July–Sept.	3	4
60 +	0	2	0	2	Oct.–Dec.	2	4
Total	3	12	8	9		15	17

Duration of asthma			Severity of asthma before present attack		
Duration (yr.)	Cortisone	Control	Severity	Cortisone	Control
Under 1	0	1	Discomfort	6	8
1–10	7	7	Unable to work	5	7
11–20	4	7	Confined to bed	1	2
21 +	4	2	Not recorded	3	0
Total	15	17		15	17

standard treatment (antispasmodics, &c.) received by each patient.

Results

32 patients from twelve hospitals were admitted to the trial : 15 in the cortisone group and 17 in the control group. These relatively small numbers were undoubtedly because of the requirement that only patients in whom " standard " methods of treatment had failed over a period of 24 hours could be accepted. In practice, the majority of patients admitted in status asthmaticus to the participating hospitals showed sufficient improvement during this initial treatment period to exclude themselves from the trial—i.e., they were no longer in status asthmaticus.

Details of the patients by age, sex, duration of asthma, severity of asthma before present attack, and time of year in which they were admitted to hospital are given in table I. There was, by chance, some difference in the sex composition of the two groups, 12 of 15 patients in the cortisone group being females, as opposed to 9 of 17 in the control group. For each of the other characteristics, however, there was close similarity between the two groups on admission to the trial.

Clinical Assessment

The results of clinical assessment of the patients are presented in table II for the day preceding the trial (day 0) and at successive intervals therafter. On the day before trial therapy commences all trial patients are in status asthmaticus (i.e., grades 4 or 5), but some improvement is apparent as early as day 1, though at this stage there is little to choose between the two treatment groups. By day 2 the cortisone group begins to show an advantage, and this advantage is more marked by day 4, when 10 of the 15 cortisone patients have reached the two highest clinical grades (1 and 2), compared with 4 of 17 in the control group. This considerable difference between the effects of the two treatments, when the proportion of patients free from any serious degree of bronchial obstruction is considered, remains evident at all later stages of the fortnight trial period ; even though the numbers are small the difference is technically significant from day 4 onwards. At the end of the period 11 of 15 patients (2 of 3 males and 9 of 12 females) have achieved complete freedom from their attack of asthma on cortisone plus standard treatment, whereas only 4 of 17 (1 of 8 males and 3 of 9 females) have done so on the combination of standard treatment and placebo tablets.

Controlled trial of effects of cortisone acetate in status asthmaticus. *Medical Research Council*

THE LANCET]   ORIGINAL ARTICLES   [OCT. 20, 1956   805

The final two columns of table II record the number of patients removed from the trial either because of treatment changes (i.e., stopping of cortisone or placebo tablets) or death. Treatment was changed in 5 patients in the control group and in 1 cortisone patient. The single death during the first 14 days occurred in a patient receiving cortisone. Notes from the case-histories of the patients concerned are given below :

Death

Cortisone :

1. Male, aged 47 years, cough since pertussis at one year, asthma since early childhood, 3–4 attacks a year lasting 2–7 days, present attack began 8 days before admission, no benefit from tablets, overwhelming infective element present, died day 4, necropsy showed bronchiectasis, bronchopneumonia, and cor pulmonale.

Treatment Changes

Cortisone :

1. Female, aged 54 years, asthma 7 years, mitral stenosis with no history of rheumatic fever, mild degree of heart-failure 1 year ago, present attack began 14 days before admission. *On admission* liver palpable but no suggestion of heart-failure. Digitalis and penicillin given prophylactically. Asthma improved after 3 days, but œdema and auricular fibrillation appeared. By day 6 liver was enlarged and patient had ascites. Tablets withheld. Three months later patient was readmitted from convalescence in severe status asthmaticus and died in spite of corticotrophin therapy. Necropsy showed death to be due to status asthmaticus, chronic bronchitis and emphysema, and mitral stenosis.

Control

1. Male, aged 54 years, asthma 2 years, present attack 3 weeks, condition desperate on day 1, and it was feared patient might die. Changed to cortisone with good response.

2. Male, aged 47 years, asthma 3 years, present attack 1 week before admission, trial discontinued during day 2 because of failure of patient to respond to treatment. Constantly passing into clinical grade 5 and eventually being maintained thus. Corticotrophin gel given with excellent effect.

3. Female, aged 60 years, asthma 10 years, present attack 2 weeks, no response to tablets. Deterioration of condition led to treatment with corticotrophin on day 6. Rapidly improved.

4. Male, aged 47 years, asthma 10 months, present attack 2 days. After 9 days was showing no benefit from treatment,

TABLE II—NUMBER OF PATIENTS WITH GIVEN CLINICAL GRADES AT DIFFERENT POINTS OF TREATMENT

Time of assessment	Treatment group	Clinical grade* 1	2	3	4	5	Treatment discontinued or changed	Deaths
Day 0 :								
1st 12 hr.	Cortisone	..	..	..	7	8	..	..
	Control	..	..	..	11	6	..	..
2nd 12 hr.	Cortisone	..	..	..	7	8	..	..
	Control	..	..	..	14	3	..	..
Day 1 :								
1st 12 hr.	Cortisone	..	..	3	7	5	..	..
	Control	..	2	2	11	2	..	..
2nd 12 hr.	Cortisone	..	1	8	3	3	..	..
	Control	..	3	1	10	3	..	..
Day 2	Cortisone	2	3	4	4	2	..	..
	Control	..	1	6	6	3	1	..
Day 4	Cortisone	4	6	3	1	..	..	1
	Control	..	4	5	5	1	2	..
Day 6	Cortisone	8	2	3	1	..	..	1
	Control	3	..	7	4	..	3	..
Day 8	Cortisone	9	3	..	1	..	1	1
	Control	3	..	5	6	..	3	..
Day 10	Cortisone	9	3	1	..	..	1	1
	Control	3	2	6	2	..	4	..
Day 14	Cortisone	11	..	2	..	..	1	1
	Control	4	1	4	3	..	5	..

*Clinical grades :
  Grade 1 : no clinical evidence of bronchial obstruction.
  Grade 2 : able to get about, wheezing audible only on auscultation.
  Grade 3 : patient comfortable in bed, wheezing respiration heard at bedside.
  Grade 4 : wheezing respiration, accessory muscles in use, discomfort intermediate between grades 3 and 5.
  Grade 5 : severe distress, able to talk only in gasps.

TABLE III—TEMPERATURE, RESPIRATION, AND PULSE-RATE

Day of trial	No. of patients with temp. above 99°F Cortisone	Control	No. of patients with resp.-rate greater than 25 per min. Cortisone	Control	No. of patients with pulse-rate greater than 100 Cortisone	Control	No. of "failures" —i.e., deaths and treatment changes Cortisone	Control
Day 0 :								
1st 12 hours ..	1	2	10	8	12	15	..	..
2nd 12 hours..	3	4	12	10	12	12	..	..
Day 1 :								
1st 12 hours ..	2	2	7	11	11	13	..	..
2nd 12 hours..	3	4	8	9	12	12	..	..
Day 2 ..	4	5	3	9	10	11	..	1
Day 4 ..	2	2	2	6	5	10	1	2
Day 6 ..	1	2	0	6	1	9	1	3
Day 8 ..	0	2	1	4	0	11	2	3
Day 10 ..	0	1	0	3	1	6	2	4
Day 14 ..	0	0	0	1	1	5	2	5

was becoming desperately ill, and was given corticotrophin. Made a dramatic recovery but relapsed later.

5. Female, aged 53 years, asthma 20 years, present attack 7 months. By day 10 patient had become very exhausted and was threatening to leave hospital. Cortisone given and patient improved.

It should be noted that each of the 5 patients who did not respond to the control treatment showed considerable, even dramatic, improvement under treatment with either cortisone or corticotrophin. In addition, 2 of the 3 control patients who were still in clinical grade 4 at the end of the trial period were recorded as having received cortisone and corticotrophin immediately afterwards (day 15), and again both patients showed a good response to hormone therapy. Thus there were 7 control patients who failed to make any worthwhile response to their allocated treatment but showed a rapid and substantial improvement on being changed to treatment with either cortisone or corticotrophin.

Temperature, Respiration, and Pulse-rate

The assessment presented for each of these three characteristics is the number of patients with recordings above an arbitrarily chosen level at different stages of the trial (table III). Few patients experienced any rise of temperature, and there is little evidence of any difference between the cortisone and control patients. For both respiration and pulse-rate, however, it is evident that the cortisone group have the more favourable experience. The numbers of patients with a respiration-rate greater than 25 a minute before treatment and during the first day of the trial are closely similar in the two groups. On day 2 the cortisone group show a comparatively sharp decrease in this respect, and by day 6 all in the group have respiratory rates lower than the level chosen for assessment. Among the control group, on the other hand, the decline is delayed and more gradual, and on days 6, 8, and 10 there remain 6, 4, and 3 patients respectively whose respiration-rates are above 25 a minute. A similar pattern is displayed by the column giving numbers of patients with a pulse-rate greater than 100. The number of cortisone patients remaining in this category declines considerably on day 4, and by day 8 pulse-rates of all patients in the group are below 100, whereas 11 of the control patients still have pulse-rates above this level.

The final column repeats the number of patients who, having been removed from the trial by death or treatment change, were excluded from the assessments at various stages. These patients were those showing little or no response to treatment, and control patients predominate among the group. It therefore seems likely that, had it been possible, their continued inclusion would, if any-

Controlled trial of effects of cortisone acetate in status asthmaticus. *Medical Research Council*

TABLE IV—STANDARD THERAPY RECEIVED BY PATIENTS IN CORTISONE AND CONTROL GROUPS AT DIFFERENT STAGES OF TRIAL

Day of trial	No. of patients receiving anti-spasmodics		No. of patients receiving oxygen		No. of patients receiving sedatives		No. of "failures" —i.e., deaths and treatment changes	
	Corti-sone	Con-trol	Corti-sone	Con-trol	Corti-sone	Con-trol	Corti-sone	Con-trol
0	15	17	9	3	13	12	..	..
1	12	13	6	4	10	11	..	..
2	10	9	4	2	10	9	..	1
4	7	8	1	2	7	9	1	2
6	4	8	1	1	8	8	1	3
8	3	8	0	0	7	7	2	3
10	2	5	0	0	5	6	2	4
14	3	5	0	0	5	4	2	5

thing, have increased the differences noted between the two treatments.

Standard Therapy

The numbers of patients receiving antispasmodics, oxygen, and sedatives are given separately and for different times in table IV. All the patients received antispasmodic drugs on the day before treatment with the trial tablets was started, and there is a successive decline therafter in the numbers requiring them. The cortisone group again show an advantage in this respect, and by the end of the first week only 3, compared with 8 control patients, are receiving antispasmodics. The control group shows some subsequent improvement, and by day 14 the numbers are 3 and 5 respectively.

The experience of the two treatment groups as regards the number of patients receiving either oxygen or sedatives was very similar at all stages of the trial.

Follow-up

There was no evidence at follow-up three months later, available for 11 cortisone and 14 control patients, that cortisone therapy had decreased the chances of a subsequent attack of status asthmaticus. Of the patients followed up 9 in the cortisone group and 7 in the control group were recorded as having further attacks. The chronic asthma of both the remaining cortisone patients was said to be better compared with its state before the trial, whereas the comparable assessments in the other 7 control patients were 3 better, 3 with no change, and 1 worse.

Discussion

The results of the trial show clearly that in this group of patients in status asthmaticus, in whom treatment with the usual antispasmodic drugs for 24 hours had failed to produce relief, cortisone in the dosage used is effective treatment. By day 4 of treatment 10 of the 15 patients treated with cortisone no longer had disabling bronchial obstruction, whereas only 4 of the 17 control patients were in this satisfactory condition. This difference between the two groups was maintained to the end of the 14-day period of treatment.

It had been agreed, before the trial began, that any patient whose condition caused serious concern should be withdrawn from the trial and treated by any method which the clinicians thought advisable. It is interesting and supports the general result that 5 patients were withdrawn from the trial because they were not doing well and were all effectively treated with either cortisone or corticotrophin. These patients were, in fact, in the control group, although this was not known to the clinicians in charge of their treatment.

The 1 patient having cortisone who was withdrawn from the trial had mitral stenosis and developed signs of cardiac failure on day 6 of the trial. During the trial

there was 1 death of a patient in the cortisone group. He was a middle-aged man who had had asthma for many years and had considerable bronchial infection and bronchopneumonia. The results of treating these 2 patients emphasise two of the difficulties of cortisone treatment : the danger of precipitating cardiac failure, especially in patients who are known to have had it previously ; and the possibility that, in patients with severe bronchial infection, the treatment will not be effective and may be dangerous.

One of the interesting features of the trial was the relatively small numbers of patients who were admitted to it at each of the centres which took part. This was the result of the decision that all patients should first be treated with antispasmodic drugs according to the usual method of the clinician in charge. Only when these methods failed after being used for 24 hours was the patient accepted for the trial. In fact, in the majority of patients this " standard " treatment was successful, and after 24 hours of it the patients were no longer in status asthmaticus and so were not admitted to the trial. Because of the dangers and difficulties of cortisone treatment it should be used only after other methods have been tried vigorously and have failed. Except for the occasional patient who is extremely exhausted and dehydrated it seems advisable and satisfactory to use first of all treatment with antispasmodic drugs.

Observation of patients over a period of three months after the conclusion of the trial showed that most reverted to their usual asthmatic condition, and that the period of cortisone treatment did not prevent this. This is in agreement with the findings of other authors (Davies and Williams 1955). As regards recurrence of attacks of status asthmaticus, it is worthy of comment that 9 out of 11 patients in the cortisone group had further attacks in the three months after the trial, whereas in the control group 7 out of 14 had further attacks.

Summary

A comparison is made between the results of treating patients in status asthmaticus with antispasmodic drugs alone and with cortisone in addition to antispasmodic drugs.

All the patients were first treated for 24 hours with antispasmodics, and only those who were still in status asthmaticus were admitted to the trial.

32 patients in twelve hospitals were admitted to the trial, of whom 15 were in the cortisone group and 17 in the control group.

The patients in the cortisone group were without doubt more effectively treated than the others. By the 4th day 10 of the 15 patients treated with cortisone no longer had disabling bronchial obstruction, whereas only 4 of 17 in the control group were as well as this. At the end of the 14-day period 11 of 15 in the cortisone group, but only 4 of 17 in the control group, were free from bronchial obstruction.

Observation of the patients for three months after the trial showed that those in both groups reverted to their usual asthmatic condition ; and attacks of status asthmaticus recurred in 9 out of 11 patients in the cortisone group and in 7 out of 14 in the control group.

We wish to thank the physicians who referred cases for inclusion in the trial, and Messrs. Roussel Laboratories Limited, who very generously provided the large number of placebo tablets.

REFERENCES

Ball, K. (1954) *Lancet*, i, 1162.
Carryer, H. M., Koelsche, G. A., Prickman, L. E., Maytum, C. K., Lake, C. F., Williams, H. L. (1950) *Proc. Mayo Clin.* **25**, 482.
Davies, B. M., Williams, D. A. (1955) *Brit. med. J.* ii, 293.
Medical Research Council (1956) *Lancet*, ii, 798.
Pearson, J. E. G. (1955) *Brit. med. J.* i, 189.

Controlled trial of effects of cortisone acetate in status asthmaticus. *Medical Research Council*

BRITISH MEDICAL JOURNAL   4 MARCH 1972

585

PAPERS AND ORIGINALS

Beclomethasone Dipropionate: A New Steroid Aerosol for the Treatment of Allergic Asthma

H. MORROW BROWN,   G. STOREY,   W. H. S. GEORGE

British Medical Journal, 1972, 1, 585-590

Summary

Beclomethasone dipropionate was used in pressurized aerosols for the treatment of 60 cases of chronic allergic asthma for up to 15 months. Twenty-eight out of 37 cases were transferred to this treatment after being dependent on oral steroids for up to 16 years. Nineteen out of 23 other asthmatics not dependent on steroids were also completely controlled. No biochemical evidence of adrenal suppression was found. Steroid withdrawal symptoms were often a problem, suggesting absence of systemic absorption. The precise mode of action and metabolic fate of this corticosteroid are not yet known.

Introduction

It has been obvious since the very early days of steroid therapy for allergic asthma that the deposition of the active drug directly on to the bronchial mucosa by means of an aerosol could be an advantageous method of treatment. The drug would be delivered only at the site where it was required. The local concentration could be high, yet systemic absorption minimal and the side effects of steroid therapy avoided.

Attempts to establish this method have been the subject of reports by many investigators from Gelfand (1951) onwards, including studies by Brockbank *et al.* (1956), Brockbank and Pengelly (1958), Helm and Heyworth (1958), Herxheimer *et al* (1958), Smith (1958), Bickerman and Itkin (1963), Brown (1963), and a further publication, including a review of nine others, by Kravis and Lecks (1966). Hydrocortisone was used as powder by early investigators, and later dexamethasone phosphate in pressurized aerosols by others, with varying degrees of success. However, systemic absorption of dexamethasone with

typical steroid side effects was noted by Siegel *et al.* (1964), Novey and Beall (1965), and Toogood and Lefcoe (1965). Biochemical evidence of adrenal suppression was reported by Linder (1964). Systemic absorption of dexamethasone thus proved an insuperable problem which rendered administration of this steroid by aerosol rather pointless.

Beclomethasone dipropionate, which has already been used for some years as a topical ointment for eczema, does not suffer from this defect. This compound was used in aerosol form for the present trial.

Case Selection

Sixty patients were selected for the trial from both National Health Service and private practices. All except one were stable perennial asthmatics, as shown by observation over a period of from six months to 16 years. Sputum examination in 59 cases showed a significant excess of eosinophil cells. Intensive investigation of allergic factors and treatment, when indicated, using the methods described by Brown (1970) had been ineffective or unhelpful. Thirty-seven of the patients had been continuously dependent on steroid therapy for from 1 to 16 years, taking total daily doses of from 0·5 to 1·5 mg of betamethasone or 5 to 15 mg of prednisolone. Repeated attempts at steroid withdrawal had resulted in relapse. Thirty-five of the steroid-dependent group had previously taken part in a trial (unpublished) of disodium cromoglycate but only four had improved.

The cases were not classified as intrinsic or extrinsic, but simply as perennial allergic asthma. The extent of the reversibility of the airways obstruction in each case varied widely, and steroid-dependent patients were well indoctrinated to take the minimum dose possible. As shown in Table I 14 patients were

---

Derwent Hospital and Derby Chest Clinic, Derby
H. MORROW BROWN, M.D., F.R.C.P., Consultant Chest Physician and Allergist
G. STOREY, M.B., B.S., B.SC., Medical Registrar

Derby Hospitals
W. H. S. GEORGE, F.R.C.P., M.R.C.PATH., Consultant Chemical Pathologist

---

TABLE I—*Steroid-dependent Group (37 Patients)*

		Response to Aerosol		
Steroid withdrawal symptoms	17			
Worsening of eczema	4		Better	25
Unmasking of allergic rhinitis	5	Peak flow { No change	7
Disodium { Not tried	2	Worse	4
cromoglycate { Ineffective	31	Successful transfer to aerosol	28
{ Helpful	4	Occasionally needed short-term	
Steroid therapy side effects		steroids	13
evident	28	Failed transfer	9
{ Ineffective		Failed on account of frequent	
{ (200 units)	14	infections	2
Corticotrophin { Responsive	10		
{ Not known	13		

586   BRITISH MEDICAL JOURNAL   4 MARCH 1972

known not to respond to doses of 200 units of corticotrophin gel because of adrenal suppression. They were considered almost certainly steroid-dependent for life and this fact influenced their selection for a trial of a new mode of treatment.

The patients were therefore a miscellaneous group of proved allergic asthmatics. In 37 there was serious anxiety regarding their future because of dependence on steroid therapy and in 23 control by bronchodilators was regarded as inadequate and steroid therapy was considered inadvisable on a long-term basis.

The importance of sputum examination for eosinophils was brought home to us by the patient (Case 60) who did not have this investigation before entry to the trial. He was a 36-year-old ex-marine commando who gave a history so suggestive of mild allergic asthma of several years' duration that a search for causative allergens lasted over six months. It was then decided to give up attempts to find a cause and, as he was already using a peak flow meter, he was given the aerosol steroid. Two weeks later one of us (H. M. B.) was surprised to find that the expected increase in peak flow had not occurred. The sputum was belatedly examined and the cytological examination showed typical bronchitis with no eosinophils. The true diagnosis was, of course, early chronic bronchitis.

This case illustrates the value of examination of the sputum for eosinophils, so long as the methods described by Brown (1958) are strictly adhered to. It must be emphasized that the routine laboratory examination for eosinophils is not worth while unless the technician has been shown the simple method described.

Material and Methods

Beclomethasone dipropionate was administered by means of a metered aerosol delivering 50 μg of micronized powder per puff. The average size of the particles delivered is 5 μm, so they will penetrate to the smaller bronchi. The structural formula of this compound is:

$$CH_2 \cdot O \cdot CO \cdot C_2 H_5$$

9-α-chloro-11β,17α, 21-trihydroxy-16 -β-methylpregna-1, 4-diene-3, 20-dione, 17, 21-dipropionate

Two puffs four times daily, giving a total of 400 μg, was the usual dose, occasionally increased to three puffs four times a day. In 56 cases 400 μg was the optimum dose but four remained well controlled on 150 to 200 μg daily. This dosage regimen is empirical, and may not be optimal. Three patients changed to 200 μg twice a day and had a gradual decrease in peak flow rate, suggesting that it is best to use the aerosol at least four times daily.

Most of the patients had used pressurized aerosols for long periods. Nevertheless, it was felt necessary to give practical instruction on their use before beginning the trial. Particular emphasis was placed on preliminary complete expiration and on firing the aerosol at the very beginning of inspiration, ensuring that particles of steroid are carried on the airstream as far down the bronchi as possible. It soon became obvious that many patients had never been instructed properly.

Each patient was supplied with a Wright Peak Flow Meter for personal use four times a day, fully instructed in its use, and shown how to keep a graph of the results. In addition, a very comprehensive symptoms diary was kept which included a daily record of all types of therapy. This is shown in Fig. 1. A control

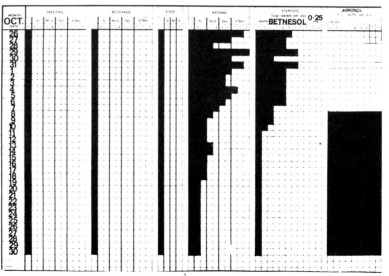

DERBY CHEST AND ALLERGY CLINIC, GREEN LANE, DERBY

Allergy Symptoms Chart, 1971

This is a new type of symptoms diary and we hope you will help us to help *you* by filling it up every day with great care.

We want you to decide how severe your symptoms are on a number scale from 0, meaning no symptoms, to 9, meaning very, very severe symptoms. As long as you do not change your mind every day, it should make sense when it is analysed by the laboratory.

For example, 1 or 2 would be slight, 3 or 4 moderate, 5 or 6 severe and 7, 8 or 9 very severe. This rating is deliberately biased to exaggerate the bad patches.

Put a cross in the correct square every night before bed, and please remember to mark the '0' squares if you have *no symptoms* or are having *no medicines*. Please keep on filling it up even on holiday. The NOTES section at the end is for entering where you are, or if you have a cold, bronchitis, etc. Please ask your doctor to enter name of tablets if not known.

FIG. 1—Child aged 9 years. This symptoms and treatment chart was introduced two years ago. It has been found that most patients are surprisingly careful in filling it in, and that the correlation with the daily counts of airborne seasonal allergens with either symptoms or treatment requirements is often remarkably close. In this case the transfer from oral steroids to aerosol is well documented. Only half the chart is shown here, other symptoms, treatment, and weather also being provided for.

ALWAYS BRING THIS CHART ON EVERY VISIT TO THIS CLINIC

Beclomethasone dipropionate: a new steroid aerosol for the treatment of allergic asthma. *Brown HM, Storey G, George WHS*

BRITISH MEDICAL JOURNAL 4 MARCH 1972 587

period of at least two weeks preceded the introduction of the aerosol. Many patients had already been keeping peak flow records for long periods as part of an intensive investigation. When the patient was seen again, if record-keeping was good aerosol therapy was started, but if record-keeping was inadequate the case was rejected as unsuitable.

In steroid-dependent patients the aerosol, 100 µg four times a day, was added to the usual daily dose of oral steroids for four days, after which the oral steroid was gradually phased out over the next three to four days. For example, a patient taking 10 mg of prednisolone daily would reduce the dose by 2·5 mg/day, or if on betamethasone 1 mg daily, by 0·25 mg/day.

Peak flow readings were averaged over at least two weeks before the aerosol was introduced, readings over periods of many months being available in those patients who were being studied intensively. The average readings after the introduction of the aerosol were taken from a two-week period beginning from two weeks after the transfer to the aerosol or from the point at which the peak flow rate had become stabilized.

Results

STEROID-DEPENDENT GROUP (37 CASES)

These 37 cases are summarized in Fig. 2 and Table I, which also shows the "side effects" encountered in introducing the aerosol. Seventeen steroid-dependent patients experienced withdrawal symptoms to a greater or lesser degree. These consisted of tiredness, lassitude, headache, aches and pains, depression, and occasionally emotional instability, lasting for a week or longer. All but three were already known not to respond to cortico-

trophin. This was so common that we soon began to warn ...ents in advance that they might have to endure all the discomforts of relative adrenal insufficiency even though their peak flow meter readings might be the same or even much better than before. No serious episodes of adrenal insufficiency occurred in any case.

Five patients complained bitterly of allergic rhinitis and four of a worsening of eczema after transfer to the aerosol steroid. This surprising finding suggests that lack of exogenous oral corticosteroid in the blood stream, contrasting with local suppression of the bronchial allergy, had unmasked latent allergic symptoms in the nasal mucosa or skin. This finding contrasts markedly with the reports of Novey and Beall (1965) and of Toogood and Lefcoe (1965), who observed (and photographed) pronounced Cushingoid effects from dexamethasone phosphate aerosols. Moonface became less evident in those in whom this side effect was prominent. One patient who had been on steroids for 10 years was delighted by the fact that many of her friends failed to recognize her in the street. On their own these effects suggest that systemic absorption of the steroid is negligible, quite apart from the results of tetracosactrin and insulin tests shown in Fig. 3.

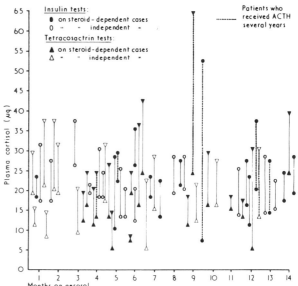

FIG. 3—Adrenal function tests in 29 patients, at up to over a year on aerosol steroid, showing the rise in plasma cortisol achieved as a result of direct and of indirect adrenal stimulation. There is no evidence of decrease in response with duration of treatment. Twelve patients had serial tests at wide intervals, again with no evidence of adrenal suppression.

We are particularly interested in this surprising effect because nasal provocation tests can still be carried out without the usual difficulty of the masking of positive results by oral steroids. Previously it had been necessary to omit steroids on the day of a provocation test.

If the patient cannot inhale enough air it follows that he cannot inhale enough aerosol of any kind for it to be effective. This simple fact should be obvious, but surprisingly this is not always so. Thus if a patient had severe airways obstruction, whether on or off steroids, it was essential to use high-dosage steroid therapy for a short time to clear the bronchi and thus allow the aerosol to become fully effective.

The best example of this type of case is illustrated in Fig. 4 which refers to a case of late-onset asthma of three years' duration in a man aged 45. During the control period he became progressively worse. As shown, the aerosol was first introduced in an attempt to gain control without using oral steroids, but it had an irritant effect, causing severe bronchospasm lasting half an hour or more, and it became obvious that oral steroids were essential. However, once his peak flow had risen markedly on oral steriods

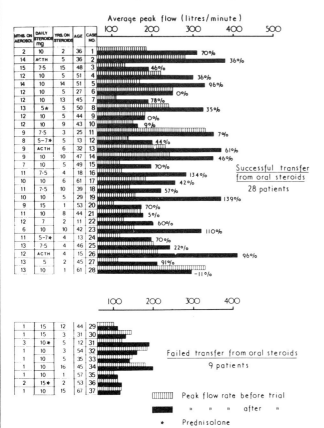

FIG. 2—Steroid-dependent group. The steroid usually preferred was betamethasone but the dosage has been expressed as an equivalent dose of prednisolone to render evaluation easier; 0·5 mg of betamethasone has been taken to equal 5 mg of prednisolone. Cases treated with prednisolone are indicated by an asterisk. Comparative averages of peak flow readings taken from two-week periods before and for two weeks after established on aerosol.

Beclomethasone dipropionate: a new steroid aerosol for the treatment of allergic asthma. *Brown HM, Storey G, George WHS*

H

BRITISH MEDICAL JOURNAL   4 MARCH 1972

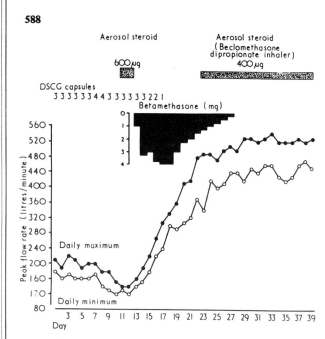

FIG. 4—Man aged 45. Late-onset asthma—allergens unknown. A good example of the uselessness of aerosol therapy until airways cleared by high-dosage steroids. Disodium cromoglycate (DSCG) had been used for a year but was no longer effective. High level maintained to date on aerosol alone. The aerosol actually caused bronchospasm when first introduced. This case is not included in the present series as the patient was seen subsequently, but it is shown on account of its outstanding interest.

it became possible to phase them out and take over control with aerosol alone.

It is relevant to mention that our normal practice in recent years has been to assess reversibility of allergic asthma under peak flow meter control by giving 4 mg of betamethasone, or 40 mg of prednisolone, daily until no further increase in readings takes place. Betamethasone has been preferred for many years for most cases, mainly because of freedom from peptic ulceration, as reviewed by Brown (1961). To assess reversibility with isoprenaline aerosols has not, in our hands, been a useful manoeuvre.

Three cases were transferred from corticotrophin and 10 were known to respond well to corticotrophin gel or long-acting tetracosactrin. It was notable that none of them had any with-

drawal symptoms. In contrast, all 14 of those known not to respond to these hormones had severe withdrawal symptoms.

The failures in both groups, as can be seen from the relatively poor peak flow, were rates in cases where a good result would have been surprising as they were already known to be almost completely irreversible. Careful exclusion of such cases would obviously have produced a much better result in this trial, but it was considered more ethical to give them a chance. Other cases of this type (Cases 6, 9, 11, 21, and 28) did not show objective improvement on aerosol, but the fact that they became independent of oral steroids was regarded as most gratifying and they were considered successful transfers.

STEROID-INDEPENDENT GROUP (23 CASES)

There were seldom difficulties in establishing these patients on the aerosol, except in the failures. The results are shown in Table II and Fig. 5. No side effects whatever were noted in this

TABLE II—23 Patients Requiring Occasional Steroid Therapy or Never Required Steroid Therapy

Intermittent steroids	16	Completely established on	
Never given steroids	7	aerosol	19
Disodium cromoglycate { Never tried ..	6	Occasional loss of control during	
Helpful ..	2	infections	4
Ineffective ..	15	Failure to transfer	4

group of cases. The failures were undoubtedly due to lack of reversibility and a dominant factor of permanent structural damage or chronic infection. Stricter selection of patients would have excluded these unfortunate patients from the trial.

A striking feature which is not illustrated or counted, and which applies to all successful cases, is the very remarkable reduction in requirement for bronchodilator drugs and aerosols. Most patients finally required only the steroid aerosol on its own. One patient commented that when he found that he had forgotten his bronchodilator one evening he did not panic as he would previously have done, and thereafter never bothered to carry it at all.

EFFECTS OF AEROSOL ON PEAK FLOW READINGS

Extreme examples of one of the major differences between the effects of oral and aerosol administration of steroids are given in

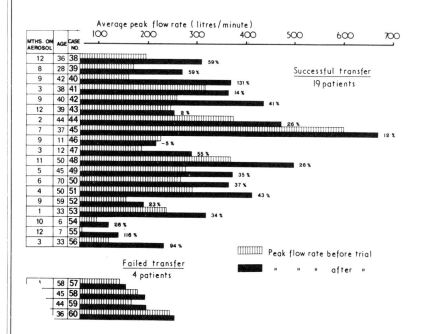

FIG. 5—Steroid-independent cases. Comparison of average peak flow readings for 14 days before and 14 days after establishment on aerosol. Case 45 would not seem severe enough to justify this treatment, but the main complaint was incessant cough which responded only to oral steroids. The cough was completely suppressed by the aerosol in 24 hours.

BRITISH MEDICAL JOURNAL   4 MARCH 1972   589

Figs. 6 and 7. This is the virtual abolition of the violent diurnal variations in peak flow which commonly occur in the labile asthmatic.

Many cases are certainly much better controlled by this aerosol than by oral steroid, a surprising finding that is possibly related to the effects of this compound on the bronchial mucosa. It should be clear that the increases in average peak flow are in many cases surprisingly great, suggesting that the local effect of the aerosol was much greater than that of their usual dose of oral steroid. The dosage which would have been required to maintain an equivalent peak flow could not have been continued on a long-term basis without serious side effects.

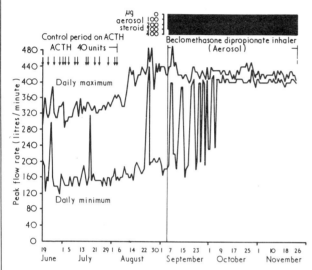

FIG. 6—Boy aged 14. Perennial asthma since age of 3. Steroid therapy for five years and transferred to corticotrophin (ACTH) two years previously. Example of abolition of diurnal variation on aerosol. Known allergens—penicillium and aspergillus. Desensitization only partly successful.

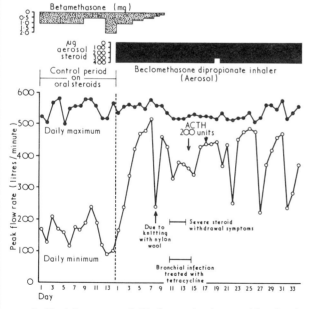

FIG. 7—Married woman aged 28. Severe chronic perennial asthmatic. Frequent episodes of status asthmaticus. Steroid-dependent six years. Usual maintenance dosage 1-1·5 mg of betamethasone. Moonface, osteoporosis, and bruising. Marked withdrawal symptoms and no response to 200 units of corticotrophin gel. Allergens unknown, but coal-tar derivatives strongly suspect. Swings of peak flow from 60 l./min at 6 a.m. to 600 l./min at 6 p.m. were a constant feature of this patient on oral steroids. Subsequently proved difficult to maintain on aerosol alone because of frequent infections.

USE OF AEROSOL STEROID IN CHILDREN

We are most impressed with the results in nine children who were trained to use a pressurized aerosol from the age of 6. Five had been on oral steroids, with serious effects on growth, for periods of some years before referral, and attempts to identify the responsible allergens were unsuccessful so that there was no prospect of cessation of steroids. Resumption of growth was remarkable, two children gaining 2 in (5 cm) in six months and another 3 in (7·5 cm) in a year. Measurements on the others were unfortunately omitted but growth had obviously been resumed. Control of the asthma was complete in four of the cases; the other child was liable to frequent infections. Unmasking, or increase in, atopic manifestations such as eczema has been troublesome in two cases.

The four children who were not steroid-dependent were all markedly improved and completely controlled. One of the striking examples is illustrated in Fig. 8, where serial records of

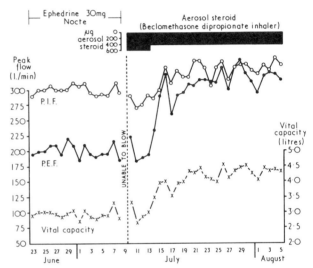

FIG. 8—Boy aged 12. Chronic perennial asthma five years. Never required steroids but seemed likely to do so just before aerosol began. Allergens unknown in spite of extensive investigation. Wright Respirometer used for serial vital capacity measurements. Peak inspiratory flow obtained by use of peak flow meter modified according to Nairn and McNeill (1963). Note the effects of the aerosol on the peak expiratory flow which soon becomes almost equal to the peak inspiratory flow.

peak inspiratory and expiratory flow, using a meter modified according to Nairn and McNeill (1963), and also vital capacity, using a Wright Respirometer, were obtained, thanks to the very high degree of co-operation from his mother. The relationships of these measurements as shown are of great interest.

EVIDENCE OF LACK OF SYSTEMIC ABSORPTION

Tetracosactrin tests and insulin hypoglycaemia stress tests, as described by Landon et al. (1963), were carried out in 27 cases and the results are presented in Fig. 3. Plasma cortisol was estimated by the method of Mattingly (1962). Two or more serial adrenal function tests were carried out at intervals of from 6 to 14 months in 12 patients. We would have preferred to do more serial tests, but for a multiplicity of reasons this was impossible. However, in none, whether steroid-dependent or not, was there any evidence of adrenal suppression with either type of test.

Apart from the biochemical data, the steroid withdrawal symptoms and the unmasking of allergic manifestations can be reasonably assumed to indicate absence of significant absorption

Beclomethasone dipropionate: a new steroid aerosol for the treatment of allergic asthma. *Brown HM, Storey G, George WHS*

590   BRITISH MEDICAL JOURNAL   4 MARCH 1972

of the aerosol steroid. Serial liver function and full blood examinations have disclosed no abnormality in any of the cases.

In order to obtain further evidence regarding possible adrenal suppression three volunteer subjects inhaled excessive quantities of the aerosol daily for two days, following several daily basal cortisol estimations. The results are shown in Fig. 9, and from

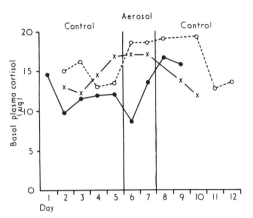

FIG. 9—Effects of inhaled beclomethasone dipropionate on the morning basal cortisol. An aerosol delivering 250 µg per puff was used eight times a day, for two days, in one healthy volunteer (X-X) and a patient (●-●), who had already been on 400 µg daily for six months. Another volunteer (O - - - O) took 4 mg daily for two days.

this it is clear that in at least three subjects there is no evidence whatever of the occurrence of adrenal suppression in higher dosages than have been used normally in the treatment of patients.

Conclusions and Discussion

Beclomethasone dipropionate aerosol would seem to provide an alternative to long-term oral steroid therapy in many cases of chronic perennial asthma. Effective control of the asthma is achieved with no evidence of systemic absorption or of steroid side effects. The exact mode of action of this compound remains to be fully elucidated.

The best results are in the younger and more reversible cases. The abolition of diurnal fluctuation is a surprising feature. It is possible to substitute this therapy for long-term oral steroids even when taken for many years. Steroid withdrawal symptoms, and unmasking of hitherto suppressed allergic manifestations, have presented interesting problems.

Selection of pure allergic asthmatics, or cases where the allergic factor is dominant, is a sine qua non of this, or any other,

trial of a steroid preparation in allergic asthma Care has been taken to exclude seasonal cases, where daily fluctuations of airborne allergens can cause wide variation in peak flow.

It cannot be overemphasized that these patients are in a precarious condition in the event of trauma or infection. It is essential that they be instructed to resume oral steroids in high dosage without delay, when obviously necessary, without waiting for medical advice. They must carry warning cards clearly indicating their potentially dangerous situation.

Such serious problems do not arise in relation to patients who have had only occasional steroid therapy, or have never required it. On the data presented here there seems to be no contraindication to the use of this preparation by mild asthmatics who would not normally be considered for the use of corticosteroids. As many of them had already failed to respond to disodium cromoglycate this new therapeutic approach may have much to offer, especially in paediatrics. In all types of case considerable clinical expertize and experience of the management of allergic asthma may be required during the transfer period.

This method of treatment has no place whatever in status asthmaticus. Those unable to inhale air surely cannot inhale enough aerosol to have any effect. The presence of excess bronchial mucus and often pus must also form a barrier the aerosol cannot penetrate. The future role of aerosol therapy is clearly confined to maintenance of airway patency and prevention of attacks.

Thanks are due to Dr. David Harris, of Allen and Hanburys Limited, for the supply of aerosols and for much additional help, and to the Midlands Asthma and Allergy Research Association, Derby, for facilities and help with the illustrations.

References

Bickerman, H. A., and Itkin, S. E. (1963). *Journal of the American Medical Association*, **184**, 533.
Brockbank, W., Brebner, H., and Pengelly, C. D. R. (1956). *Lancet*, **2**, 807.
Brockbank, W., and Pengelly, C. D. R. (1958). *Lancet*, **1**, 187.
Brown, H. M. (1958). *Lancet*, **2**, 1245.
Brown, H. M. (1961). *British Journal of Clinical Practice*, **15**, 1001.
Brown, H. M. (1963). *Lancet*, **2**, 147.
Brown, H. M. (1970). *British Journal of Clinical Practice*, **24**, 513.
Gelfand, M. L. (1951). *New England Medical Journal*, **245**, 293.
Helm, W. H., and Heyworth, F. (1958). *British Medical Journal*, **2**, 765.
Herxheimer, H., McAllen, M. K., and Williams, D. A. (1958). *British Medical Journal*, **2**, 762.
Kravis, J. P., and Lecks, H. I. (1966). *American Journal of Diseases of Children*, **3**, 343.
Landon, J., Wynn, V., and James, V. H. T. (1963). *Journal of Endocrinology*, **27**, 183.
Linder, W. R. (1964). *Archives of Internal Medicine*, **113**, 655.
Mattingly, D. (1962). *Journal of Clinical Pathology*, **15**, 374.
Nairn, J. R., and McNeill, R. S. (1963). *British Medical Journal*, **1**, 1321.
Norman, P. S., *et al.* (1967). *Journal of Allergy*, **39**, 57.
Novey, H. S., and Beall, G. (1965). *Archives of Internal Medicine*, **115**, 602.
Siegel, S. C., *et al.* (1964). *Pediatrics*, **33**, 245.
Smith, J. M. (1958). *Lancet*, **2**, 1248.
Toogood, J. H., and Lefcoe, H. M. (1965). *Journal of Allergy*, **37**, 321.

INHIBITION OF EXPERIMENTAL ASTHMA BY A NEW COMPOUND
—DISODIUM CROMOGLYCATE "INTAL". (R) *by* R. E. C. ALTOUNYAN,
Fisons Pharmaceuticals Limited, Holmes Chapel, Cheshire.

Asthma was induced in an atopic subject (RECA) by the inhalation
of mixed pollen antigens. The dose of antigen inhaled was adjusted so
that the FEV_1 fell by a maximum of approximately 45 per cent in
control experiments.

The activities of anti-allergic compounds were assessed by comparing
the FEV_1 changes which occurred during control and test experiments
conducted at intervals of 3–4 days.

Over the past nine years a large number of compounds have been
examined for anti-allergic activity by this method; of these disodium
cromoglycate, Intal ®, showed outstanding protective activity when inhaled before antigen challenge.

The maximum protection (70 per cent) occurred at an estimated
dose of 1.0 mg or more inhaled as an aqueous aerosol ten minutes before
antigen; some protection (40 per cent) was, however, observed at a
dose as low as 0.15 μg.

When the time interval between drug inhalations and antigen challenge was extended to 2 hours no protection was observed with the
lower dose although some protection was still evident following a dose
of 1.0 mg. A single clinical dose (20 mg) inhaled as a micronised powder from a specially designed appliance afforded greater than 50 per
cent protection for at least 6 hours.

By contrast, inhalation of the compound even one minute after
antigen was less effective and no protective effect could be detected
when Intal was inhaled 15 minutes after antigen challenge.

Inhibition of experimental asthma by a new compound
disodium cromoglycate "intal". *Altounyan REC*

J

SEPTEMBER 9, 1967   ORIGINAL ARTICLES   THE LANCET   539

A DOUBLE-BLIND TRIAL OF DISODIUM CROMOGLYCATE IN THE TREATMENT OF ALLERGIC BRONCHIAL ASTHMA

J. B. L. HOWELL
M.B., Ph.D. Lond., F.R.C.P.
CONSULTANT PHYSICIAN, ROYAL INFIRMARY, MANCHESTER, AND SENIOR
LECTURER IN MEDICINE, UNIVERSITY OF MANCHESTER

R. E. C. ALTOUNYAN
M.B. Cantab.
OF THE RESEARCH DEPARTMENT, FISONS PHARMACEUTICALS LIMITED,
HOLMES CHAPEL, CHESHIRE

Summary   A double-blind cross-over sequential trial of a new antiallergic compound, disodium cromoglycate (' FPL670 ', 'Intal ') was carried out over a period of 6 weeks in ten patients severely disabled with allergic bronchial asthma. There was a significant clinical improvement during administration of FPL670 plus isoprenaline in all patients compared with two periods in which isoprenaline alone was given. Spirometric improvement occurred in only four patients. Subsequent experience over periods up to 26 months with these and other patients has confirmed the therapeutic value and safety of FPL670 in the management of allergic bronchial asthma.

Introduction

IN 1965 a new compound, disodium cromoglycate (' FPL 670 ', ' Intal ', 1,3-bis[2-carboxychromon-5-yloxy]-2-hydroxypropane, disodium salt), was found to be effective in reducing the asthmatic response to inhaled antigen in sensitised individuals (Altounyan 1967). The protective effect, which persisted for several hours, was greatest when the compound was inhaled before the antigen challenge; the drug was ineffective when inhaled a few minutes after the antigen challenge. FPL670 has no intrinsic bronchodilator-type or corticosteroid-type activity and it does not antagonise histamine, slow-reacting substance of anaphylaxis (S.R.S.-A.), or other known spasmogens. A preliminary report of the pharmacology and toxicology of FPL670 will be published elsewhere (Cox 1967).

These observations suggested that FPL670 might be useful in the prophylaxis and treatment of allergic asthma. The short-term effect was investigated in twelve patients with severe chronic allergic asthma, whose symptoms were poorly controlled by even high doses of corticosteriods, and in whom the dangers of side-effects were causing serious concern. In this pilot study there was rapid, and in some cases striking, symptomatic improvement, particularly in the severity and frequency of acute attacks, cough, and sputum volume. However, in only five patients was this improvement accompanied by an increase in the forced expiratory volume in the first second (F.E.V.$_1$) greater than 20% of control values.

In view of this lack of consistent correlation between the apparent symptomatic improvement and spirometric measurements, it was considered desirable to carry out a double-blind trial to reduce bias both of patient and of observer.

Patients and Methods

Patients

Patients were considered suitable for the trial if: (1) severe symptoms persisted despite conventional bronchodilator and corticosteroid therapy; (2) a smear of sputum, stained by the method of Lendrum (1944), contained one or more clumps, each containing at least five eosinophils; (3) they were willing to cooperate in the trial, which necessitated regular and fre-

L3

A double-blind trial of disodium cromoglycate in the treatment
of allergic bronchial asthma. *Howell JBL, Altounyan REC*

540   SEPTEMBER 9, 1967   ORIGINAL ARTICLES   THE LANCET

TABLE I—DETAILS OF TEN PATIENTS IN DOUBLE-BLIND TRIAL OF FPL670

Case no.	Age (yr.)	Sex	Height (in.)	Weight (lb.)	Duration of severe symptoms (yr.)	Family history of atopy	Hospital admissions for asthma during past year	Minimum maintenance dose of prednisone (mg. per day)
1	35	M	70	155	15	+	0	12·5
2	47	M	67½	154	3½	−	0	10
3	45	M	72	167	1¼	+	2	15
4	55	M	70	132	1½	−	3	20
5	30	F	62	118	24	+	1	10
6	48	M	72	202	½	−	0	15
7	62	M	66½	164	¾	−	4	20
8	42	F	65	112	1	−	2	20
9	48	F	65½	131	6	+	4	15
10	45	F	62	118	½	+	4	15

quent attendances for assessment; and (4) they were able to assess carefully and record symptoms twice daily on a specially designed questionary.

Patients fulfilling these criteria were invited to participate in a trial of a new treatment for asthma. They were told that while short-term toxicity trials of the new compound in animals and in twelve volunteers had shown no toxic effects, long-term investigation had not yet been completed.

Of the patients approached, one refused the invitation and one patient who accepted was not included in the final analysis because of a severe exacerbation during the control period. Details of the ten patients in the trial are shown in table I.

Experimental Design

Statistical.—The restricted sequential procedure employed (Armitage 1960), was designed on the following basis: (1) that the result obtained would be significant at the 5% level ($p < 0.05$); (2) that there was a high probability ($1 - \beta = 0.95$) of detecting a true difference between the response to routine treatment and the response to drug; (3) that, in nine cases out of ten, the response would be in favour of drug: ($\theta_1 = 0.90$); (4) that patients who showed no preference for either drug or routine treatment would be excluded; (5) that the maximum number of preferences needed to give a result in favour of drug, or in favour of routine treatment, or to show no significant difference between the two is nineteen ($N = 19$).

Procedure.—The trial extended over three consecutive periods, each of 2 weeks. The patients were instructed to continue their usual treatment throughout the trial and not to alter their steroid dosage other than by increasing it appropriately should a severe exacerbation occur. They were told that they would receive, in addition, capsules containing powder to be inhaled at approximately 6-hourly intervals (4 daily) from a special inhaler ('Spinhaler'). In the first 2 weeks the powder would contain only a known bronchodilator and the purpose of this initial practice period was to enable them to become proficient in the use of the spinhaler and in the completion of their daily record charts. The capsules for this period were of clear gelatine and contained 0·1 mg. isoprenaline sulphate diluted with lactose. The control period will hereafter be referred to as isoprenaline (control). During each of the next 2-week periods (periods A and B) they would receive pink-coloured capsules which were identical in appearance, but would contain a different preparation. Patients were asked not to comment on any difference which they might notice in the taste or physical properties of each preparation lest this should influence the assessor. Both preparations contained 0·1 mg. isoprenaline in lactose but only one contained FPL670 (20 mg.). The order in which patients received each preparation was randomised. These two periods will hereafter be referred to as isoprenaline (test) and FPL670, respectively.

Clinical and laboratory assessment.—Each morning and evening patients assessed the severity of breathlessness on exertion, frequency of attacks at rest during the day and night, morning tightness, cough, sputum volume and its character, and the number of times they had used their usual broncho-

dilator aerosol. Each week the patients were interviewed individually about their symptoms and any untoward effects. They also received a full physical examination. In a separate laboratory the resting PCO_2 was measured by a rebreathing method (Campbell and Howell 1960), followed by the vital capacity (V.C.), and F.E.V.$_1$, before and after isoprenaline. Sputum smears were examined for eosinophils and polymorphonuclear leucocytes. Blood was taken before and after the trial for routine hæmatological examination, hepatic-function tests, and determination of serum-electrolytes and blood-urea.

Assessment of Response to Treatment

The design of the trial required one of us (J. B. L. H.) to decide whether each patient was better during period A or period B, or whether there was no significant difference between the two. His decision was based on evidence obtained from interview and from examination of the patient, together with inspection of the daily record charts. It is important to note that the objective laboratory measurements which were made throughout the trial were not known to the physician at the time of his assessment and therefore did not influence his decision.

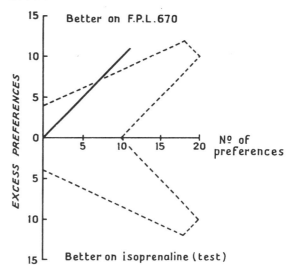

Fig. 1—Sequential analysis of results of trial.

Results

Physician's Assessment

In each case, the assessing physician had no difficulty in deciding that the patient's condition was better during one period than the other. When ten patients had completed the trial the first analysis was made. It was then found that all the preferences were in favour of FPL670 and it will be seen from the sequential analysis graph (fig. 1) that the sample path crossed the upper boundary at the seventh preference. The exact probability of this result, being due to chance, is 0·016. The trial was therefore terminated.

Analysis of Changes in Symptoms

Each subjective symptom was recorded on a 5-point scale, except for attacks of breathlessness at rest and bronchodilator-aerosol usage, where actual numbers were recorded. The total score for each item was found for each 2-week period. A difference in the score of 7 or more was arbitrarily chosen as indicative of significant change, except for bronchodilator usage for which a difference of 28 doses was considered to be significant.

Results are shown graphically in figs. 2–4 where the number of patients recording a significant change in symptom scores during the three periods of the trial are

SEPTEMBER 9, 1967   ORIGINAL ARTICLES   THE LANCET   541

TABLE II—F.E.V.₁ MEASUREMENT IN TEN PATIENTS

Case no.	F.E.V.₁ (l.) in week* no.:						% change in F.E.V.₁ during administration of FPL670	No. of symptoms improved during FPL670 administration compared with placebo iso-prenaline (test)
	1	2	3	4	5	6		
1	0·51	0·54	*0·49*	*0·51*	0·47	0·49	+4	5
2	0·74	0·76	0·60	0·56	*0·87*	*0·98*	+60	1
3	0·84	0·95	*1·16*	*1·57*	1·41	1·38	−2	2
4	0·65	0·43	*1·44*	*1·14*	0·85	0·89	+48	4
5	1·43	1·68	*1·65*	*1·68*	1·76	1·53	+1	3
6	0·68	1·00	*0·98*	*1·06*	0·89	..	+14	4
7	0·83	1·03	0·79	0·78	*0·87*	*1·08*	+24	2
8	..	0·56	1·05	0·81	*1·00*	*0·89*	+2	6
9	1·68	2·06	2·39	1·97	*2·33*	*8·63*	+15	4
10	0·54	0·62	0·89	0·44	*0·81*	*0·95*	+32	6

* Weeks 1 and 2 are control period, weeks 3 and 4 are period A, and weeks 5 and 6 are period B. Figures in italics refer to the period in which FPL670 was given.

† % change is calculated from the mean values obtained during each of the two periods:

$$\% \text{ change} = \frac{\text{FPL670} - \text{Isoprenaline (test)}}{\text{Isoprenaline (test)}} \times 100.$$

compared. There was no significant difference between the symptom scores during isoprenaline (control) and isoprenaline (test) periods. The ten patients had a total of 19 items which improved during the isoprenaline (test) period and 23 items improved during the control period (fig. 2).

By contrast, a striking difference in the patient's condition was observed during the period on FPL670 compared with both the isoprenaline periods. Comparing FPL670 with isoprenaline (control) (fig. 3), 39 items improved during FPL670 administration and only 4 items improved during the control period. Similarly, comparing FPL670 with isoprenaline (test) (fig. 4)=37 items improved during drug period and only 1 during the test period.

No single patient showed improvement in all of the items assessed, neither did any patient fail to show any improvement in at least 1 item. Morning tightness, nocturnal attacks, attacks at rest during the day, and use of bronchodilator aerosol were the items most frequently improved during FPL670 administration.

Analysis of Laboratory Measurements

Spirometry.—F.E.V.₁ measurements are shown in table II. V.C. measurements showed corresponding changes, and are not recorded. Only four of the ten patients showed a change greater than 20% in the F.E.V.₁. However, these patients did not show a greater number of symptoms improved during drug administration, when compared with those patients showing little or no change in F.E.V.₁.

Other tests.—Pco₂ values showed no significant change throughout the trial. There were no abnormal changes in the biochemical and hæmatological results obtained before and after completion of the trial.

Untoward Events

No untoward event was reported by any patient or observed by the physician during the trial.

Discussion

Initially we were concerned lest the difference in taste between isoprenaline (test) and FPL670 (which is slightly bitter) should influence the result. However, we believe that this did not happen, because: by chance, half of the patients received FPL670 in period A yet there was no difference in their symptom response to isoprenaline (test) compared with that in patients receiving FPL670 during period B; the patients derived an immediate subjective response from the isoprenaline content of both preparations, and this was consistent with their original briefing that they were comparing two forms of treatment, both of which were active; and, when questioned after completion of the trial three patients (cases 3, 4, and 5) had not detected any difference in taste between capsules

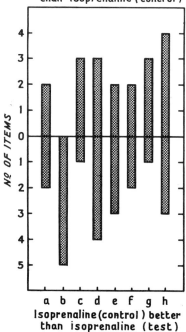

Fig. 2—Number of patients showing significant changes in symptom scores while receiving isoprenaline (test and control).

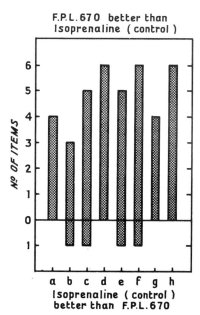

Fig. 3—Number of patients showing significant changes in symptom scores while receiving isoprenaline (control) and FPL670.

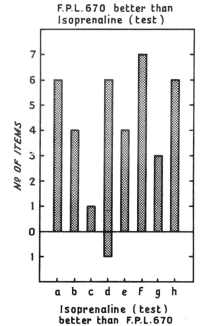

Fig. 4—Number of patients showing significant changes in symptom scores while receiving FPL670 and isoprenaline (test).

A double-blind trial of disodium cromoglycate in the treatment of allergic bronchial asthma. *Howell JBL, Altounyan REC* and there was no difference in their pattern of symptomatic improvement from the other patients.

The consistent improvement in subjective symptoms during FPL670 administration contrasts with the variable objective spirometric changes. This disparity implies that the symptoms of asthma are not due solely to increase in airways resistance; indeed, there is no *a priori* reason why such symptoms as cough, sputum, morning tightness or intermittent attacks of breathlessness at rest should be reflected in a change in isolated " spot check " values of the F.E.V.$_1$. Furthermore, the persistence of reduced F.E.V.$_1$ values, despite full bronchodilator, corticosteroid, and FPL670 therapy, suggests that factors other than allergy were causing residual airways obstruction.

The results of this study indicate that reliance on simple spirometry alone would have led to a failure to recognise the therapeutic value of FPL670 in six of the ten patients.

Although the primary aim of the trial was to study whether FPL670 was active in the treatment of asthma, it became evident that the compound was of considerable therapeutic value to these patients, at least in the short term. This was confirmed when all of the patients elected to continue with FPL670 therapy, which they received continuously for the next 12 months. A placebo was then substituted on a single-blind basis, deterioration occurred in all cases, which was reversed when FPL670 therapy was recommenced.

Since completing this double-blind trial we have used FPL670 for the treatment of over two hundred patients with mild to severe allergic and non-allergic airway disease. In over a hundred of these patients treatment has extended for periods of 6 to 26 months. The degree of benefit afforded to individual patients has varied considerably. No toxic effects have been noted and we believe that FPL670 is a major advance in the management of allergic airway disease.

We thank Dr. A. Adelstein for his help and advice with the statistical aspects of the trial; Dr. J. E. McIver and Mr. H. Varley and their staff at Manchester Royal Infirmary for the hæmatological and biochemical measurements; Miss Bernice Coombs for her technical assistance and Dr. J. S. G. Cox, research director, Fisons Pharmaceuticals Limited for his interest and support throughout the study.

REFERENCES

Altounyan, R. E. C. (1967) *Acta allerg.* (in the press).
Armitage, P. (1960) Sequential Medical Trials. Oxford.
Campbell, E. J. M., Howell, J. B. L. (1960) *Br. med. J.* i, 458.
Cox, J. S. G. (1967) Unpublished.
Lendrum, A. C. (1944) *J. Path. Bact.* **56**, 441.

A double-blind trial of disodium cromoglycate in the treatment of allergic bronchial asthma. *Howell JBL, Altounyan REC*

1328   NATURE. VOL. 216, DECEMBER 30, 1967

Disodium Cromoglycate (FPL 670) ('Intal'*): a Specific Inhibitor of Reaginic Antibody–Antigen Mechanisms

CHROMONE derivatives exhibiting unusual biological activity have been studied in these laboratories for several years. One of these, disodium cromoglycate (FPL 670), has been found to inhibit specifically the liberation of the mediators of anaphylaxis initiated by the interaction of antigen with reagin type antibodies. It is neither a bronchodilator nor an anti-inflammatory agent and its action is distinct from that of corticosteroids.

In experiments on an asthmatic volunteer, inhaling the compound inhibited the acute effect of subsequent antigen inhalation[1]. In patients suffering from allergic asthma, inhalation of this compound was followed by clinical improvement[2].

Disodium cromoglycate is the sodium salt of 1,3-bis-(2-carboxychromon-5-yloxy)-2-hydroxypropane. It is an odourless, white, hydrated crystalline powder moderately soluble in water but practically insoluble in alcohol. Physical investigations (elementary analysis, infrared, ultraviolet, nuclear magnetic resonance and mass spectra) were consistent with the assigned structure

The compound inhibited the passive cutaneous anaphylactic (PCA) reactions in monkeys, sensitized with human reaginic serum, when the compound was given intradermally with the antigen, but did not affect the skin reactions to intradermal histamine, 5-hydroxytryptamine or bradykinin. Antigen induced bronchoconstriction in anaesthetized marmosets, sensitized intravenously with human reaginic serum, was substantially reduced by disodium cromoglycate.

Homologous PCA reactions with reagin-like antibody in rats, using both the egg albumen/B. pertussis[3] and Nippostrongylus brasiliensis[4] systems, showed substantial inhibition in the presence of the compound. Although the compound inhibited the PCA reaction it failed to affect the skin lesions induced by compound 48/80.

In contrast, in guinea-pigs, homologous PCA reactions with precipitating antibody were unaffected, as were aerosol or intravenous antigen induced bronchospasm and the release of histamine and SRS-A (slow reacting substance–anaphylaxis) from actively or passively sensitized lung in vitro.

The release of histamine and SRS-A from portions of chopped human lung, passively sensitized with human reaginic serum, has been measured after exposure to specific antigen(s) in vitro[5]. Inhibition with disodium cromoglycate was found over a narrow range of concentrations.

In an in vitro system in which contractions of human bronchial chain, exposed to passively sensitized and shocked human lung, were used to simulate the supposed events in an attack of allergic asthma, FPL 670 at 10 μg/ml. caused a significant reduction (40 per cent) in the contractile response.

It was considered important to study the effect of the compound on those antibody systems concerned with immunity. No adverse effect was found on several in vitro virus/antibody neutralizing systems including influenza A, polio virus type II, vaccinia and herpes simplex with human and rabbit antisera.

Likewise no effect was found on the LD_{50} in mice of mouse adapted polio virus, nor on their protection by

* Trade mark—Fisons Pharmaceuticals, Ltd.

Disodium comoglycate (FPL 670) ('Intal'*): a specific inhibitor of reaginic antibody-antigen mechanisms. *Cox JSG*

NATURE, VOL. 216, DECEMBER 30, 1967 1329

Salk vaccine. No effect was observed on the neutralization of *Clostridium welchii* type A α-toxin by specific antiserum nor on the cytotoxic behaviour of rabbit anti-HeLa on HeLa cells *in vitro*. Nor did it interfere with any of the several bacterial agglutinating systems tested.

Further *in vivo* work was carried out on the effect of the compound on the passive protection of guinea-pigs with diphtheria antitoxin, on the development of immunity and response of immune mice to pneumococcus and on the development of experimental tuberculous lesions in guinea-pigs. In addition, an examination was made of the rate of production of antibody and the titre achieved in monkeys to T_1 coliphage. In all these *in vivo* systems no change in the normal pattern was observed over the range of doses administered.

Disodium cromoglycate has few general pharmacological effects. Relatively large doses (up to 100 mg/kg) given intravenously, intraperitoneally or to the cerebral ventricles in conscious animals from a wide range of species produced negative or only weak non-specific effects in various behavioural studies. Only in the dog were marked effects observed, intravenous injection of moderate doses (for example, 8 mg/kg) causing immediate collapse and transient apnoea with rapid recovery.

In studies of anaesthetized animals, large doses of disodium cromoglycate had only weak inconsistent effects on the cardiovascular and respiratory systems of the cat, pig, monkey, guinea-pig and rat. In anaesthetized dogs, doses as small as 10 μg/kg elicited reflex mechanisms originating in the pulmonary and coronary circulations producing bradycardia, hypotension and in some cases apnoea. In marmosets, however, the compound caused a rise in blood pressure and heart rate with little effect on respiration.

Studies with the new compound on bronchial tone in anaesthetized guinea-pigs demonstrated little activity. It had no direct action on human bronchial chain nor did it antagonize the responses to histamine, SRS-A or acetylcholine. The compound showed no significant effect in several anti-inflammatory tests nor did it have any consistent influence on the anti-inflammatory activity of hydrocortisone.

Disodium cromoglycate had no significant effect on several other functions studied including steroid metabolism, gastrointestinal mobility and urine and bile flow. It had little effect on the ciliary activity of either isolated frog oesophagus or human bronchial epithelium. The compound had no direct action on Trendelenburg's reflex of isolated guinea-pig ileum, neither did it antagonize the response of the ileum to histamine, 5-hydroxytryptamine, acetylcholine, nicotine, substance P, bradykinin or SRS-A.

The absorption, distribution and excretion of disodium cromoglycate have been studied in a variety of laboratory animals. Following oral administration, only a very small proportion (less than 0·5 per cent) of the dose was absorbed. After inhalation of the powder aerosol, only a small proportion of the dose reached the peripheral lungs, a major part being trapped in the upper respiratory tract. Plasma and lung tissue levels indicated that the powder reaching the peripheral lungs was rapidly and completely absorbed. The compound was rapidly eliminated, the major portion unchanged, via the urine and bile; no accumulation could be detected in any tissue even after repeated daily intramuscular injections. Studies of the urinary excretion and plasma levels in human volunteers have suggested that the same general pattern applies in man.

Disodium cromoglycate has been shown to be relatively non-toxic. Thus in *in vitro* tests a concentration of at least 5 mg/ml. was required to produce effects on the morphology of HE$p2$ cells and chick embryo fibroblast cells, and on the migration of guinea-pig macrophages. In acute toxicity tests in small laboratory animals, the LD_{50} on parenteral administration was usually between 2,000 and 4,000 mg/kg, while in a prolonged test in rats no toxic effect resulted from ninety daily subcutaneous injections, except at doses greater than 30 mg/kg. The only pathological lesion produced in any of these tests was an inflammation and degeneration of the renal tubules. Neither this nor any other toxic effect was found in 90-day inhalation studies.

No teratogenic effects were seen in rabbits in which the compound was given intravenously daily throughout pregnancy in doses up to 250 mg/kg.

Disodium cromoglycate had few general pharmacological effects, was rapidly excreted and seemed to have a low order of toxicity. The compound appeared to inhibit specifically the anaphylactic process initiated by reaginic antibody–antigen interactions. This novel property may permit a more specific treatment of allergic disease, especially of the lung, and will undoubtedly contribute to basic knowledge in these areas.

The results given here represent the combined efforts of the staff of the Research Departments at Holmes Chapel too numerous to name individually.

I wish to thank Dr Geoffrey Taylor, of Manchester Royal Infirmary, for valued advice and work on immunological problems, and Dr A. J. O'Hea, Robroyston Hospital, and Dr L. G. Bruce, Victoria Infirmary, Glasgow, who performed the study on tuberculous infection.

J. S. G. Cox

The Research Laboratories,
Fisons Pharmaceuticals, Ltd.,
Holmes Chapel,
Cheshire.

Received October 5; revised October 30, 1967.

[1] Altounyan, R. E. C., *Acta Allergologica* (in the press).
[2] Howell, J. B. L., and Altounyan, R. E. C., *Lancet*, ii, 539 (1967).
[3] Mota, I., *Life Sci.*, 1, 465; ibid., 917 (1963).
[4] Ogilvie, B. M., *Nature*, 204, 91 (1964).
[5] Sheard, P., Killingback, P. G., and Blair, A. M. J. N., *Nature*, 216, 283 (1967).

PROPHYLACTIC INOCULATION AGAINST HAY FEVER.

BY L. NOON, B.C. CANTAB., F.R.C.S. ENG.

(*From the Laboratory of the Department for Therapeutic Inoculation, St. Mary's Hospital.*)

HAY fever is a form of recurrent catarrh affecting certain individuals during the months of May, June, and July. It is caused by a soluble toxin found in the pollen of grasses. The patients present the idiosyncrasy of being sensitive to this toxin, which is innocuous to normal individuals. The idiosyncrasy may be detected during any season of the year by dropping a little of an extract of grass pollen into the eye of the suspected individual ; a reaction, described more fully below, will be obtained in the case of a hay fever patient, but a normal man will show no effect.

Bostock (1819)[1] recognised the seasonal recurrence of hay fever as separating it from other forms of catarrh. Blackley (1873)[2] advanced much evidence in favour of the pollen theory of its causation, but we owe chiefly to Dunbar (1903)[3] the exhaustive scientific proof of this theory. Dunbar showed that not only all the mucous membranes but even the skin of hay fever patients is sensitive to pollen toxin in a way not shown by normal individuals. He also proved that the injection of the pollen toxin gives rise in animals to the production of an antitoxin having a specific power of neutralising this toxin. Further, in hay fever patients, he showed the occurrence of some of the reactions associated with the production of immunity :—namely, a specific precipitation of pollen extracts by the patient's serum, and the phenomenon of complement deviation, during the hay fever season, and persisting for a short time after this. Pollen toxin is, therefore, a body capable of giving rise to the production of antibodies in animals and even in hay fever patients, subjected to its action. It is also undoubted that hay fever patients sometimes become cured of their idiosyncrasy. The most reasonable explanation of this phenomenon would seem to be, that the cured patients have had the good fortune to develop an active immunity against the toxin, to the action of which they have been liable for so long.

The repeated absorption of toxin at short intervals is, however, more likely to induce a condition of hypersensibility, and this is the more usual fate of the patient, who becomes only more sensitive during each succeeding season. The local application of a specific serum, such as pollantin, offers a reasonable method of treatment, but one which is difficult and laborious, and which is not calculated to bring about a permanent cure. Cures are, indeed, ascribed to the use of this remedy, but admittedly in exceptional cases ; and where the conditions are not understood and the experience is not constantly repeated, one must hesitate to attribute the result to the cause cited. On general grounds a much more satisfactory result would be expected from the induction of an active immunity, and it seemed worth while to put this expectation to the test of experiment. The questions to be answered are as to what degree of immunity can be induced in hay fever patients by inoculations of pollen toxin, how these inoculations may best be regulated, and whether the affection can by this means be permanently cured.

With this end in view the experiments here described were undertaken in the past autumn, winter, and spring to study the reaction of hay fever patients towards inoculations of pollen toxin. The off season of the year, when the patients were not exposed to spontaneous inoculations, was favourable to this investigation, as the scheme of dosage was then not liable to be upset by spontaneous absorption of toxin from the air, laden with actively poisonous pollen grains. The plan of experiment was to obtain a numerical measure of the sensitiveness of the patients to the pollen toxin and to observe whether this was increased or decreased by subcutaneous inoculations of various quantities of pollen toxin. These observations can be conveniently carried out by the method described below, and it was found that, with well-regulated dosage, it was possible in every case to raise the patient's resistance, to a marked degree, within the lapse of a few months, while, on the other hand, ill-regulated dosage was at once made evident by a decrease in the resisting power.

The pollen extract used was prepared by Dunbar's method of extraction with distilled water, aided by freezing and thawing several times. The extracts were boiled for ten minutes after having been sealed in glass tubes ; this treatment was not found to decrease their activity at all. The pollens tested were grass pollens of different species— *Phleum pratense*, *Poa trivialis*, *Holcus lanatus*, and *Agropyrum caninum*. These pollens were all found capable of exciting an energetic reaction when instilled into the conjunctival sac of hay fever patients. Timothy grass (*Phleum pratense*) was found to yield the most active extract, and this extract was consequently used throughout the rest of the experiments. One gramme of pollen was extracted with 50 c.c. of water. The activity of this extract may be judged from the fact that one drop of a five thousand-fold dilution is sufficient to excite a distinct reaction in the conjunctiva of the more sensitive patients.

In order to express the strengths of pollen extracts used in testing patients and the doses of pollen toxin given subcutaneously, a unit of pollen toxin has been arbitrarily chosen. This unit is the quantity of pollen toxin which can be extracted from the thousandth part of a milligramme of Phleum pollen, and it has the advantage that all the quantities used can be expressed in whole numbers. The strength of a pollen extract is given below in terms of the number of such units contained in a cubic centimetre of the extract. Extracts of other pollens have been standardised against the Phleum extract by comparative tests on the eyes of hay fever patients.

A measure of the patient's resistance during the experiments is obtained by observing the strength of pollen extract necessary to excite a conjunctival reaction. One drop of the diluted extract is instilled into the eye. The reaction obtained consists in a reddening of the caruncula and, to a lesser degree, of the palpebral conjunctiva, together with a slight injection of the vessels of the ocular conjunctiva and some lacrymation. The patient experiences a feeling of burning and itching. These signs reach a maximum in about five minutes, and a little later there may be a slight attack of sneezing. The reaction lasts as a rule about half an hour. The strength of the extract, which is just sufficient to give this reaction, is used to describe the resistance of the patient. The most sensitive patients examined gave before treatment a distinct reaction with a dilution containing only 4 units per c.c., their resistance is described as 4 ; the least sensitive reacted to a strength of 70 units per c.c., or, in other words, had a resistance of 70. Normal individuals fail to react with the strongest extract (strength 20,000 units) and even resist the application of fresh pollen dust to the conjunctiva. Their resistance is therefore, by our scale, more than 20,000, but it is not infinite as a cubic centimetre of this extract injected beneath the skin of a normal man has been

[1] John Bostock : Medical and Chirurgical Transactions, vol. x., 1819, p. 161.

[2] C. H. Blackley : Experimental Researches on the Causes and Nature of Catarrhus Aestivus, London, 1873.

[3] W. P. Dunbar : Zur Ursache und specifischen Heilung des Heufiebers, München, 1903.

found to give rise to a slight local swelling and tenderness, lasting for about 24 hours.

Course of immunisation.—Patients received subcutaneous injections of pollen extract. At first very minute doses were given at intervals of three or four days (Fig. 1), and the resistance of the patients rose rapidly; on increasing the dose, however, it was found that the resistance ceased to rise and even went back towards its original value. Longer intervals were then allowed to elapse between successive

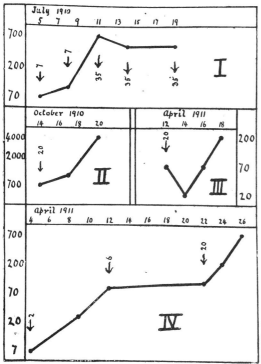

The numbers at the sides denote the resistance of the patient, given in terms of the strength of pollen extract, one drop of which was sufficient to excite a conjunctival reaction. The arrows indicate subcutaneous inoculations of pollen extract, quantities given in the units described in the text. Figs. 1 and 2 refer to one patient at different periods of treatment; Fig. 3 shows the response obtained after about a month's treatment in another case; and Fig. 4 the early stages of treatment.

inoculations. The patient to whom Fig. 1 refers had a three months' respite and, after that interval, responded to a moderate dose in the way shown in Fig. 2. It is not necessary, however, to leave such a long interval as this between the doses: ten days or a fortnight are, as a rule, sufficient, and at the beginning of treatment, when small doses are being given, a week is enough (Fig. 4). After some time, when the resistance has been considerably raised, small doses cease to have any effect. On increasing the dose it is found that the first effect of the inoculation is to lower the resistance for a few days, giving a *negative phase*, after which the resistance rises again and passes beyond its former maximum (Fig. 3). Ultimately a stage is reached at which the resistance, as measured by the ocular test, ceases to rise, or rises so slowly that the alteration is only obvious after prolonged observation. At this stage the patients will withstand gradually increasing subcutaneous inoculations without showing a negative phase. In the early stages of immunisation it is possible, by an overdose, to induce a severe attack of hay fever lasting nearly 24 hours; this has not been observed in the later stages.

The result of these experiments so far is to show that the sensibility of hay fever patients may be decreased, by properly directed dosage, at least a hundredfold, while excessive or too frequent inoculations only serve to increase the sensibility. It still remains to be seen whether the immunity thus attained is sufficient to carry the patients through a season without suffering from their annual attacks of hay fever. Patients are under observation who have undergone treatment for periods varying from a few weeks to eight months.

It is hoped that these cases will afford material for a

further report after the present hay fever season. This work is now in the hands of my colleague, Dr. J. Freeman, who very kindly came to my assistance and carried on the observations during my enforced absence of some months.

Devonshire-place, W.

814 THE LANCET,]   DR. J. FREEMAN: THE TREATMENT OF HAY FEVER, ETC.   [SEPT. 16, 1911.

FURTHER OBSERVATIONS ON THE TREATMENT OF HAY FEVER BY HYPODERMIC INOCULATIONS OF POLLEN VACCINE.

BY J. FREEMAN, M.D. OXON.

(*From the Laboratory of the Department for Therapeutic Inoculation, St. Mary's Hospital.*)

THIS paper is the sequel to Mr. L. Noon's paper on Hay Fever in THE LANCET of June 10th, 1911, in which was described research work for treatment by hypodermic inoculations of pollen toxin.

Previous Work.

Dunbar had described a simple ophthalmo-reaction as a diagnostic test for that susceptibility to pollen which constitutes hay fever; a watery extract of pollen of a certain strength dropped into the eyeball of a normal man produces no effect, but will cause a miniature attack of hay fever in susceptible persons. The test is quantitative in nature, and by noting the dilution of pollen which will just cause the eye to react it is possible to obtain some measure of the patient's susceptibility. Changes in susceptibility presumably have an inverse correlation with changes in immunity to the pollen toxin, and Noon applied this quantitative test to the study of changes in immunity produced by subcutaneous inoculations of pollen vaccine. In this way he demonstrated that *suitable* doses of pollen toxin increased the patient's immunity, while unsuitable doses either did not affect, or even decreased, this immunity; this brings the pollen inoculation work into line with the bacterial inoculation work of Wright and his school. These points established, Noon set to work to immunise hay fever patients during the off season in preparation for the season which we have just passed through. Unfortunately, circumstances compelled him to give up work last February, and the research passed into my hands; it is now possible to tabulate some laboratory data about these and subsequent inoculated hay fever cases, and also to give the clinical results of the treatment as disclosed by the past summer season.

Laboratory and Clinical Evidence in Table.

Explanation of table.—Adjoined is the tabulated list of the 20 cases treated on this system by hypodermic inoculations of pollen toxin; it is important to note that the list is not a collection of flattering "unsolicited testimonials," but gives an account of every case which had any systematic treatment, excluding only one or two people who were seen once and then lost sight of.

The first column gives the reference number of each case. The cases are arranged in the order in which they arrived for treatment; those who were already suffering from hay fever when they first presented themselves are marked with an asterisk.

The second column gives the dates of the beginning and end of treatment; these dates refer especially to the parallel figures in the next two columns.

The third column gives the state of pollen-immunity as judged by the ophthalmo-reaction at these dates. The unit of measurement here employed was explained fully by Noon in his paper last June; it is convenient shortly to redescribe it here. The quantitative measurement of the ophthalmo-reaction is made by noting the weakest dilution of pollen extract of which one drop, when dropped on the eyeball, will just produce a slight flushing of the inner canthus of the eye. The unit of measurement is a one-millionfold dilution of Phleum pratense pollen in water—which is spoken of as one unit of pollen, or shortly as 1 U.P. Thus, a hundred-thousandfold dilution of pollen would equal 10 U.P., a thousandfold dilution would equal 1000 U.P., and so on.

The fourth column gives the hypodermic doses of pollen extract which were used at these two dates respectively; these doses are also given in terms of pollen units, 1 U.P. being 1 cubic centimetre of the millionfold extraction, or, to put it another way, the amount of pollen toxin extracted from one-millionth of a gramme of Phleum pratense pollen.

The fifth column gives a short summary of the fate of the patients during the hay fever season this year as reported by the patients or their friends.

In the sixth column I sum up my own impression of the case.

Laboratory evidence in table.—In studying this tabulated list of inoculated cases, the first point to be noted is the increased tolerance of pollen toxin which was produced by the inoculations in every case. This is shown in Column 3 by the ophthalmo-reaction which the patient gives at the beginning and end of treatment; and as the personal equation, the "functional error," of the observer enters very little into the results of this reaction, it is claimed that this change in the ophthalmo-reaction represents an undoubted change in the immunity of the patient.

Then, again, it is clear from Column 4 that the doses also were increased. Now, it was found by experiment that it

THE LANCET,]　　　DR. J. FREEMAN: THE TREATMENT OF HAY FEVER, ETC.　　[SEPT. 16, 1911.　815

was impossible at the commencement of treatment to give much larger inoculations than those indicated in the list without producing symptoms of an overdose—symptoms clinically, and as noted in the laboratory by a falling off in the ophthalmo-reaction. If the dose *were* increased markedly, one might produce even in mid-winter such unpleasant things as swelling, pain, and urticaria at the site of inoculation, a general malaise, and all the nose and eye symptoms of a thorough attack of hay fever. Yet as immunisation progressed it was found by repeated ophthalmo-reactions that larger doses could be given with advantage, and though some of these were enormously greater than the initial dose, they were given without any clinical symptoms and without lowering the ophthalmo-reaction.

As denoted by the asterisks, most of the people, at the end of the list were already suffering from hay fever when they came, but it was found that in these cases also there was an increase in immunity and an increase in the dose employed. The original scheme was one of prophylactic immunisation, and this was much more suitable for the preliminary research work because the effects of each dose could not be obscured by chance doses of pollen from the atmosphere; but clearly phylactic inoculations are of more use if only they will answer reasonably well. At first thought it might be argued that phylactic doses of pollen toxin will only add poison to an already poisoned patient, but this objection is no more valid in the treatment of hay fever than it is in the treatment of boils by staphylo-

Case.	Month and year.	Resistance.	Dose.	Patient's opinion.	Writer's opinion.
1	July, 1910. May, 1911.	40 U.P. 5000 U.P.	4 U.P. 2000 U.P.	Extremely bad with hay fever for last four years. Inoculated persistently during the off season; stopped treatment in May. Tested well, but absolutely immune.	Eminently satisfactory.
2	July, 1910. (Did not continue.)	40 U.P.	2 U.P.	Refused treatment owing to article on anaphylaxie. Had hay fever worse than ever this year.	(Satisfactory.)
3	Sept., 1910. May, 1911.	20 U.P. 400 U.P.	4 U.P. 120 U.P.	Inoculated irregularly and also with two bacterial vaccines. Had hay fever, but probably not so bad as formerly, and was sooner over.	Disappointing.
4	Feb., 1911. May, ,,	20 U.P. 170 U.P.	6 U.P. 25 U.P.	Certainly much better, though not clear of hay fever.	Fairly satisfactory.
5	March, 1911. June, ,,	40 U.P. 400 U.P.	18 U.P. 20 U.P.	Has been practically free from hay fever this season, but has felt "on the verge of it" once or twice. Went in hay fields, motored, &c. (which was impossible formerly).	Satisfactory.
6	March, 1911. June, ,,	40 U.P. 1000 U.P.	12 U.P. 100 U.P.	"Have had no hay fever this year, except one attack lasting an hour after walking through a hay field, and no asthma. In former years had bad hay fever for at least six weeks and asthma at night."	Eminently satisfactory.
7	April, 1911. July, ,,	6 U.P. 1000 U.P.	2 U.P. 18 U.P.	"I think I may fairly say that though I had it pretty badly occasionally, it was not in so severe a form nor so easily excited. Susceptibility diminished, perhaps one-third. Effects less pronounced in the same proportion."	Inconclusive.
8	May, 1911. June, ,,	13 U.P. 170 U.P.	4 U.P. 20 U.P.	"Quite a marked improvement, if not an absolute cure."	Moderately satisfactory.
9	May, 1911. June, ,,	40 U.P. 500 U.P.	4 U.P. 25 U.P.	This case was handicapped by the inoculations being given rather irregularly. "The attacks were less violent on the whole, and certainly did not last so long."	,,
10*	May, 1911. June, ,,	130 U.P. 170 U.P.	4 U.P. 10 U.P.	Did not improve after several inoculations, and as he could with difficulty spare the time he decided to postpone the treatment for prophylaxis in the winter.	Failure.
11	May, 1911. July, ,,	13 U.P. 170 U.P.	1½ U.P. 10 U.P.	Had a little sneezing, but was clear of hay fever most of the time—probably not a very severe case. He reported, "the cure still continues to work marvellously."	Satisfactory.
12	May, 1911. June, ,,	40 U.P. —	4 U.P. 10 U.P.	"I do not want to boast, but I think I am quite done with the accursed thing for this year. There can be no sort of doubt, seeing the kind of season it has been, that I should have suffered, and that severely, if I had not had these inoculations."	,,
13*	May, 1911. June, ,,	5 U.P. 17 U.P.	1 U.P. 5 U.P.	"I *did* have a return of the hay fever after the cure" (i.e., three inoculations), "but only slight, and have not had it for over three weeks now."	,,
14*	May, 1911. July, ,,	170 U.P. 500 U.P.	10 U.P. 15 U.P.	"Since the inoculations began I have had practically no running at the eyes and nose, nor do my eyes get bloodshot."	Fairly satisfactory.
15	June, 1911. June, ,,	170 U.P. 500 U.P.	10 U.P. 300 U.P.	A Canadian who gets bad hay fever in August, but not earlier. Has had none this year up to date.	No test.
16*	June, 1911. June, ,,	17 U.P. 170 U.P.	1 U.P. 6 U.P.	"She is certain that the condition improved after the third, and she thinks it was better after the second dose. Afterwards she had very little return of symptoms till treatment was discontinued, when there was a slight return."	Satisfactory.
17*	June, 1911. July, ,,	5 U.P. 50 U.P.	1 U.P. 6 U.P.	Reported a distinct improvement after the second and third doses, and had no hay fever after the fourth.	,,
18*	June, 1911. July, ,,	170 U.P. 1700 U.P.	10 U.P. 50 U.P.	Reported himself very much better after the second dose, and was clear of hay fever from June 16th onwards.	,,
19*	June, 1911. June, ,,	5 U.P. 17 U.P.	1 U.P. 3 U.P.	"The hay fever inoculations, although I came to you having hay fever rather severely, did me an immense amount of good, and I intend next spring … "	Fairly satisfactory.
20*	June, 1911. July, ,,	17 U.P. 150 U.P.	1 U.P. 5 U.P.	"First inoculation (given during severe attack) gave immunity for two days. Second gave complete immunity from Monday till Sunday. Third (rather stronger than before) brought on attack which lasted three days. I have perfect confidence in its power of giving immunity if the right strength is found."	Satisfactory.

Thus, Columns 3 and 4 both denote an increase in pollen immunity during treatment. This increase as here shown varies partly no doubt with the individual, but also with the thoroughness with which the inoculations were undertaken. It might be thought that both an increased ophthalmo-reaction and tolerance of an increased dose were tests of the same thing, and that therefore they must run parallel; this was not the case. At the commencement of treatment the dose could not with advantage be increased as rapidly as the increase of the ophthalmo-reaction, while at the end of treatment there was a tendency to a sticking-point in the ophthalmo-reaction, but the dose could gradually be made larger without producing symptoms either clinical or laboratory.

coccus vaccine; the answer is the same in both cases. Though it may or may not be true that at the seat of the disease the tissues are over-poisoned, yet the rest of the body may, under the stimulus of an inoculated vaccine, respond by an increased production of antibodies; this surmise is justified when it is found that such an inoculation *is* followed by a demonstrable increase in immunity.

It is claimed that this increase in immunity produced by pollen vaccine is in itself the best proof of the soundness of this line of treatment, whether prophylactic or phylactic. It is true that one does not know if this increase is sufficient for all purposes, but the change is certainly in the right direction, and must be doing good.

Further observations on the treatment of hay fever by hypodermic inoculations of pollen vaccine. *Freeman J*

Clinical evidence in table.—In judging a system of treatment by "results" there are obvious sources of error which should be taken into account; and in criticising Column 5 let us give due weight to (1) the natural bias of the operator; (2) the bias of the patient; and (3) outside circumstances—i.e., luck, affecting the result. Every medical man so desires that his patient's condition shall be improved by his treatment that there is a constant tendency to detect such improvement in adventitious fluctuations of health. To avoid this danger most of the results were summarised for me either by the patients or their friends. On the patient's side there is also the desire for improvement, reinforced by the impression made on the mind by a rather novel system of treatment and a certain atmosphere of "science." As a set-off to such faith-healing, most of the patients had undergone several "cures" which they had been told were infallible, and they therefore submitted themselves to treatment in a critical, sceptical, or even hostile spirit. There is another point: any one who works at hay fever research will have a highly intelligent and critical material to work with—a very high proportion of the people in the above list have been accustomed by their position or employment to give discriminating judgments. Lastly, luck, or outside circumstances; was this year a better year for hay fever patients? Apparently not. The general, though not universal, opinion seems to be that the season was, on the contrary, more severe than usual—that it began and ended earlier. As some test of the season many of the patients were urged to select another hay fever case as similar as possible to themselves as a control case for observation; all these controls had much worse hay fever than the inoculated patient.

Considering all the cases generally, there seems little doubt that there has been a distinct amelioration of symptoms. This improvement took several forms; a greater freedom from attack, the attack not so bad as in former years, and the attack sooner over, the constitutional disturbance not so great, less asthma. The people who had already developed hay fever when they commenced treatment were, perhaps, the most generous in their comments, possibly because they had recently had a reminder of what hay fever was like.

Application of Treatment.

Diagnosis.—It remains to be considered how this treatment is to be turned to account prophylactically next winter and spring, and phylactically next summer. Whatever the treatment, the diagnosis is important; though an uncomplicated case will usually present no difficulty, yet it is sometimes convenient to have a test of susceptibility to pollen toxin, and this is almost a necessity when prophylactic inoculations are to be commenced in the off season. But there are many reputed cases of hay fever which are partly, and even wholly, caused by a bacterial infection; indeed, it seems probable that an attack of hay fever may be the starting point of a bacterial infection, or that a catarrh of the air passages may predispose to hay fever, and before treatment of any kind it is essential to disentangle these two factors. During the present research several so-called hay fever cases were excluded from treatment because the eyeball was unaffected by pollen toxin—one of these confessing to malingering, and the remainder being the victims of bacterial infections. A case treated by a colleague is a good illustration of the value of a diagnostic test. A lady reported to have hay fever had slightly inflamed eyes which streamed with clear tears; as she did not react to pollen toxin hay fever was excluded. The tears were found to be swarming with staphylococci, a vaccine was made, and in a short time the symptoms disappeared.

In the list of cases treated last season the first ophthalmo-reaction will be seen to vary between 5 U.P. and 170 U.P.; those who did not react to 5000 U.P. were said to give a negative test; there were no unaccountable cases—i.e., people whom subsequent events proved to have been negative giving a positive result, and *vice versâ*.

Initial dose.—Whether or no the help of such a test is required in fixing the diagnosis, it will at any rate be required in fixing the initial dose, should vaccination treatment be decided on. Noon suggested as a suitable initial dose one-third of a cubic centimetre of that dilution of pollen toxin which gives the ophthalmo-reaction. On this plan a man giving a diagnostic reaction of 6 U.P. would receive 2 U.P. hypodermically, and a man who reacted to 100 U.P. would receive 33 U.P. This seems to be about correct, or perhaps to err on the side of over-dosing, especially when hay fever is already developed. In this connexion it should be said that the cases in the tabulated list are not all to be taken as models, as experience was being gathered all the time. In addition, there were several deviations from the ideal course to suit special circumstances.

Subsequent doses.—The patient was, as a rule, re-inoculated every week or ten days: the larger doses were given after a longer interval, while the very small doses were repeated after three or four days. Those cases which were being treated phylactically usually finished treatment with the fifth or sixth dose, the prophylactic inoculations were naturally much more numerous, as an attempt was being made to produce as high an artificial immunity as possible.

All these doses were determined on with the assistance of ophthalmo-reactions. These were taken not only at the time of inoculating but also frequently between the doses; and it is urged that whenever this is possible it enables the operator to mark the success of his treatment, to detect mistakes, and, if necessary, to adapt his doses to the idiosyncrasies of his patient. Clearly that dose should be selected which will give the greatest increase to the immunity of the patient; if a dose or a series of doses fails to increase the patient's immunity as measured by the ophthalmo-reaction, then it is to be presumed that the dose is either too small to be efficient or so large as to be over-dosing the patient, and this latter will be the case if the resistance of the patient is not only not increased but is even diminished after the doses. As a result of such tests it was generally found advisable not to increase the dose quite as rapidly as the increase in the ophthalmo-reaction, at any rate at first. Later in the process of immunisation the ophthalmo-reaction ceased to rise so quickly, and it was sometimes possible to regain the 1 : 3 ratio between the dose and the reaction. Lastly, in the case of very highly immunised patients—e.g., Case No. 1—the ophthalmo-reaction at last became stationary, but the dose was still increased.

It is, perhaps, possible by the ophthalmo-reaction to detect three stages in immunisation. In the first stage favourable doses are followed by an immediate rise in resistance, but should not be followed by a corresponding increase in the size of the next inoculation. In the second stage a larger dose is required, giving first a slight negative phase followed by a slow rise in immunity. In the final stage the eye reaction becomes stationary, but apparently the doses may be increased with advantage so long as there is no evidence, either laboratory or clinical, of an overdose.

Rule-of-thumb inoculations.—Owing to the nature of hay fever there is no danger to life and only temporary danger to health by inoculating "blindly"—i.e., without controlling the doses by ophthalmo-reactions; but it is thought that in order to make a diagnosis and to fix the first dose, at least one eye-testing will be necessary. As a rule-of-thumb, the second and third doses seemed to be usually half as much again as the first dose, while the fourth, fifth, and sixth are perhaps twice as much as the first, though in several cases the size of the dose was increased more rapidly than this.

Pollen supply.—With regard to the pollen extract necessary for testing the eye and for injecting as a vaccine, Dunbar's method of extraction is to be followed. The brief directions given by Noon in the previous paper should enable anyone, who has sufficient time and a laboratory, to construct his own pollen dilution. This will prove inconvenient to many, and it is proposed that the Inoculation Department of St. Mary's Hospital shall make arrangements to put these dilutions of pollen toxin on the market through Messrs. Parke, Davis, and Co., the proceeds to go to the upkeep of the department as in the case of their bacterial vaccines.

A final word as to the species of pollen employed. Noon selected that of timothy grass (Phleum pratense), because the pollen of this grass gave in his hands the strongest extract as tested on the eyes of the patients. This spring I tested various pollens as they matured, rushes, sedges, grasses, &c., but none gave so strong an extract as this timothy grass. The pollen of Alopecurus pratensis gave good results, but only possessed one-quarter the strength of Phleum pratense. The grasses and flowers dreaded by the hay-fever patients differ considerably in different cases, and the question arises—Is one kind of pollen more active in one case and another in another case? Though the question cannot be regarded as settled, apparently this is not so. For one reason, the ratio between the strength of, say, a phleum extract and an alopecurus extract remains about the same with different patients—i.e., 4 : 1. Furthermore, a patient inoculated with alopecurus pollen vaccine is found to become immune to the phleum pollen extract as tested by the ophthalmo-reaction. Apparently, therefore, we need not select different types of pollen for treating different patients.

Devonshire-place, W.

MAXIMUM FORCED EXPIRATORY FLOW RATE AS A MEASURE OF VENTILATORY CAPACITY

WITH A DESCRIPTION OF A NEW PORTABLE INSTRUMENT FOR MEASURING IT

BY

B. M. WRIGHT, M.A., M.B.

National Institute for Medical Research, Mill Hill, London

AND

C. B. McKERROW, M.D., M.R.C.P.

Pneumoconiosis Research Unit (Cardiff),
Llandough Hospital, Penarth, Glam

The use of a single forced expiration as a method of assessing ventilatory capacity is becoming increasingly popular, mainly because, as pointed out by Kennedy (1953), it is a much simpler and less tiring procedure than the maximum voluntary ventilation (M.V.V.).

The basis of most of the various single-breath methods is the same: the volume of air expired is measured against time by means of a spirometer with either a recording drum or a timing device. There are some differences of opinion about the most suitable interval of time over which to measure the volume and about the relative merits of a recording drum or a timing device, but it is generally agreed that methods of this kind are clinically valuable and give results which are comparable

Maximum forced expiratory flow rate as a measure of
ventilatory capacity with a description of a new portable
instrument for measuring it. *Wright BM, McKerrow CB*

with those of the M.V.V. All the methods, however, suffer from the disadvantage that the necessary apparatus is cumbersome and normally requires connexion to an electric supply. Attention has therefore been directed to the possibility of using the maximum forced expiratory flow rate (or "peak flow rate"), instead of what is in effect the average for a limited time, as a measure of ventilatory capacity; such a measurement seemed likely to lend itself to the use of a simpler instrument, consisting merely of a flowmeter with a device for recording the maximum.

According to Donald (1953) the empirical use of a measurement of this kind is very old. "The physician of the last century who asked a patient with respiratory disease to whistle or blow a candle out was crudely assessing the maximum respiratory velocities" (sic). Donald suggested that a "simple, whistle-like instrument" might be developed and might become a standard clinical tool.

In this paper an instrument of this kind is described, but first it may be useful to give an account of the maximum forced expiratory flow rate as a physiological measurement.

Historical

Apart from the rather vague reference quoted by Donald the earliest systematic attempt to use the peak flow rate as a physiological index was that of Hadorn (1942), who measured the flow rate on expiration by means of an aneroid manometer connected across a simple orifice. The resistance of the system was high, as much as 32 cm. of water at a flow of 500 l./min., and no provision was made for recording the maximum deflection of the manometer pointer except judging it by eye. The highest flow rates he recorded were about 500 l./min. Wyss (1950) used the same type of orifice as Hadorn, but recorded the pressures photographically, using a membrane manometer and an optical lever. This gave a permanent record and a higher frequency response. He registered flow rates as high as 720 l./min.

The basic method used by both these workers has the disadvantage that the pressure drop across a simple orifice varies as the square of the flow rate, with the result that the higher flows are considerably reduced, thus cramping the scale of the measurement. In addition the sensitivity of the method at low flow rates is low, giving an unsatisfactory logarithmic scale. Nevertheless, an instrument of this kind has been produced commercially and has been the basis of a number of studies of the relationship between the maximum forced expiratory flow rate and the vital capacity (Hildebrandt and Hanke, 1956). The instrument, called a "pneumometer," incorporates an aneroid manometer fitted with a device for recording the maximum flow rate. Rates up to about 700 l./min. can be recorded.

Of recent years the use of improved forms of pneumotachograph (Silverman and Whittenberger, 1950; Lilly, 1950) has led to many observations of the expiratory flow pattern, but no systematic attempt to use the peak flow rate as a physiological measurement in its own right appears to have been made. Moreover, although the pneumotachographs themselves have had very low resistances (of the order of 2 mm. $H_2O/100$ l./min.) which gave a linear relationship between flow and pressure, for some reason which is not clear they seem to have sometimes produced a considerable reduction in peak flow rate in healthy normal men. For instance, Shephard (1955), measuring peak flow rates during a forced expiration in "healthy young adults," recorded none higher than 427 l./min., and one of only 183 l./min. in an apparently healthy man of 25. Similarly, Leuallen and Fowler (1955) found no flows higher than 660 l./min. in a group of normal males; and Comroe, Forster, Dubois, Briscoe, and Carlsen (1955) quote 500 l./min. as a "typical figure" for a "maximum expiratory flow rate." In their table of "normal values," however, they quote a figure of 400 l./min. and make it clear that this is averaged over a volume of one litre. In contrast, as will be seen, we have found that peak flow rates over 700 l./min. are common in adult males and flows up to nearly 1,000 l./min. by no means rare. To measure such flows it has been necessary to make use of an enlarged version of the Lilly pneumotachograph with connexions of very wide bore. Details of this instrument are given later.

For two reasons it is desirable to measure the peak flow rate in such a way as to get the maximum possible figure. In the first place, the higher the figures given by normals the more clearly they are differentiated from the abnormals, whose relatively low flow rates are less affected by resistance, especially if it is non-linear in type. Secondly, one important advantage of the peak flow rate as a physiological index is that it is relatively easily understood and defined. Respiratory physiology is beset with measurements which are peculiar to the instrument and the laboratory where it is made (Comroe et al., 1955), and therefore it is highly desirable that, if possible, a measurement should be absolute, and clearly defined, so that it will be the same however and wherever it is measured.

Both the earlier and the latest forms of pneumotachograph suffer from the disadvantage of being fairly complicated and not easily portable. A much simpler and more robust and portable instrument, designed specifically for measuring the peak flow rate, has been described by Goldsmith and Young (1956) and called by them the "puffmeter." It is of basically the same design as the Lilly and Silverman pneumotachographs, but uses a robust ceramic grinding wheel as a linear resistance and an aneroid manometer to measure pressure.

It appears to suffer from two disadvantages; the pressure drop across the resistance is relatively high, about 1 cm. $H_2O/100$ l./min., and the maximum reading has to be read off from a presumably rapidly moving hand on a dial. Nevertheless, Goldsmith (1958) has used it extensively, and by calibrating it empirically against a pneumotachograph he has obtained a considerable body of data about peak flow rates. Unfortunately, his results are all given in "puffmeter" units, which are admitted to be much lower than the actual flow measured with a pneumotachograph. He calibrated the puffmeter by connecting it to the outlet of a Lilly pneumotachograph, using peak flows varying from 100 to 700 l./min. produced voluntarily by one individual; from this he claimed to be able to estimate the true figures. His mean values for a "normal reference population" aged 40–65 and free of all apparent respiratory disability, translated into absolute units in this way, were about 600 l./min. for men and 450 l./min. for women. These results are difficult to compare with our own because of the very wide age group for which they are given, but they appear to be compatible with them.

Before we became aware of the pneumometer or of Goldsmith's work with the puffmeter, a quite different

Maximum forced expiratory flow rate as a measure of ventilatory capacity with a description of a new portable instrument for measuring it. *Wright BM, McKerrow CB*

type of instrument was developed for the same purpose. It seems to have some advantages over the pneumometer and the puffmeter in that it is simpler and more easily portable, and has a lower resistance at high flow rates.

The Peak Flow Meter (P.F.M.)

This instrument operates on different principles from any used hitherto for this purpose, being of the class of flowmeter known as a " variable area orifice meter," of which the best-known example is the rotameter (see Linford, 1949).

This type of meter has a number of advantages for respiratory measurements. It can make use of the fact that, although only a small resistance can be tolerated, an expiration has large volume, so that a very simple and robust instrument can measure rapidly changing flows with quite sufficient accuracy. Although the pressure drop at low flow rates is higher than that of plain orifice-type instruments it rises only ten times over the whole range from 100 to 1,000 l./min., so that at high flow rates the resistance is comparable to that of Goldsmith's puffmeter.

The principle of operation of the instrument is illustrated diagrammatically in Fig. 1. A cylindrical cavity about 5 in. (12.7 cm.) in diameter and 1⅜ in. (3.6 cm.) deep has a radial inlet nozzle (1), and contains a movable vane (2) pivoted in the centre of the cylinder and fitted closely without touching. A fixed partition (3) extends from one side of the inlet orifice to within a short distance of the boss of the vane, but again does not touch it. A spiral spring (4) attached to one end of the spindle of the vane tends to rotate it towards the

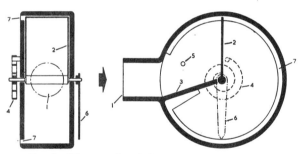

FIG. 1.—Diagram of peak flow meter. For key see text.

inlet orifice, a stop (5) preventing it from passing the orifice. A pointer (6) on the other end of the spindle indicates the position of the vane on a dial (not shown) and also serves to counterbalance it. An annular orifice (7) extends round the periphery of the cylinder at the back, from one side of the inlet orifice to the other.

It can be seen that when air is blown into the instrument it cannot escape (except for a small amount which leaks past the vane) until the vane has moved and uncovered part of the annular orifice. When the area of orifice uncovered is such that the pressure behind the vane is just sufficient to balance the force of the spring, the vane will come to rest in a position which will depend on the flow rate. Since for a given pressure the rate of flow is proportional to the area of the orifice, the deflection of the vane would be proportional to the air flow if the tension of the spring were constant. In practice, the tension of the spring increases with the deflection, so that the deflection is proportionately less at high flows than at low. This has the effect of

increasing the range of the instrument without loss of sensitivity at the lower end of the range, so that flows from 50 to 1,000 l./min. can be covered in one instrument.

The instrument is fitted with a ratchet which holds the vane and pointer in the position of maximum deflection. They can be returned to zero by pressing a release button.

The general appearance of the instrument, which weighs about 2 lb. (900 g.), and its method of use are shown in Fig. 2. The subject is asked to take a deep breath, as for a vital capacity, to place the mouthpiece in his mouth, and then to blow into the instrument as hard as he can. It is not necessary to try to empty the lungs, and it is undesirable to do so, because it is unpleasant and tiring, but a certain amount of "follow through" is required. After a couple of practice blows, three attempts in succession are recorded and the average is taken. This is statistically a more satisfactory procedure than

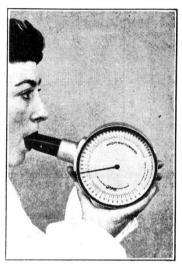

FIG. 2.—Peak flow meter, showing method of use.

simply taking the highest reading, although logically the latter would be preferable, since a maximum is being measured. Most subjects will give three readings which agree within 10% after the practice tries, but the observer must ensure that the subject is really trying his hardest. As with all ventilatory tests of this kind, including the M.V.V., failure to produce reasonably concordant readings usually indicates lack of co-operation.

The instrument is supplied with a plastic mouthpiece, which can be easily removed for washing and sterilization. Disposable cardboard mouthpieces are also available. A removable coarse-mesh gauze in the inlet nozzle prevents the ingress of large particles of sputum, etc.

Performance Tests

The P.F.M. was originally developed as a largely empirical device, and it has only recently been possible to arrange for satisfactory physical and physiological testing. Two forms of calibration have been used—with steady and with transient flows.

Steady-flow Calibration

Because of its low resistance the instrument can be easily calibrated by simply blowing air through it in series with a rotameter. Calibration in this way of an instrument with a dial graduated in degrees gives a curve of the form shown in Fig. 3. The curve does not pass through the origin, because even when the annular orifice is completely shut off there is some leakage round the vane ; a certain minimum flow is therefore needed to deflect the vane against the spring. The exact

Maximum forced expiratory flow rate as a measure of
ventilatory capacity with a description of a new portable
instrument for measuring it. *Wright BM, McKerrow CB*

calibration of the instrument in this range is thus liable to be much affected by the accuracy of construction, so that steady-flow calibration is a convenient method of checking this point. Fig. 3 also shows the relationship between flow rate and pressure

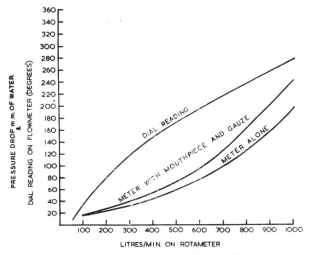

FIG. 3.—Steady flow calibration curve of peak flow meter and pressure/flow curves with and without inlet gauze and mouthpiece.

drop through the instrument. At low flow rates the pressure drop is relatively high, but it rises only slowly with increasing flow rate. At high flow rates the fixed orifice component of the resistance comes more and more into play and the pressure drop increases more steeply. The additional resistance of the mouthpiece and gauze, of which the latter is the main component, is also more important at higher flow rates; this additional resistance has been found to be an advantage in practice, as it makes the instrument more comfortable to blow into, and it does not appreciably affect even high peak flows.

Transient-flow Calibration

The only instrument which can be used to test the ability of the P.F.M. to measure very transient flows is a pneumotachograph. As already noted, the one we have used is an enlarged version of that described by Lilly (loc. cit.), and gives an approximately linear response to flows up to 1,000 l./min. It has a resistance of 400-mesh gauze, 4 in. (10.2 cm.) in diameter, giving a pressure drop of 1 mm. $H_2O/100$ l./min. The entry and exit cones connect to tubes $1\frac{1}{4}$ in. (3.2 cm.) internal diameter, and the subject blows through a mouthpiece connected to the instrument by 10 in. (25.4 cm.) of hose of $1\frac{1}{2}$ in. (3.8 cm.) internal diameter. The overall pressure drop through the complete instrument, including the mouthpiece, is 1.5 cm. H_2O at 700 l./min.

A capacitance manometer is used to convert the pressure into an electric signal, which is suitably amplified and recorded by a "mingograf" spray writing pen. This instrument has a high-frequency response which sometimes makes its records difficult to interpret owing to the amount of "noise" recorded. It is therefore used with a 1 μF condenser connected across its input.

For technical reasons it is not convenient to connect the P.F.M. in series with the pneumotachograph. It has

also proved impossible so far to produce artificial peak flows of sufficiently smooth wave form for satisfactory recording by the pneumotachograph. The procedure, therefore, has been to ask a series of subjects to blow alternately into the P.F.M. and the pneumotachograph. Usually three blows into each instrument are used and the instrument to be blown into first is alternated between subjects.

Although this procedure is rather laborious and time-consuming it has the two great advantages that the calibration is carried out on actual human peak flows, and that the question of whether the resistance of the P.F.M. modifies the peak flow does not arise. On the other hand, the scatter of readings is increased because the two instruments are in fact measuring different peak flows; this scatter can be reduced by taking a large number of readings and averaging them, but with any practicable design of experiment the scatter from this cause is inevitably considerable.

Another difficulty that arises when an attempt is made to use pneumotachograph recordings to measure the peak flow rate is the practical definition of the term "maximum expiratory flow rate." Fig. 4 shows a drawing of a pneumotachograph recording of a typical normal forced expiration. It will be seen that in this case the definition and measurement of the maximum expiratory flow rate present no difficulty. Fig. 5, on the other hand, shows a type of record that is sometimes obtained from abnormal subjects, where the maximum

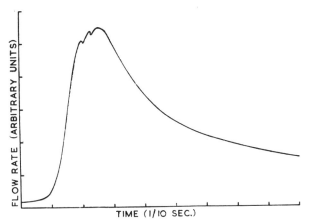

FIG. 4.—Normal type of forced expiratory curve.

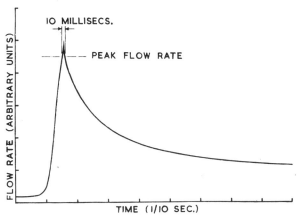

FIG. 5.—Abnormal type of forced expiratory curve, showing method of deciding level of peak.

Maximum forced expiratory flow rate as a measure of ventilatory capacity with a description of a new portable instrument for measuring it. *Wright BM, McKerrow CB*

is in the form of a sharp " peak " which is sustained for only a very short time.

To take the top of a peak of this kind as the maximum is unsatisfactory for two reasons. First, the actual height of the peak is critically dependent on the characteristics of the recording instrument. Secondly, the volume of air represented by quite a large change in peak level is very small, so that it is likely to have little physiological significance. On both instrumental and physiological grounds, therefore, it has seemed to us better to ignore the top of the peak and to take a level of flow which is sustained for a definite time as being what we call the " peak flow rate " (P.F.R.). An interval of 10 millisecs was chosen as being the shortest which lent itself to reasonably accurate measurement of the peak on a pneumotachograph record. The P.F.R. is therefore defined as the highest flow rate sustained for at least 10 millisecs (cf. McKerrow *et al.*, 1958).

As can be seen from Fig. 5, although this definition is fairly easy to understand, the actual measurement of peak levels defined in this way sometimes presented some difficulty, owing to the steepness of the sides of the peak, even when recorded on paper moving as fast as 10 cm./sec. There was thus room for considerable observer error in making the measurement, but by averaging the results of a number of recordings fairly stable figures could be obtained.

A number of calibrations of different models of P.F.M.s were carried out in the way described, using a variety of subjects ranging from children of 4 years to healthy male adults capable of peak flows up to nearly 1,000 l./min. and also including many seriously disabled patients. It soon became apparent that, although the P.F.M. tended to underestimate the P.F.R. as recorded by the pneumotachograph, the relationship between its reading and that of the pneumotachograph was remarkably consistent.

The reason for the underreading of the P.F.M. is rather obscure. It is probably due chiefly to the fact that the instrument is highly damped and therefore fails to reach equilibrium in the short time available.

In view, however, of the high correlation obtainable between the P.F.M. and the pneumotachograph it seemed legitimate to aim at producing an instrument with a dial graduated in litres/min. peak expiratory flow rate. This would conceal to some extent the fact that the relationship between the P.F.R. recorded by the P.F.M. and that recorded by the pneumotachograph was not perfectly constant, and in particular the fact that it was liable to vary at different levels of flow and with different patterns of expiration, but such a loss of information seemed amply compensated by the simplification in the use of the instrument that would result. To have an instrument with a dial calibrated in degrees, or in " peak flow units," and supply various calibration curves to the user did not seem reasonable in view of the relatively small differences involved, especially for an instrument intended primarily for clinical use.

When carrying out the final calibration of the proto-type production instrument, therefore, the procedure was as follows: A group of 20 normal subjects (male and female, ranging in age from 15 to 69), 10 children (male and female, ranging in age from 5 to 11), and 20 male patients (mostly suffering from pneumoconiosis, ranging in age from 30 to 70) was used. A much larger

and more heterogeneous group would obviously have been desirable, but the time and labour available for carrying out the calibration were unfortunately limited. Each subject made two practice blows, and then three blows into the P.F.M. and the pneumotachograph alternately, the order of starting being reversed after each subject. The calibration of the pneumotachograph was checked against a rotameter after each subject, and also by integrating some of the curves and comparing them with the forced expiratory volume (F.E.V.) recorded with a Gaensler (1951) type of apparatus. The overall accuracy of the instrument was considered to be $\pm 5\%$.

The steady-flow calibration of the P.F.M. was also checked at intervals, and was found to be constant within the limits of accuracy with which it could be determined—that is, about $\pm 2\%$.

Fig. 6 shows the result of the P.F.M./pneumotacho-graph calibration. The P.F.M. results are recorded in degrees, and each point is the average of the three readings. It can be seen that there is considerable scatter in the results, which for the reasons given above is inevitable, but a simple curve cutting the abscissa at 50 l./min., the point at which the P.F.M. ceases to record, can be quite easily fitted. The equation of this curve, for which we are indebted to Miss S. Findley, is $y = -20.6 + 0.39x - 0.000068x^2$, and the 5% confidence

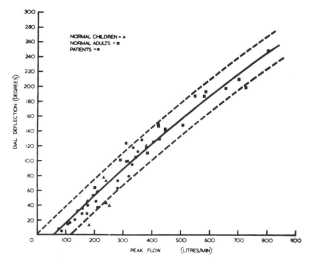

FIG. 6.—Calibration curve of prototype peak flow meter, using human subjects.

limits are as shown on the graph. It will be noted that the points for the different types of subject tend to be grouped together, but the error resulting from assuming that the points are homogeneous is not large.

A curve of this form was used to prepare a dial reading directly in litres per minute peak expiratory flow rate, as shown in Fig. 2.

The instrument has now been in commercial production in various forms for about two years. When the final design incorporating the new dial had been in production for about three months, two instruments were taken from stock and rechecked against the pneumotachograph, using exactly the same procedure as before, except that a rather smaller number of subjects were used and the patients were different. Fig. 7 shows the results for one instrument, and it can be seen that the agreement is satisfactory. The results for the other

Maximum forced expiratory flow rate as a measure of ventilatory capacity with a description of a new portable instrument for measuring it. *Wright BM, McKerrow CB*

instrument were so similar that they have been omitted for the sake of clarity.

A batch of 100 instruments were made at an early stage for a nation-wide survey of bronchitis organized

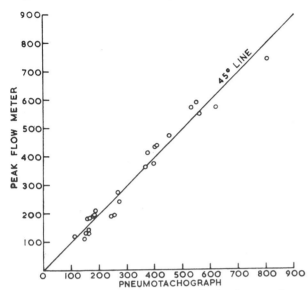

FIG. 7.—Recheck calibration on production instrument.

by the College of General Practitioners. Many of these were rather unsatisfactory, owing to " teething troubles," but the faults were mainly mechanical and did not affect their calibration. The stability of this is illustrated in the Table, which shows single readings taken on 17 subjects with six instruments which had been in use for a year. (We are indebted to Dr. C. M. Fletcher for these figures.)

Peak-Flow-Meter Readings in Litres per Minute

Subject	Instrument Number					
	107	125	135	158	173	217
1	780	780	770	760	740	780
2	820	750	780	760	760	740
3	730	690	720	700	690	670
4	730	640	680	620	640	610
5	490	470	450	420	440	440
6	440	430	430	380	420	420
7	750	740	720	700	700	680
8	620	600	660	600	600	560
9	490	460	440	400	440	430
10	530	530	550	500	530	550
11	740	690	680	700	650	640
12	590	600	570	560	550	520
13	152	136	140	140	112	120
14	190	164	170	180	147	140
15	450	420	460	430	440	400
16	320	300	290	320	310	310
17	120	140	130	130	100	120
Mean ..	526	501	508	488	486	478

Clinical Value of P.F.R. and Relation to Other Tests

It is not the purpose of this paper to enter into a detailed account of the clinical use of the instrument, because our experience of its use in this way has been rather limited.

The prototype instrument was constructed in 1954, and since that time has been used continuously by Dr. C. M. Fletcher, of the Postgraduate Medical School, London, for clinical and survey work. Another early model of the instrument has been used in several surveys conducted by the Pneumoconiosis Research Unit ; an account of one of these has been given by Higgins (1957).

Using an early but quite satisfactory model of the instrument, Higgins carried out some extensive studies amongst a normal population in an agricultural district. In a restricted group of males aged 55 to 64 he found that the correlation coefficient between the P.F.R. and the F.E.V. (0.75 sec.) was 0.86, and he also obtained figures for the distribution of normal values for men and women aged from 25 to over 65 years. These figures are of interest for comparison with those quoted earlier which were given by other workers using other methods, but two points must be borne in mind. (1) As the instrument he used was an early model it had not been calibrated against actual peak flows. The figures he quotes were obtained by using the steady-flow calibration, which was quite consistently 17% too low. His figures, therefore, have all been multiplied by 1.17 to convert them to true peak flows. (2) The population he studied was a sample of a complete population and so included a number of disabled persons. Even so, the average value for males aged 25 to 34 with no history of exposure to dust was over 700 l./min. About 25% have P.F.R.s over 800 and about 3% over 900 l./min. At the other end of the scale, he recorded flows below 50 l./min. in very disabled elderly women, but otherwise flows below 100 l./min. were uncommon.

The only data at present available for children (given in Fig. 6) suggest that they can produce flows over 100 l./min. as soon as they will co-operate sufficiently to give reproducible results—that is, usually at about 4 years of age.

Initially, the P.F.M. was looked upon as a more convenient but substandard method of measuring the F.E.V., which in turn is usually regarded as bearing the same sort of relationship to the M.V.V.

An attempt was made to study directly the relationship between the peak expiratory flow rate and the M.V.V., but the results were not very satisfactory. Since then the use of the M.V.V. has been practically abandoned by the Pneumoconiosis Research Unit, so no further opportunity of carrying out a direct correlation study has occurred.

Meanwhile, however, it has become apparent that the P.F.R. is quite a stable and reproducible measurement —so much so that it has been customary to check both the P.F.M. and the pneumotachograph by using the known values of subjects who have had a reasonable amount of practice.

As a result, the relationship of the test to others such as the M.V.V. or the F.E.V. has become of less interest. It is obvious that no single factor can be used to translate the P.F.R. into the M.V.V., any more than the same can be done for the F.E.V., although numerous attempts have been made to do so.

In this paper, therefore, the P.F.M. is put forward as a simple and reliable device for measuring the maximum expiratory flow rate during a forced expiration, which in turn is put forward as a stable and useful measure of ventilatory capacity. Only clinical experience can eventually decide whether it is as generally useful as the M.V.V. or F.E.V., or whether, if it is not, its lesser usefulness is to some extent compensated for by the greater simplicity and portability of the instrument used for measuring it.

Summary

The advantages of the maximum forced expiratory flow rate as a measure of ventilatory capacity are

Maximum forced expiratory flow rate as a measure of ventilatory capacity with a description of a new portable instrument for measuring it. *Wright BM, McKerrow CB*

considered and the history of the use of the measurement is reviewed.

A new instrument, the peak flow meter, for making the measurement is described, and an account given of the method of calibration.

The available figures for the range of normal values are reviewed, and it is noted that the figures obtained with the peak flow meter are much higher than those recorded by most previous observers using other methods.

It is suggested that the maximum forced expiratory flow rate (" peak flow rate ") measured with the peak flow meter may be found to be a convenient and reliable way of estimating ventilatory capacity.

This instrument has been developed over a period of several years, and it is impossible to acknowledge the help of all those who have assisted us. We should, however, specially like to thank the following: Dr. J. C. Gilson and the staff of the Pneumoconiosis Research Unit who have assisted in innumerable ways, including offering themselves and their children as subjects on a number of occasions ; Mr. V. Gubb, who made two of the early models ; and Messrs. Fred Ferraris, who started commercial manufacture and contributed a number of useful features to the design. Mrs. M. McDermott gave much valuable advice and assistance on the physical problems involved in the testing of the apparatus. The calibrations against the pneumotachograph were carried out by Miss M. Collins and Miss P. Edwards, and the drawings were made by Mr. C. W. Couling, Miss M. B. Wilson, and Miss M. Jenkins. Finally, we thank Dr. C. M. Fletcher for arranging numerous clinical trials of the instrument and for his constant help and encouragement. The instrument is distributed by Messrs. Airmed Ltd., of 16, Wigmore Street, London, W.1, who also supplied the photograph.

REFERENCES

Comroe, J. H., Forster, R. E., Dubois, A. B., Briscoe, W. A., and Carlsen, E. (1955). *The Lung*, p. 130. Year Book Publishers, Chicago.
Donald, K. W. (1953). *Brit. med. J.,* **1**, 415.
Gaensler, E. A. (1951). *Science,* **114**, 444.
Goldsmith, J. R. (1958). *Amer. Rev. Tuberc.,* **78**, 180.
—— and Young, A. C. (1956). *J. appl. Physiol.,* **8**, 562.
Hadorn, W. (1942). *Schweiz. med. Wschr.,* **23**, 946.
Higgins, I. T. T. (1957). *Brit. med. J.,* **2**, 1198.
Hildebrant, G., and Hanke, O. (1956). *Ärztl. Wschr.,* **11**, 439.
Kennedy, M. C. S. (1953). *Thorax,* **8**, 73.
Leuallen, E. C., and Fowler, W. S. (1955). *Amer. Rev. Tuberc.,* **72**, 783.
Lilly, J. C. (1950) In *Methods in Medical Research,* edited by J. H. Comroe, **2**, 113. Chicago.
Linford, A. (1949). *Flow Measurement and Meters.* Spon, London.
McKerrow, C. B., McDermott, M., Gilson, J. C., and Schilling, R. S. F. (1958). *Brit. J. industr. Med.,* **15**, 75.
Shephard, R. J. (1955). *Thorax,* **10**, 258.
Silverman, L., and Whittenberger, J. L. (1950). In *Methods in Medical Research,* edited by J. H. Comroe, **2**, 104. Chicago.
Wyss, F. (1950). *Helv. med. Acta,* **17**, 516.

Maximum forced expiratory flow rate as a measure of ventilatory capacity with a description of a new portable instrument for measuring it. *Wright BM, McKerrow CB*

BRITISH MEDICAL JOURNAL   9 DECEMBER 1978

1627

Contemporary Themes

A miniature Wright peak-flow meter

B M WRIGHT

British Medical Journal, 1978, **2**, 1627-1628

Summary and conclusions

A new miniature Wright peak-flow meter has been designed and produced. The meter is tubular with a spring-loaded piston and a longitudinal slot through which air escapes. Its dynamic characteristics have been carefully designed to make it respond only to peak flow and not to rate of rise. Performance tests on early instruments showed fairly close correlation with the Wright peak-flow meter but with a constant error of + 38 l/min. On later models the correlation was increased to 0.990 and the error reduced to +3%.

The mini-meter correlates as well with the standard instrument as two standard instruments correlate with each other and should prove useful clinically.

Introduction

The Wright peak-flow meter, which was designed as a "simple and reliable device for measuring the maximum expiratory flow rate during a forced expiration,"[1] is now in worldwide use as a measure of ventilatory capacity.

The instrument's popularity has been due partly to its portability and simplicity: patients taking part in therapeutic trials could take the instrument home and make their own measurements and so avoid admission to hospital. This practice was largely responsible for showing the value of disodium chromoglycate in asthma; occasional tests in clinics had previously shown the drug to be of little value.[2]

Nevertheless, the instrument is rather expensive, cumbersome, and unnecessarily precise for these clinical uses as it was originally designed for epidemiological studies. This paper describes a simpler version of the meter.

Evolution of the new instrument

The first attempt at a simplified design was the "de Bono whistle."[3] Described in 1963, this was a tube with a longitudinal slot and a whistle in the end. It fitted inside a standard cardboard mouthpiece, and the length of slot uncovered was adjusted until the subject could only just blow the whistle. The device did not survive because it was difficult to hear the short, faint whistle produced when near the end point and because the test usually required several attempts and some disabled people can give only one peak expiration at a time.

Bioengineering Division, Clinical Research Centre, Harrow HA1 3UJ
B M WRIGHT, MA, MB, visiting worker

I adopted the idea of a tubular instrument in 1965, when a prototype was constructed with a light spring-loaded piston and a longitudinal slot as the variable orifice, in which was carried a rider as peak indicator. Clinical tests showed that readings from the new instrument correlated well with those from the standard peak-flow meter and that it was acceptable to patients, particularly young children, because of its smaller size. When it was produced commercially in 1973, however, as the Peak Flow Gauge changes in its design had altered its dynamic properties so that its readings did not correlate well with those of the standard model.[4]

Meanwhile development continued and the instrument reached its present form in 1969, though it has been in commercial production only since 1977 as the mini Wright peak-flow meter (figs 1 and 2).

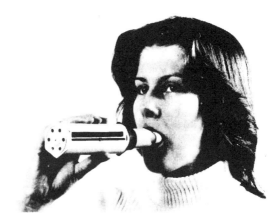

FIG 1—Mini-Wright peak-flow meter showing correct method of use.

Operation and use

Air blown into the instrument cannot escape (except for a small amount which leaks past the piston) until it has moved and uncovered part of the slot. When the area of slot uncovered is such that the pressure behind the piston is just enough to balance the force of the spring, the piston comes to rest in a position that depends on the flow rate. Thus, under steady-flow conditions the instrument's calibration depends only on its geometry and the characteristics of its spring. Under dynamic conditions with rapidly changing flow rates, as during a peak expiration, the mass of the piston is equally important. Unless it is light enough in comparison with the controlling forces the piston may overshoot, so that the reading is affected not only by the magnitude of the peak flow but also by its rate of rise. The mass of the piston has therefore been reduced to the minimum possible.

The instrument is used in the same way as the standard model. It may be held in either hand, but the slot must face away from the hand (as shown in fig 1), so that air can escape freely. As it is not affected by gravity it need not be held horizontally. The valve prevents the return of the piston blowing back into the subject's mouth.

Cleaning and disinfection—The instrument may be cleaned easily in running water or in a detergent solution. The mouthpiece may be

1628 BRITISH MEDICAL JOURNAL 9 DECEMBER 1978

FIG 2—Diagram of mini-Wright peak-flow meter. The cylindrical body (1) and one end of the instrument are moulded in one piece with a slot (2) down one side. The other end (3) carries a tapered socket (4) which accepts a sterilisable mouthpiece (5) or a disposable cardboard mouthpiece. It has a central hollow boss (6) which houses a tension spring (7). The mouthpiece end is held to the body by a knurled nut (8) screwed on to the threaded end of a central rod (9), the other end of which is secured in the fixed end of the body.

Both ends are hexagonal in section to prevent the instrument from rolling and are pierced by a ring of six holes (10, 11) to allow free passage of air. A thin PTFE disc valve (12) is secured to the boss inside the mouthpiece end. The piston (13), which is a light plastic disc with a short sleeve, rides freely on the rod and just clear of the cylinder bore. The scale, which is read vertically, is marked in l/min from 60-800, but a scale in l/s to conform with SI units will be available if required. The rider (14) is spring-loaded in the slot with sufficient friction to prevent it overshooting without appreciably affecting movement of the piston.

The meter is 5·0 cm in diameter and 15 cm long, and weighs 75 g.

autoclaved but the instrument itself must not be heated above 75°C. Details of sterilisation methods are supplied with each instrument.

Calibration—As all parts are moulded in plastic, except for the spring, which is calibrated by its makers, and the metal central rod and nut, only steady-flow calibration is required; this is carried out before the scale is attached. For most purposes two operators with widely differing but stable PEFRs can check the calibration for themselves using a standard peak-flow meter as reference.

Performance

The instrument has been tested by several workers. Perks et al[10] found a correlation coefficient of 0·970 with the standard instrument on a hundred pairs of PEF measurements ranging from 100 to 700 l/min, but with a constant error of +38 l/min. They noted that this error was being corrected in later instruments. Pride (N R Pride, personal communication) in a study of 14 paired observations over a similar range found a correlation coefficient of 0·990. McDermot and Oldham (M McDermot and H G Oldham, personal communication) studied the mini-meter at various times during its production. With early models they found the same high readings as Perks et al but with later models the error was reduced to +3%, and the correlation coefficient was 0·990 on a group of 44 comparisons.

In all these studies subjects blew alternately through the two instruments in a randomised fashion. This was the procedure followed by Wright and McKerrow and was unavoidable because of the nature of the standard peak-flow meter and the pneumotachograph with which it was compared. It does, however, inevitably increase the scatter, as the breaths measured are not the same.

The mini-meter, however, being small and tubular, lends itself to being enclosed in a case and connected in series with a standard peak-flow meter. When this was done the correlation coefficient rose to 0·995, which was a significant improvement. For practical purposes therefore the performance of the mini-meter is identical with that of the standard instrument.

Discussion

When the peak-flow meter was first described the importance of a physically correct measurement was emphasised: the measurement should be absolute and clearly defined so that it would be the same however and wherever it was measured.[1]

Since the peak-flow meter was developed several similar devices have been produced in addition to the de Bono whistle. The Floscope[5] and Pneumometer[6] both measure the pressure drop through a fixed orifice. Results with the Floscope seem to correlate well with those of the peak-flow meter, but the need to

change orifices to get the right range for the patient means that, like the de Bono whistle, more than one attempt may have to be made before a reading can be obtained. The Airflometer[7] is a rather complex instrument in which a turbine is driven round and the peak flow recorded depends on the amount of over-run. Measurements with this device are likely to be affected by friction and workmanship, and the instrument does not seem to measure any definable physical value. The most recent device, the Pulmonary Monitor[8] is similar to the mini-meter but is calibrated in arbitrary units and its mouthpiece is too small to take peak flows from a healthy adult.

The peak expiratory flow rate, as defined by Wright and McKerrow,[1] is now such a well-established clinical and epidemiological measurement that it seems a pity that devices purporting to measure it should be described without adequate consideration of their physical properties and without carefully controlled correlation studies against the standard instrument or some more nearly absolute instrument such as a pneumotachograph. When the original peak-flow meter was being developed it was first calibrated on steady flows, but when used for PEFRs it gave figures that were much higher than those in published reports. The rotating parts were therefore made as light as possible to eliminate overshoot, and tests against a Lilly pneumototachograph showed that the instrument actually underestimated PEFRs by about 17%; allowance was made for this in the instrument's calibration, which was carried out on actual PEFRs.

The commercial version of the instrument was developed by Mr J McNaughton of Clement Clarke, and I am grateful to him for keeping as closely as possible to the original design while making valuable contributions that were necessary for commercial production. I am also grateful to Dr C M Fletcher for making many clinical tests of prototypes and to Mrs M McDermot and her colleagues for organising and carrying out a full laboratory evaluation.

The instrument is the subject of British Patent No 1463814 dated February 1977, the rights in which are vested in the National Research Development Corporation. The instrument is made and marketed by Clement Clarke International Ltd, Airmed House, Edinburgh Way, Harlow, Essex, CM20 2ED, from whom it may be obtained.

References

[1] Wright, B M, and McKerrow, C B, *British Medical Journal*, 1959, **2**, 1041.
[2] Robertson, D G, Epstein, S W, and Warrell, D A, *British Medical Journal*, 1969, **2**, 552.
[3] de Bono, E F, *Lancet*, 1963, **2**, 1146.
[4] Wright, B M, *Lancet*, 1974, **1**, 1151.
[5] Spitzer, S A, and Neuman, E, *Chest*, 1974, **66**, 440.
[6] Hildebrant, G, and Hanke, O, *Ärtzliche Wochenschrift*, 1956, **11**, 439.
[7] Friedman, M, and Walker, S, *Lancet*, 1975, **1**, 310.
[8] Haydu, S P, Chapman, T T, and Hughes, D T D, *Lancet*, 1976, **2**, 1225.
[9] Anderson, J P, *British Journal of Clinical Practice*, 1966, **20**, 635.
[10] Perks, W H, et al, *Thorax*. In press.

(Accepted 1 November 1978)

A miniature Wright peak-flow meter. *Wright BM*

10 February 1968

BRITISH
MEDICAL JOURNAL 335

Papers and Originals

Observations on Recent Increase in Mortality from Asthma

F. E. SPEIZER,* M.D.,; R. DOLL,† M.D., F.R.C.P., F.R.S.; P. HEAF,‡ M.D., F.R.C.P.

Brit. med. J., 1968, 1, 335–339

An increase in the mortality from asthma, particularly in children, has been reported from Australia (Gandevia, 1967). the United States (Richards and Patrick, 1965), and Britain (Smith, 1966), and suggestions have been made that the increase is due to the introduction of new methods of treatment (Ford, 1966 ; Kessler and Geller-Bernstein, 1966 ; Greenberg and Pines, 1967). We have therefore examined the trends in mortality from asthma throughout the world and have sought evidence to account for the increase in England and Wales.

Trends in Mortality at All Ages

Before 1948 deaths classified as asthma ranged from various forms of bronchitis and influenza to deaths associated with a variety of cardiovascular, renal, and allergic diseases. In 1948, with the sixth revision of the *International Classification of Diseases,* asthma was given a more specific category (List No. 241), but it was still classified with several conditions in which asthma may have played only a subsidiary part. These included " asthmatic bronchitis " and other forms of bronchitis where asthma was mentioned without specifying that it was allergic. When the seventh revision of the *Classification* was undertaken in 1955 these types of " bronchitis " were removed and the asthma category began to correspond to a single disease entity (Table I).

These changes reflect, in part, changes in the clinical concept of the disease, and further revisions may be expected as diagnostic precision and knowledge of causation improve. Meanwhile the available statistics can be used only as initial guides to trends in mortality.

TABLE I.—*International Classification of Causes of Death : Description of Deaths Attributed to Asthma Between 1938 and 1966*

1938–1947— *5th Revision of I.C.D.*

112	Asthma	
	Asthmatic bronchitis	Hay asthma
	Bronchial asthma	Hay fever
	Bronchitic asthma	Spasmodic asthma
	Catarrhal asthma	
112.1	With influenza as a contributory or secondary cause	
112.2	With chronic endocarditis as a contributory or secondary cause	
112.3	With myocardial disease as a contributory or secondary cause	
112.4	With arteriosclerosis as a contributory or secondary cause	
112.5	With chronic nephritis as a contributory or secondary cause	
112.6	Without any of the complications here specified (1–5)	

1948–1957— *6th Revision of I.C.D.*

241	Asthma (bronchial)	
	Allergic (any cause)	Bronchitis, allergic
	Sporadic	Hay asthma
	Asthmatic bronchitis	Hay fever with asthma

This title excludes cardiac asthma (434.2) and pneumoconiotic asthma (523–524)

1958– —*7th Revision of I.C.D.*

241	Asthma (bronchial)	
	Allergic (any cause)	Bronchitis, allergic
	Sporadic	Hay asthma
		Hay fever with asthma

This title excludes cardiac asthma (434.2) and pneumoconiotic asthma (523–524.). It also excludes asthma not indicated as allergic with mention of bronchitis (acute) (chronic) (500–502).

In England and Wales the number of deaths decreased progressively from 1,879 in 1952 to 1,507 in 1957, dropped with the new classification to 1,214 in 1959, and rose subsequently to 2,040 in 1966. Between 1959 and 1966 the death rate increased by 56%, from 2.7 to 4.2 per 100,000 persons.

The trends in 19 countries between 1951 and 1964 have been summarized by the World Health Organization (1966). These show that:

(1) In virtually every country there was a sharp decline in the crude mortality rate between 1957 and 1959 which presumably reflected the change from use of the sixth revision of the *International Classification* to the seventh revision.

(2) With the exception of Venezuela, every country with data available before 1958 showed an excess mortality in males, and since 1958 this excess has been reduced. Before 1958 the excess is likely to have been due to the inclusion of a high proportion of deaths from bronchitis, a condition which is appreciably commoner in males.

(3) In 1964 the crude mortality varied between the countries from 1.1 to 9.7 per 100,000 persons, a variation which is likely to be due, in part, to variation in diagnostic criteria.

(4) Between 1959 and 1964 several countries showed sporadic increases in mortality, but the general picture is of a constant rate with a slight tendency to decrease.

(5) England and Wales alone showed a steady increase.

Trends in Age-specific Mortality

Not all the deaths attributed to asthma are likely to have been due to asthma, and this is particularly true for deaths that occurred in infancy and old age. Under 5 years of age asthma may be confused with bronchiolitis or bronchitis which has led to airway obstruction and presented as overinflation with wheezing. Over 65 years of age asthma is commonly complicated by bronchitis and heart failure, which may be the result of the underlying respiratory disease or of independent heart disease. In both these age groups the selection of asthma as the underlying cause of death is partly subjective, and many deaths attributed to asthma could more properly be attributed to other causes.

A more accurate picture of the trend in mortality attributable to the disease may therefore be obtained by confining the comparison to ages 5 to 64 years. At these ages the increase in mortality in England and Wales is even more pronounced ; the annual number of deaths increased from 720 in 1959 to 1,401 in 1966, and the corresponding death rate nearly doubled (from 2.0 to 3.7 per 100,000 persons).

* U.S. Public Health Service Special Fellow, Medical Research Council's Statistical Research Unit.
† Director, Medical Research Council's Statistical Research Unit.
‡ Chest Physician, University College Hospital, London W.C.1.
Requests for reprints should be addressed to Dr. R. Doll, University College Hospital Medical School, 115 Gower Street, London W.C.1.

336   10 February 1968   Asthma—*Speizer et al.*   BRITISH MEDICAL JOURNAL

Figs. 1 and 2 show that the rates have been approximately equal in both sexes in three age groups—10 to 14 years, 5 to 34 years, and 35 to 64 years. Between 1957 and 1960 the rates fell at ages 35 to 64 years, due largely to the change in the method of classification, but there was little consistent change at younger ages. Since 1960–61 the rates have increased.

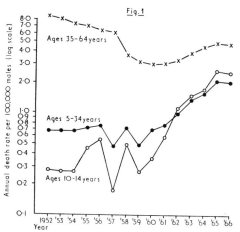

FIG. 1.—Asthma mortality in males aged 10 to 14 years, 5 to 34 years, and 35 to 64 years in England and Wales from 1952 to 1966.

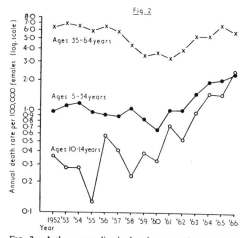

FIG. 2.—Asthma mortality in females aged 10 to 14 years, 5 to 34 years, and 35 to 64 years in England and Wales from 1952 to 1966.

Table II shows the changes since 1959 in greater detail. Since the male and female rates have been approximately equal the figures for both sexes have been combined to reduce the effect of random fluctuation due to small numbers. From Table II it is evident that an increase in mortality began to occur in about 1961 and that all ages between 5 and 64 years of age have been affected. The greatest increase in mortality has taken place at ages 10 to 14 years, at which ages the rate has increased eight times, from 0.3 to 2.5 per 100,000 persons. The increase has, however, been substantial at all ages from 5 to 34 years, and at these ages the annual number of deaths increased by 308 and the death rate trebled from 0.7 to 2.2 per 100,000 persons.

In the rest of this paper we have confined our observations to mortality at ages 5 to 34 years, partly because this age group has shown a large increase in mortality, partly because asthma which develops under 35 years of age is usually classed as

"allergic" and can be distinguished clinically from the disease which develops at a later age, and partly because the mortality from bronchitis begins to exceed that from asthma at about 35 years of age and the possibility of confusing these conditions as the cause of death increases rapidly with advancing years.

TABLE II.—*Number of Deaths and Death Rates from Asthma per 100,000 Persons, by Age : England and Wales, 1959 to 1966**

Age in Years		Deaths	1959	1960	1961	1962	1963	1964	1965	1966
5–9	{	No.	6	12	6	6	9	23	18	17
	{	Rate	0·18	0·37	0·18	0·18	0·27	0·67	0·51	0·47
10–14	{	No.	12	13	24	29	41	53	66	80
	{	Rate	0·33	0·35	0·65	0·84	1·21	1·60	2·02	2·46
15–19	{	No.	19	17	24	39	36	62	73	91
	{	Rate	0·64	0·55	0·77	1·11	0·99	1·67	1·96	2·45
20–24	{	No.	24	27	28	32	56	51	79	83
	{	Rate	0·85	0·94	0·97	1·09	1·87	1·66	2·49	2·52
25–29	{	No.	32	28	39	38	45	69	90	79
	{	Rate	1·12	0·98	1·37	1·31	1·53	2·33	3·00	2·64
30–34	{	No.	30	31	48	47	83	84	77	81
	{	Rate	0·99	1·04	1·61	1·57	2·79	2·85	2·63	2·78
5–34	{	No.	123	128	169	191	270	342	403	431
	{	Rate	0·66	0·68	0·89	1·00	1·40	1·76	2·05	2·18
35–64	{	No.	597	594	568	655	845	903	1,072	970
	{	Rate	3·32	3·29	3·13	3·60	4·64	4·96	5·89	5·34
5–64	{	No.	720	722	737	846	1,115	1,245	1,475	1,401
	{	Rate	1·96	1·96	1·99	2·26	2·97	3·30	3·90	3·69
All ages	{	No.	1,214	1,188	1,269	1,352	1,655	1,800	2,080	2,040
	{	Rate	2·67	2·60	2·75	2·89	3·52	3·80	4·35	4·24

* From the *Registrar General's Statistical Reviews of England and Wales for* 1959 *to* 1965, the *Quarterly Return for England and Wales,* 3rd Quarter 1966, and personal communication.

The relative importance of the increase in mortality between 1959 and 1966 is indicated by the change in the proportion of all deaths attributed to asthma over the same period. In 1959 and 1960 approximately 1% of all deaths at ages 5 to 34 years were attributed to asthma; in 1966 the proportion was 3.4%. At ages 10 to 14 years the proportional mortality increased from 1% to 7.2%.

Data are not yet available for the numbers of deaths due to other causes in 1966; but in 1965, when asthma accounted for 5.7% of all deaths at ages 10 to 14 years, it ranked sixth in the list of causes of death (Table III). The only categories with

TABLE III.—*Ten Major Causes of Death in England and Wales in Children Aged 10–14 Years for the Year 1965**

Cause of Death (I.C.D.)	No. Male	No. Female	Total	Percentage of Total Deaths in Age Group
1. All motor accidents (E810–E825)	127	66	193	16·6
2. Malignant neoplasms other than leukaemia (I.C.D. 140–203, 205)	85	39	124	10·7
3. All congenital malformations (I.C.D. 750–759) ..	50	51	101	8·7
4. All diseases of nervous system (I.C.D. 330–398) ..	53	37	90	7·8
5. Leukaemia and aleukaemia (I.C.D. 204)	39	35	74	6·4
6. Asthma (I.C.D. 241) ..	43	23	66	5·7
7. All pneumonia (I.C.D. 490–493)	27	36	63	5·4
8. Drowning (E929)	44	9	53	4·6
9. All gastrointestinal diseases (I.C.D. 530–587) ..	31	19	50	4·3
10. All genito-urinary diseases (I.C.D. 590–637) ..	14	33	47	4·1
All other diseases	190	109	299	25·8
Total all diseases	703	457	1,160	100·0

* *Registrar General's Statistical Review of England and Wales for the Year* 1965.

substantially higher rates were motor accidents (I.C.D. List Nos. E810 to E825), malignant neoplasms other than leukaemia (List Nos. 140–203, 205), congenital malformations (List Nos. 750–759), and diseases of the nervous system and sense organs (List Nos. 330–398). Other diseases whose rates were of the same order as asthma were leukaemia (List No. 204) and pneumonia (List Nos. 490–493).

Observations on recent increase in mortality from asthma. *Speizer FE, Doll R, Heaf P*

Trends in Other Countries

Mortality rates and trends in mortality in other countries fall into two fairly distinct groups. Those countries whose death rate for asthma at ages 5 to 34 was less than 0.5 per 100,000 persons in 1959 to 1960 and those whose rate ranged between 0.5 and 1 per 100,000 persons. The United States and virtually all western European countries apart from Britain (including Belgium, France, Italy, Netherlands, Spain, West Germany, Denmark, and Sweden) fall into the first group, and none of these showed any appreciable increase in mortality up to 1964, irrespective of whether or not they showed any change in total asthma mortality at all ages.

The remaining countries need to be considered individually. *Scotland's* death rate for asthma at ages 5 to 34 years was generally lower than in England and Wales. After 1962, however, the increase in the number of deaths was similar. The increase became appreciable in 1963, and in 1964 the rate was approximately three times the average for 1961 and 1962. At ages 35 to 64 years there has also been some increase, but less pronounced.

Before 1964 *Australian* death rates at ages 5 to 34 years were higher than in England and Wales; and until then they were relatively stable. A substantial increase took place from 1963 to 1964 (from 0.9 to 1.8 per 100,000 persons), but there was no further increase in 1965. In contrast to England and Wales and Scotland, comparable increases also occurred at ages 10 to 14 years and at ages 35 to 64 years.

In *Japan* the rates have shown a somewhat different trend. At ages 5 to 34 years there has been a steady but rather slow increase in mortality, which in 1964 had risen by about 40%, in contrast to the rise of over 250% in England and Wales. This, however, was accompanied by a decrease in mortality at ages 35 to 64 years.

New Zealand alone had an asthma death rate at ages 5 to 34 years of over 0.5 per 100,000 persons in 1959 and showed no increase in mortality in the next six years.

Different results are obtained when the comparison is limited to ages 10 to 19 years—the decade in which the largest increase was recorded in England and Wales. Five-year age-specific rates are available for the whole period 1959 to 1964 for only 11 countries, and these are shown in Table IV. The individual

at ages 15 to 19 years. In Western Europe, Japan, and Australasia increases have occurred in the range of 85 to 103% at ages 10 to 14 years and in the range of 23 to 45% at ages 15 to 19 years. In the United States the increases have been small, but they still show the same trend. Small increases were again observed in 1965 (to 0.30 and 0.40 per 100,000), but provisional data for 1966, for which we are indebted to the Division of Vital Statistics of the Department of Health, Education, and Welfare of the U.S. Public Health Service, suggest that a substantial increase may now have occurred. From 1965 to 1966 the number of deaths attributed to asthma at ages 1 to 14 years increased by 64%, from 146 to 240.

Reasons for Increased Death Rate

One possible explanation of the increase in England and Wales is that it is an artifact brought about by changes in the diagnostic criteria used by physicians certifying the cause of death. This possibility has been investigated by comparing the trends in mortality attributed to asthma and a variety of other respiratory diseases; that is, from all forms of bronchitis (*I.C.D.* List Nos. 500–502), bronchiectasis (List No. 526), emphysema without mention of bronchitis (List No. 527.1, pneumonia (List Nos. 490–493), and other chronic interstitial pneumonias (List No. 525). The annual numbers of deaths and the death rates attributed to these causes are summarized in Table 5. Some decrease occurred in the number of deaths attributed to pneumonia, but the reduction (107 deaths between 1959 and 1965) is less than a half of the increase in asthma deaths (280 over the same period) and the pneumonia death rate oscillated while the asthma mortality increased steadily. No appreciable change took place in the death rates attributed to bronchitis or other chronic respiratory diseases, and changes in the use of these categories cannot by themselves have led to an increase in the number of deaths attributed to asthma. Moreover, the number of deaths attributed to bronchitis for which asthma was mentioned on the death certificate did not decrease at these ages—as would be expected if there had been a tendency for doctors to attribute the underlying cause to asthma alone rather than to asthma and bronchitis—but increased from 24 in 1959 to 49 in 1966.

TABLE IV.—*International Death Rates from Asthma for Ages 10-14 and 15-19 Years : 1959-61 and 1962-4**

Country	Age in Years	1959–1961 No. of Deaths	1959–1961 Average Yearly Death Rate per 100,000	1962–1964 No. of Deaths	1962–1964 Average Yearly Death Rate per 100,000	Per cent. Increase 1959–61 to 1962–4
Britain:						
England and Wales	10–14	59	0·48	143	1·26	162·5
Scotland	15–19	69	0·67	151	1·23	83·6
Australasia:						
Australia†	10–14	21	0·56	44	1·14	103·6
New Zealand	15–19	30	0·94	40	1·16	23·4
Europe:						
Germany						
Sweden						
Denmark	10–14	29	0·21	54	0·39	85·7
Netherlands	15–19	31	0·24	47	0·35	45·8
Belgium						
Japan	10–14	87	0·26	147	0·50	92·3
	15–19	107	0·38	172	0·55	44·7
U.S.A.	10–14	104	0·21	140	0·26	23·8
	15–19	124	0·30	153	0·33	10·0

* Data compiled from the Official National Vital Statistics Record for each country for the years 1959-1964, with the exception of Australia.
† Data from Dr. B. Gandevia (personal communication).

TABLE V.—*Death Rate per 100,000 Persons Aged 5-34 Years from Selected Respiratory Diseases : England and Wales 1959-1965**

Diagnostic Category	Deaths	1959	1960	1961	1962	1963	1964	1965
Acute and chronic bronchitis (*I.C.D.* 500–502)	No.	121	107	124	128	126	121	131
	Rate	0·65	0·57	0·66	0·67	0·65	0·62	0·66
Chronic respiratory† diseases (*I.C.D.* 525, 526, 527.1)	No.	84	92	73	76	73	76	78
	Rate	0·45	0·49	0·39	0·40	0·38	0·39	0·40
Pneumonias (*I.C.D.* 490–493)	No.	486	403	423	474	416	398	379
	Rate	2·61	2·15	2·24	2·47	2·15	2·04	1·93
Asthma (*I.C.D.* 241)	No.	123	128	169	191	270	342	403
	Rate	0·66	0·68	0·89	1·00	1·40	1·76	2·05

* From the *Registrar General's Statistical Review of England and Wales* for each year 1959-1965.
† See text for definition.

Further evidence is provided by the fact that the number of asthma deaths that were certified by coroners after necropsy examination increased even more rapidly than the total (from 43 at ages 5 to 34 years in 1959 to 237 in 1966). If the increase were an artifact we should have to postulate that there had been an even greater change in the diagnostic criteria used by pathologists than in those used by clinicians, or that there had been a change in the type of case referred to coroners.

We conclude, therefore, that the increase in mortality attributed to asthma at ages 5 to 34 years is, in large part, real and represents a true increase in the annual number of deaths from the disease.

results are irregular, but when the countries are grouped regionally, to reduce the effect of random fluctuation of small numbers, it is found that there has been an increase in mortality rates from 1959–61 to 1962–4 in each region. The increase has been largest in Britain—162% at ages 10 to 14 years and 84%

Observations on recent increase in mortality from asthma. *Speizer FE, Doll R, Heaf P*

Two Explanations

One explanation of a true increase in mortality could be that the number of patients suffering from asthma had risen. This cannot be tested directly, but an indication of its validity can be obtained by comparing the frequency with which patients have consulted their general practitioners. In 1955 to 1956 the Royal College of General Practitioners in co-operation with the Registrar General collected figures on morbidity from a variety of diseases, including asthma (Fry, 1962), and similar data have been made available to us for the years 1961 to 1966 for a selected group of practices covering approximately 20,000 patients (Table VI). Over this 10-year period there has, in fact, been a tendency for the number of episodes of asthma leading to consultation to decrease at ages 5 to 14 years and to stay approximately the same at ages 15 to 44 years. A reduction in the number of episodes at young ages could be due to a decrease in the incidence of the disease or to some change in therapy keeping the patients away from the doctor; but even in the latter case it would seem most unlikely that the incidence of the disease could have increased appreciably.

TABLE VI.—*Morbidity from Asthma Recorded in General Practice*

Episodes per Year per 1,000 Persons Aged (in Years):	1955-6*	1961†	1962	1963	1964	1965	1966
5–14	10	9·2	4·9	6·8	3·9	4·9	4·3
15–44	7	6·6	3·6	3·0	5·1	6·4	6·6
45–65	10	5·2	9·3	5·1	5·2	4·5	9·6
All ages	9	5·8	3·8	5·6	5·2	5·3	4·6

* Fry (1962).
† 1961 to 1966, Dr. D. L. Crombie, Royal College of General Practitioners (personal communication).

Another explanation could be that there has been an increase in the case fatality rate. We have again not been able to test this directly, but it is notable that the proportion of asthma deaths at ages 5 to 34 years that were certified by coroners increased from 35% in 1959 to 55% in 1966. The proportion of deaths from all causes certified by coroners over this period is not available separately for different age groups, but there is no reason to suppose that the proportion has increased differentially in this age group, and for all ages it has remained approximately 10%. It appears probable, therefore, that the mode of death from asthma at young ages has changed. In the absence of evidence to the contrary, it would seem that an increase in the case fatality rate is the most likely explanation of the increased mortality rate, and we have accepted this as a working hypothesis.

Environmental Hazards

Several factors could be responsible. Changes in the prevalence of environmental hazards could cause patients with asthma to be more severely affected and so could result in an increased mortality. Alternatively, new methods of management of asthmatic patients might produce temporary symptomatic relief, but increase the hazards of dying from the disease later.

Morbidity studies in New Orleans, U.S.A., have suggested that asthma can reach epidemic levels under particular conditions of atmospheric pollution (Weill *et al.*, 1965), but it is difficult to believe that this could be a factor in England. Certainly the increase could not be due to smoke pollution, which has decreased in English towns over the last decade, nor could it be attributed to pollution with sulphur gases, which has remained approximately constant (Ministry of Technology, 1967). Motor traffic has increased considerably, and one of the constituents of motor fumes could perhaps have had a harmful effect. If this were the case, however, a substantial difference in mortality would be expected between urban and rural areas, and we have failed to find any evidence of this in the national mortality data for 1966. The death rate was 2.0 per 100,000 persons aged 5 to 34 years in conurbations, 3.0 in urban areas of more than 100,000 population, 2.2 in urban areas of under 50,000 population, and 1.9 in rural districts.

Other environmental hazards are associated with smoking and occupation, but these cannot be responsible for changes that have been observed characteristically at ages 10 to 14 years in both sexes.

New Methods of Treatment

Substantial advances in the management of respiratory failure from a variety of chronic pulmonary diseases have been made in the last 15 years (Detty, 1966), and new methods of both emergency and long-term therapy have been introduced for the treatment of asthma. Corticosteroids were introduced into the management of the disease in 1952, but the increase in mortality did not begin until nine years later. This discrepancy, however, is not sufficient to exculpate them entirely. The frequent and prolonged use of corticosteroids spread slowly, and the risk of harmful effects may be at a maximum only after patients have been under treatment for several years. A much closer correlation obtains with the use of pressurized aerosols containing sympathomimetics. These were introduced in England and Wales in 1960 and began to gain wide acceptance in 1961; and in the next five years their consumption is estimated to have increased more than fourfold (Ministry of Health, unpublished data). The closeness of the correlation justifies inquiry into the possible harmful effect of the preparations, but a temporal correlation of this sort, taken by itself, is a poor basis for drawing conclusions about cause and effect.

If either of these forms of therapy is to be considered as a possible cause of an increased fatality rate, it will be necessary to inquire why a similar effect has not been recorded in other countries where they have also been widely used. It may be, however, that a large increase in mortality has not been recorded in some of those countries where the mortality from asthma was initially much lower than in Britain, because similar deaths have been, and currently still are, attributed to other causes. In New Zealand the size of the population is so small that chance factors might obscure the evidence of even a substantial increase in risk. It is notable, however, that since 1959 an increase in the mortality has been recorded at ages 10 to 19 years widely throughout the world. At these ages children have begun to act independently and may be particularly prone to misuse a self-administered form of treatment.

Summary

The mortality attributed to asthma has increased annually in England and Wales from 1960 to 1965. The increase is more pronounced at ages 5 to 34 years than at older ages and is most pronounced at ages 10 to 14 years. In this last age group the mortality increased nearly eight times in seven years, and in 1966 asthma accounted for 7% of all deaths.

No comparable increase has been observed in any other country, but smaller increases at ages 10 to 19 years have been observed in Australasia, Japan, western Europe, and the United States.

There is no evidence to suggest that there has been any change in diagnostic habits, certification of deaths, or methods of classification which could account for the increase in Great Britain, and it is concluded that the increase is real.

General practitioners' records provide no evidence of an increase in prevalence and it seems probable that there has been an increase in case fatality.

No environmental hazards are known which could have increased the severity of the disease, and the possibility has to be considered that the increase may be due to new methods of

10 February 1968   Asthma—*Speizer et al.*   BRITISH MEDICAL JOURNAL   339

treatment. Corticosteroids have been used increasingly since 1952, and in Great Britain the use of pressurized aerosols containing sympathomimetics has increased rapidly since 1960.

ADDENDUM.—Since this paper was submitted figures for 1966 in New Zealand supplied by the Public Health Statistician for New Zealand have been made available to us by Dr. Gandevia. These reveal an apparent increase in deaths attributed to asthma for the age group 9–54 years. Age-specific death rates are not yet available, but Dr. Gandevia suggests that an upward trend in mortality may now be occurring (Gandevia, personal communication).

We are grateful to the Registrar General of England and Wales for supplying many of the data, and for supplying them with minimal delay. We are grateful also to the Ministry of Health for information about the sale of aerosol bronchodilators ; and to Miss A. M. Hetzel, Chief of the Statistical Resources Section of the Division of Vital Statistics, U.S. Public Health Service, Dr. B. Gandevia, Associate Professor in Thoracic Medicine, the Prince Henry Hospital, Little Bay, New South Wales, Professor S. Koller, Professor of Medical Statistics, University of Mainz, and Dr. D. L. Crombie, Director of the Records and Statistics Unit of the Royal College of General Practitioners, for information about the mortality from asthma in the United States, Australia, and the German Federal Republic, and for morbidity data in Britain.

Dr. F. E. Speizer was supported by the National Center for Air Pollution, Bureau of Disease Prevention and Environmental Control, U.S. Public Health Service.

REFERENCES

Detty, T. L. (1966). *Management of Chronic Obstructive Lung Diseases*, Public Health Service Publication, No. 1457, Washington.
Ford, R. M. (1966). *Med. J. Aust.*, 2, 196.
Fry, J. (1962). *Morbidity Statistics from General Practice*, Vol. 3, pp. 15-33. H.M.S.O., London.
Gandevia, B. (1967). *Brit. med. J.*, 2, 441.
Greenberg, M. J., and Pines, A. (1967). Ibid., 1, 563.
Kessler, A., and Geller-Bernstein, C (1966). *J. Amer. med. Ass.*, 196, 458.
Ministry of Technology (1967). *The Investigation of Atmospheric Pollution 1958-1966 : 32nd Report*. H.M.S.O., London.
Richards, W., and Patrick, J. R. (1965). *Amer. J. Dis. Child.*, 110, 4.
Smith, J. M. (1966). *Lancet*, 1, 1042.
Weill, H., Ziskirdj, M. M., Derbes, V. J., Horton, R. J. M., McCaldin, R. O., and Dickerson, R. C. (1965). *Arch. environm. Hlth*, 10, 148.
World Health Organization (1966). *Epidem. vital Statist. Rep.*, 19, 525.

Observations on recent increase in mortality
from asthma. *Speizer FE, Doll R, Heaf P*

10 February 1968   Asthma—*Speizer et al.*   BRITISH MEDICAL JOURNAL   339

Investigation into Use of Drugs Preceding Death from Asthma

F. E. SPEIZER,* M.D. ; R. DOLL,† M.D., F.R.C.P., F.R.S. ; P. HEAF,‡ M.D., F.R.C.P. ; L. B. STRANG,§ M.D., F.R.C.P.

Brit. med. J., 1968, **1**, 339–343

The annual number of deaths attributed to asthma has increased progressively in England and Wales since 1960. The increase has been substantial at all ages, but has been most pronounced in adolescence and young adult life. Between 1959 and 1966 the death rate increased three times at ages 5 to 34 years and nearly eight times at ages 10 to 14 years. Possible reasons for this change have been examined previously, when it was concluded that the increase was real and likely to be due, in large part, to changes in treatment leading to an increased case fatality (Speizer, Doll and Heaf, 1968). We have therefore sought information about the mode of death and the method of treatment used during and preceding the terminal illness in a consecutive series of deaths attributed to asthma in young persons.

Data

Copies of death certificates were provided by the Registrar General for all deaths in persons aged 5 to 34 years which were registered in England and Wales in the period 1 October 1966 to 31 March 1967, and in which asthma was described as the underlying cause. On receipt of the certificates, which was usually within two months of the date of death, we sought from the local executive councils, the coroners who had signed the certificates, or the hospitals where the deaths were recorded, the names of the general practitioners on whose lists the patients were registered. A standard questionary was then mailed to the general practitioner inquiring about the therapy the patient had received during and before the terminal illness, and whether death had been anticipated. When death was recorded at

hospital a similar questionary was also mailed to the hospital physician. At the time the inquiry was begun interest centred on the possible effect of corticosteroids and no direct questions were included about the use of pressurized aerosols. When death had been certified by a coroner, or the death certificate indicated that a post-mortem examination had been carried out, inquiries were also made about the necropsy findings.

The number of death certificates received and the number of questionaries returned are shown in Table I. In four instances no inquiries could be made as the name of the relevant general practitioner could not be ascertained. Two physicians did not respond to multiple inquiries, and one knew nothing about the patient, who had only just been entered on his list, and returned a blank questionary. In all, therefore, we obtained information relating to 96% of the deaths (177 out of 184). The forms were, in general, completed fully and carefully and many practitioners provided a great amount of detailed information. All the information requested was not, however, always available and some data refer to slightly smaller total numbers.

Fifty-two deaths were recorded in hospital and letters were sent to 52 hospital consultants. All replied. Few could provide any information beyond that associated with the management of the terminal episode, and six of the question-

* U.S. Public Health Service Fellow, Medical Research Council's Statistical Research Unit.
† Director, Medical Research Council's Statistical Research Unit.
‡ Chest Physician, University College Hospital, London W.C.1.
§ Professor of Paediatrics, University College Hospital Medical School, London W.C.1.
Requests for reprints should be addressed to Dr. R. Doll, University College Hospital Medical School, 115 Gower Street, London W.C.1.

TABLE I.—*Response to Inquiries*

Death Certified by	No. of Deaths	Questionaries to:			
		General Practitioner		Hospital Consultant	
		No. Sent	No. Returned	No. Sent	No. Returned
General practitioner	44	43	43	—	—
Coroner	109	106	104	21	21
Hospital consultant	31	31	31	31	31
All sources ..	184	180*	178†	52	52‡

* Four physicians not located.
† Including one questionary returned blank.
‡ Including six questionaries returned blank.

aries were returned blank. For most analyses we have therefore used the data provided by the general practitioners and have used the hospital data only for the analysis of necropsy findings and occasionally to amplify the practitioners' replies.

Information about the post-mortem findings was obtained for 100 of the 109 deaths certified by coroners and for 13 of the 15 other deaths which were known to have been followed by post-mortem examination. Necropsy data are therefore available for 61% of all deaths and for 91% of deaths in which a post-mortem examination is known to have been made.

Results

Clinical Characteristics

The sex and age distribution of the patients at death is shown in Table II. The total numbers of males and females were approximately equal (89 and 95 respectively). As in other data, however, there was a male excess under 20 years of age and a female excess above 25 years.

TABLE II.—*Number of Deaths by Sex and Age (Number for Which Completed Questionaries Were Received Shown in Parentheses)*

Age of Subject (in Years)	No. of Deaths in:		Total Deaths
	Males	Females	
5–9	6	1	7 (7)
10–14	12	12	24 (24)
15–19	16	15	31 (31)
20–24	16	17	33 (31)
25–29	20	25	45 (42)
30–34	19	25	44 (42)
Ages 5–34	89	95	184 (177)*

* Blank questionary omitted.

In three cases the cause of death was attributed to asthma after a coroner's post-mortem examination, but the diagnosis was disputed by the practitioner who had been looking after the patient. Brief details are as follows:

Case 1.—Man aged 24, under practitioner's care for six years without ever having attended for asthma or any other illness. No drugs prescribed. Doctor sent for because patient had "fainted"; found dead on arrival. According to wife's statement he had never had any illness previously; he suddenly complained of pain in his chest, went to sit down, and was found dead in a chair 20 minutes later. Diagnosis: coronary thrombosis. Post-mortem report: Patches of atheroma in anterior descending branch of left coronary artery, but no evidence of occlusion. Both lungs congested and moderately voluminous; small bronchi contained thick mucus. Cause of death: status asthmaticus.

Case 2.—Woman aged 29, under practitioner's care for four years. Lifelong history of bronchitis and bronchiectasis not specifically asthmatic; had been in hospital for bronchiectasis. No A.C.T.H., corticosteroids, or bronchodilators given; treated with expectorants, antibiotics, and diuretics. Terminal episode lasted half an hour. Diagnosis: right heart failure due to long-standing bronchiectasis. Post-mortem report: Fingers clubbed. Pericardiac sac contains a slight excess of fluid; the heart (320 g.) flabby and pinkish brown; both ventricles dilated, and right shows marked hypertrophy, being almost as thick as the left. Left pleural sac contains 2 oz. (57 ml.) of clear effusion and the right is largely obliterated by old adhesions. The distended lungs show generalized emphysema and are generally dry; moderate bronchiectasis in right middle and lower lobes and a general purulent bronchitis. Cause of death: cardiac failure as a consequence of bronchial asthma and bronchiectasis.

Case 3.—Woman aged 29, under practitioner's care for one year. The doctor had treated her for "mental illness" but was "not aware that she had asthma"; the only drug he had prescribed was chloral hydrate. Post-mortem report: The lungs were moderately distended with air. Bronchi congested and contained plugs of thick tenacious mucus. Gastric mucosa intensely congested. All other organs completely normal. Histological examination of lungs showed the appearance of bronchial asthma. Cause of death: status asthmaticus.

These cases have been excluded from subsequent analyses except for the analysis of the necropsy data.

Most of the remaining deaths appear to have occurred in persons with mild to moderate asthma since childhood, rather than in severe respiratory cripples. The mean duration of asthma in 159 patients for whom it was estimated was 13.1 years and the median age of onset was 7.0 years. Only five persons, all of whom died when over 15 years of age, had had asthma for less than one year. The asthma had at some time been severe enough for 81% of the patients to have been referred to a chest physician (136 out of 168), but only 59% had ever been admitted to hospital (95 out of 161).

The characteristics of the terminal illness are shown in Table III. Death was sudden and unexpected in 80% of cases (137 out of 171), and 39% of the practitioners had regarded the terminal illness as "not severe" (67 out of 171). In 133 cases the practitioners were reasonably confident that they could estimate the duration of the terminal episode. In over a quarter of these (37 out of 133) the patients died in less than one hour and only 39 (29%) survived 24 hours or more. That death was commonly sudden and unexpected is confirmed by the fact that 59% of the deaths (109 out of 184) were certified by coroners.

TABLE III.—*Characteristics of the Terminal Episode (All Patients with Asthma for Whom Questionaries were Completed)*

Assessment of Severity of Asthma	Manner of Death (No. of Deaths)		Total Deaths	No. of Patients with Terminal Episode of Estimated Duration (in Hours)				
	Sudden and Unexpected	Other		Under 1	1–5	6–23	24 or More	Not Known
Severe	95	9	104	26	19	13	23	23
Not severe	42	25	67	11	18	7	16	15
All grades	137	34	171*	37	37	20	39	38

* Severity of asthma and suddenness of death not stated for three patients.

As previously noticed, there were 31 cases in which patients had been certified by the hospital staff as dying of asthma. An additional 21 patients whose death was reported by hospitals were certified by coroners. The hospital consultant was not able to supply any information on six of these patients. Of the remaining 46 patients 10 arrived at hospital dead, and an additional four died within one hour. Twenty-two patients survived for 24 hours or more, and even among these death occurred suddenly and unexpectedly in 15 (68%).

Necropsy Findings

The classical gross pathological finding in asthma of voluminous overdistended lungs which do not collapse when removed from the chest cavity was described in 110 out of 113 post-mortem reports (97%).[1] In all but seven of these the second most important classical finding—thick tenacious mucus plugging of the smaller bronchi—was also present. Additional evidence of emphysema was described in 27 cases. Few of the protocols contained information about microscopical examination; those that did described an abundance of eosinophils in the mucoid material. The three cases not typical of asthma showed, respectively, completely normal lungs, bilateral collapse with unilateral tension pneumothorax, and advanced bronchitis.

Pulmonary findings additional to those of asthma occurred infrequently. Five cases were reported with inhalation of vomitus, four with pulmonary oedema, three with purulent pneumonia, two with bronchitis, and one each with haemorrhagic pneumonia, bronchitis and bronchiectasis, and bilateral apical pulmonary tuberculosis. The only other findings of major importance were two cases with, respectively, myocardial infarction and pericardial effusion.

[1] Including Cases 1, 2, and 3 described previously.

We attempted to compare the presence or absence of right ventricular dilatation and hypertrophy with the clinical grading of severity of the asthma. The comparison could be made in only 103 of the 113 cases.[2] In 47% of these one or other condition was described. Hypertrophy was present in 7 of the 44 not-severe asthmatics (16%) and in 15 of the 59 severe asthmatics (25%). Dilatation was present in 4 of the 18 patients who did not die suddenly and unexpectedly (22%), and in 30 out of 85 of those who did (35%). Neither of these differences is statistically significant (P in each case is approximately 0.3), but the trends are in the expected directions.

In 58 of the post-mortem reports a comment was made about the endocrine system, or specifically about the adrenal glands. Marked atrophy of the adrenals was noted in six cases in all of which the subject had been taking corticosteroids—for three and a half days in one instance, less than six months in another, and over two years in four.

Use of Corticosteroids[3]

Initially we had supposed that any patient with asthma severe enough to cause death was likely to have received corticosteroids. In fact, a substantial number of patients had not been regarded as suffering from severe asthma and more than a quarter (50 out of 173) were never given any corticosteroids at all. Thirty-one patients had received corticosteroids, but the treatment had been stopped for between a few days (three patients) and over one year (eight patients), and no corticosteroids were given in the terminal episode. In these cases the failure to give further corticosteroids can usually be attributed to the brevity of the terminal episode—21 of the 23 patients for whom its duration could be estimated (91%) dying in less than three hours. The remaining 92 patients were either receiving corticosteroids at the time their terminal episode began or were given them as emergency treatment. Details of the schedules used are summarized in Table IV. A

TABLE IV.—*Use of Corticosteroids Before and During Terminal Episode (All Patients with Asthma for Whom Questionaries were Completed)*

Treatment in Terminal Episode	No. of Patients Treated Before the Terminal Episode				Total Patients
	Without Corticosteroids	With Corticosteroids			
		Within 2 Weeks*	2–52 Weeks Previously	More than 1 Year Previously	
No corticosteroids ..	50	3	20	8	81
Corticosteroids given:					
Single injection ..	3	4	2	0	9
High dose before death:					
(a) Steady level	3	2	3	2	10
(b) Moderate or low dose increased	0	7	6	0	13
Moderate or low dose unaltered ..	0	31	8	1	40
Dose decreased before death:					
(a) High at first	0	5	0	0	
(b) Moderate or low at first	1	4	1	1	7
Regimen not known	2	3	2	1	8
All treatments ..	59	59	42	13	173‡

* Mostly on corticosteroids regularly at the start of the terminal episode.
‡ History of corticosteroids use not stated for one patient.

quarter of the patients (23) received high doses of corticosteroids immediately before death, but in the majority the dose was maintained at a moderate or low level (40 patients) or was tapered (12 patients). It may be, therefore, that many patients were given insufficient steroids to overcome adrenal suppression as a result of previous steroid therapy or the stress of the disease. It must be remembered, however, that death often

[2] The additional 10 cases were three for which the severity was unknown, four for which no questionary was completed, and three which were regarded by the general practitioners as not asthmatic.
[3] Six patients had been given A.C.T.H. For the purpose of the present analysis these have been included with those given corticosteroids.

occurred suddenly and in the absence of apparent serious respiratory distress, so that there may have been no obvious indications for increasing the dose.

Examination of the data for the patients who died at ages 10 to 19 years provides no evidence that the distribution of corticosteroid usage in this group differed from that in patients at other ages. Seventeen of the 55 patients were never given corticosteroids at any period (31%); 11 had corticosteroids before the terminal episode but not in it (20%); 1 received corticosteroids only in the terminal episode; and 26 received corticosteroids both in this episode and previously (47%). These proportions are very similar to those recorded for all patients aged 5 to 34 years in Table IV.

Use of Inhaled Bronchodilators

At the start of the inquiry we had no special concern for any particular form of therapy other than corticosteroids; doctors were therefore asked only to name other drugs that were known to have been used in the last month of the patient's life. In response to this question 130 doctors specified that inhalant preparations of bronchodilators had been so used. In the light of this evidence a further letter was sent to those doctors who had not mentioned these preparations, inquiring specifically about them, and all responded. We have, therefore, evidence that bronchodilators were being inhaled by at least 86% of the patients (150 out of 174), but we do not know how recently they had been used when the patient died. Eighteen patients had definitely not used them, and in the remaining six instances the doctors did not know for certain whether they had been used or not.

Isoprenaline was used much more commonly as an inhalant than any other sympathomimetic drug. Its use was mentioned directly or indirectly under a trade name in 108 cases (72% of specified types). Other specified sympathomimetics used in this way were orciprenaline (33 cases) and adrenaline (9 cases). In four of the cases in which adrenaline was used the preparation was in the form of a simple spray; in all other cases the sympathomimetic was given in the form of a pressurized aerosol.

The frequency with which pressurized aerosols were used in the different clinical categories is shown in Tables V and VI. Very little difference was found between those patients who were characterized clinically as severe asthmatics and those considered clinically to be not severe—89 out of 102 (87%) against 54 out of 63 (86%). The difference was somewhat larger between those who died suddenly and unexpectedly (116 out of 131, or 89%) and those who died otherwise (27 out of 34, or 79%), but it was not statistically significant (P approximately 0.2). Pressurized aerosols had also been used by nearly all patients irrespective of the duration of the terminal episode. It may be noted that only 2 of the 37 patients who died within an hour of the start of the episode had not used these preparations, and the proportion (5%) is less than that recorded for

TABLE V.—*Use of Pressurized Aerosol Bronchodilators in Different Clinical Categories (All Patients with Asthma for Whom Questionaries were Completed)*

Clinical Category	No. of Patients			Total No. of Patients
	Known to have Used Aerosols	Known Not to have Used Aerosols	Aerosol History Not Known	
Severe asthma:				
Death sudden ..	82	11*	2	95
Death not sudden ..	7	2†	0	9
Asthma not severe:				
Death sudden ..	34	4	4	42
Death not sudden ..	20	5	0	25
Category not known ..	3	0	0	3
All categories	146	22	6	174

* Three on inhalant sprays. † One on inhalant spray.

Investigation into the use of drugs preceding death from asthma. *Speizer FE, Doll R, Heaf P et al*

342   10 February 1968   Asthma—*Speizer et al.*   BRITISH
                                                                 MEDICAL JOURNAL

all other patients with known durations (13%). The difference, however, is again not statistically significant and may well be attributable to chance (P approximately 0.2).

TABLE VI.—*Use of Pressurized Aerosol Bronchodilators by Estimated Duration of Terminal Episode (All Patients with Asthma for Whom Questionaries were Completed)*

Duration of Terminal Episode (in Hours)	No. of Patients			Total No. of Patients
	Known to have Used Aerosols	Known Not to have Used Aerosols	Aerosol History Not Known	
Less than 1	35	2*	0	37
1–2	22	3	0	25
3–5	9	2	1	12
6–11	11	2†	0	13
12–23	6	1	0	7
24–47	18	1	0	19
48–167	14	2	0	16
168 or more	2	1	1	4
No estimate obtained ..	29	8*	4	41
All durations	146	22	6	174

* One on inhalant spray.   † Both on inhalant sprays.

Examination of the data for the patients who died at ages 10 to 19 years provides no evidence that the distribution of usage of pressurized aerosols in this group differed from that in patients at other ages. Nine of the 55 patients had not used them in the last month of their life (16%)—a proportion slightly greater than that shown for all patients aged 5 to 34 years in Table V (13%).

Excessive use of pressurized aerosols was reported by 29 general practitioners without specific inquiry having been made. The reports ranged from a vague implication, such as " tended to use aerosols too frequently " or " suspicion of excess aerosol at death," to direct observations such as " died clutching aerosol " and a detailed account of the amount consumed. In extreme cases the use of as many as two canisters per day or two in two hours was reported.

Other Therapy

Almost all the patients received bronchodilators by mouth during the last month of life. Ephedrine alone was used in almost 30% of patients, and it was used by most of a further 30% who used more than one preparation at a time. These preparations usually included ephedrine alone and ephedrine in combination with theophylline and a sedative. Fifty per cent. of the patients for whom information is available were given additional bronchodilators—usually in the form of parenteral adrenaline or aminophylline—in the terminal episode.

Sedatives were used, either alone or in preparations combined with bronchodilators, in 39% of the patients ; and antibiotics had been given to 46%. Neither phenothiazines, nor barbiturates, nor any other group of drugs was used by more than 15% of patients, so that it does not seem likely that any drug other than corticosteroids or bronchodilators could have been responsible for the increase in mortality.

Discussion

The results of our inquiry strongly suggest that the great majority of deaths attributed to asthma in young people are correctly ascribed. Necropsy findings were similar to those reported previously when death occurred during status asthmaticus, and there was seldom evidence of any additional pathology. Many of the patients had been regarded as only moderately affected, but the fact that two-thirds of them (114 out of 173) had received corticosteroid treatment at some time before their terminal illness indicates that as a group they were severely affected. Indeed we have to conclude that the severity of the illness was often underestimated. Deaths were frequently unexpected and occurred outside hospital, which suggests that

the patients may have been living closer to the limits of their ventilatory reserve than was realized. Certainly measurements of ventilatory capacity in asthmatics often reveal more severe degrees of impairment than are suggested from the clinical signs, and some asthmatic children simply learn not to waste their breath by complaining.

The inquiry has provided information about the circumstances in which the patients died but no clear indication of the cause for the increase in the number of deaths. Adrenal suppression due to corticosteroid treatment may have contributed to the death of some patients, but 34% (59 out of 173) had never received corticosteroids until their terminal illness ; marked adrenal atrophy was mentioned in only 6 of the 113 necropsy reports ; and there was no mention of hypotension or any other clinical feature of hypoadrenalism. The increase in mortality did not begin to appear until nearly 10 years after the introduction of corticosteroids for the treatment of asthma, and it seems unlikely that they can have been responsible for any substantial part of it.

Aerosol bronchodilators could affect the patient adversely by a number of mechanisms. Excessive amounts of a sympathomimetic, absorbed from the bronchi over a prolonged period, could cause ventricular irritability and fatal arrhythmia, or they could affect the viscosity of the bronchial mucus and lead to plugging of the bronchi. Alternatively, the inhaled bronchodilator may reduce airways obstruction without producing a corresponding improvement in arterial oxygenation (Daly and Howard, 1965 ; Field, 1967 ; Knudson and Constantine, 1967 ; Palmer and Diament, 1967). This may perhaps enable the patient to tolerate an unsatisfactory level of oxygen uptake and to come nearer to respiratory insufficiency before he, or his doctor, asks for hospital admission. The increase in the use of pressurized aerosol bronchodilators correlates closely with the increase in asthma mortality in Britain (Speizer et al., 1968), and we obtained evidence that they had been prescribed for 84% of the patients (146 out of 174). Accounts of the excess use of aerosols have been obtained in some cases, but decisive evidence to incriminate them is lacking.

Summary

Copies of death certificates were provided by the Registrar General for all deaths attributed to asthma in persons aged 5 to 34 years which were registered in England and Wales in the last quarter of 1966 and the first quarter of 1967. Information was obtained from the relevant general practitioners about 177 of the 184 subjects, and necropsy data were obtained for 113 of the 124 cases in which a post-mortem examination was known to have been made.

Ninety-eight per cent. of the subjects for whom evidence was obtained were known to have been suffering from asthma, and signs of severe asthma (overdistended lungs and small bronchi plugged with mucus) were found in 91% of necropsies (57% of all deaths). Evidence that death might have been due to any other pathological condition was rare.

Death was sudden and unexpected in 81% of the subjects (137 out of 171), and 59% of all deaths were referred to coroners. In 39% of cases (67 out of 171) the practitioner had not regarded the patient as suffering from severe asthma in his terminal episode.

Corticosteroids and sympathomimetic preparations were the only drugs to have been used by a large proportion of patients. Two-thirds of the patients had received corticosteroids before the terminal episode, but detailed information about their use provided no suggestion that excess use could have been responsible for any large proportion of the deaths. Eighty-four per cent. of the patients were known to have used pressurized aerosol bronchodilators, and several instances of their use in excess were described. Routine inquiries about their use in the

Investigation into the use of drugs preceding
death from asthma. *Speizer FE, Doll R, Heaf P et al*

hours immediately preceding death were not made, and further evidence is required before their effect can be assessed adequately.

We are grateful to the Registrar General for providing us with copies of the death entries relating to young persons who had died of asthma, to the many doctors and coroners who replied to our questions and made their records available to us, and to Mrs. Ranjana Ash for help in coding and analysing the data.

Dr. F. E. Speizer was supported by the National Center for Air Pollution, Bureau of Disease Prevention and Environmental Control, U.S. Public Health Service.

REFERENCES

Daly, J. J., and Howard, P. (1965). *Thorax*, **20**, 324.
Field, G. B. (1967). *Clin. Sci.*, **32**, 279.
Knudson, R. J., and Constantine, H. P. (1967). *J. appl. Physiol.*, **22**, 402.
Palmer, K. N. V., and Diament, M. L. (1967). *Lancet*, **2**, 383.
Speizer, F. E., Doll, R., and Heaf, P. (1968). *Brit. med. J.*, **1**, 335.

* From the Cardiac Clinic, Departments of Medicine and Surgery, Groote Schuur Hospital, and the Cardiovascular Pulmonary Research Group, University of Cape Town. Supported in the Department of Medicine by the Council for Scientific and Industrial Research.

1 Elema-Schönander, Stockholm, Sweden.
2 Devices Ltd., Welwyn Garden City, Herts, England.
3 United States Catheter Corporation, Glen Falls, U.S.A.

Investigation into the use of drugs preceding
death from asthma. *Speizer FE, Doll R, Heaf P et al*

Thorax 1988;**43**:674–678

Salmeterol, a new long acting inhaled β_2 adrenoceptor agonist: comparison with salbutamol in adult asthmatic patients

ANDERS ULLMAN, NILS SVEDMYR

From the Department of Clinical Pharmacology, Sahlgrenska University Hospital, Gothenburg, Sweden

ABSTRACT Salmeterol is a new inhaled β_2 adrenoceptor agonist, which has been shown in animal experiments to produce a more prolonged bronchodilator effect than currently available β_2 adrenoceptor agonists. It was studied in eight adult asthmatic patients. Each patient received on separate test days salbutamol 200 μg and salmeterol 50, 100, and 200 μg according to a randomised, double blind, crossover design. FEV_1, peak expiratory flow (PEF), heart rate, blood pressure, and tremor were recorded in the clinic for six hours after drug inhalation; PEF was recorded for a further six hours at home. All three doses of salmeterol produced peak increases in FEV_1 (mean 0·5–0·8 l) and PEF (71–100 l/min) similar to those produced by salbutamol 200 μg (0·5 l and 74 l/min). After salbutamol FEV_1 and PEF had returned to baseline within six hours, but after all three doses of salmeterol more than half of the maximum bronchodilator effect remained after 12 hours. The effects of salbutamol and the two lower doses of salmeterol (50 and 100 μg) on cardiovascular measurements and on tremor were similar, whereas after salmeterol 200 μg there was a small decrease in diastolic blood pressure and an increase in heart rate and tremor. Thus inhaled salmeterol has a long acting bronchodilator action in asthmatic patients. This effect may be of value in the treatment of asthma, particularly in patients with nocturnal symptoms.

Introduction

Inhaled β_2 adrenoceptor agonists have become established as first line treatment for the management of acute asthma because of their excellent bronchodilator effects, wide therapeutic range, and low level of side effects.[1–4] The major disadvantage of currently available inhaled β_2 adrenoceptor agonists is their short duration of action; none of the currently available inhaled β agonists has an effect lasting for more than six hours.[5 6] Consequently, oral bronchodilator drugs may need to be added to other treatment for patients with early morning dyspnoea or wheeze. The availability of a longer acting inhaled β_2 adrenoceptor agonist would therefore appear to be an important therapeutic advance.

Salmeterol hydroxynaphthoate is a β_2 adrenoceptor agonist that has been shown to produce long acting bronchodilatation in both in vitro and in vivo animal

Address for reprint requests: Dr Anders Ullman, Department of Clinical Pharmacology, Sahlgrenska University Hospital, S-413 45 Gothenburg, Sweden.

Accepted 20 May 1988

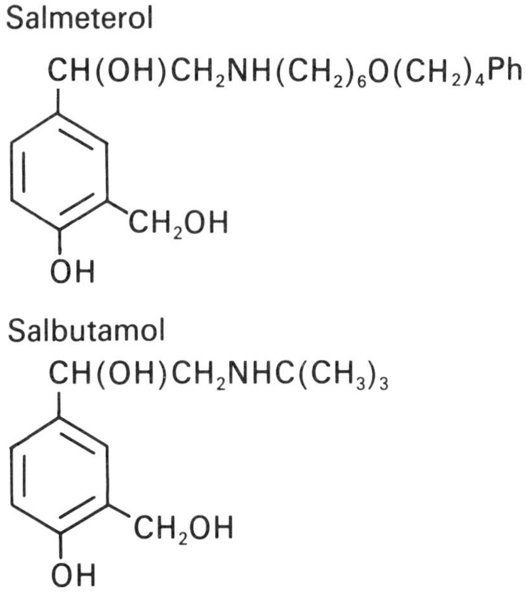
Salmeterol
CH(OH)CH2NH(CH2)6O(CH2)4Ph
CH2OH
OH
Salbutamol
CH(OH)CH2NHC(CH3)3
CH2OH
OH

Fig 1 *Chemical structures of salbutamol and salmeterol.*

Salmeterol, a new long acting inhaled β_2 adrenoceptor agonist: comparison with salbutamol in adult asthmatic patients. *Ullman A, Svedmyr N*

Salmeterol, a new β₂ adrenoceptor agonist: comparison with salbutamol $\qquad$ 675

Table 1 $\quad$ *Characteristics of the patients*

Patient No	Sex	Age (y)	Height (cm)	Smoking history	FEV₁			Treatment	
					l	% pred	Reversibility (%)	Oral	Inhaled
1	M	62	171	NS	1·51	49	23	th, tb	becl, sb
2	M	63	178	NS	1·41	42	33		becl, sb
3	M	67	183	NS	1·53	44	47	tb, pred, bh	becl, tb
4	M	67	184	ES	2·58	75	32	tb	sb
5	M	61	167	NS	2·26	77	25	sb	becl, sb
6	M	42	182	ES	3·12	76	25		becl, sb
7	M	64	172	NS	2·26	74	49	th	becl, sb
8	F	58	168	S	1·58	61	42	th, tb, pred	becl, sb

S, smoker; ES, ex-smoker; NS, non-smoker; th, theophylline; tb, terbutaline; becl, beclomethasone; sb, salbutamol; pred, prednisolone; bh, bromhexine.

studies.[7][8] The β_2 selectivity of salmeterol has been shown to be similar to that of salbutamol (Glaxo, on file). On the basis of results of oral dosing and animal studies, the plasma half life of salmeterol seems to be in the same range as that of salbutamol (Glaxo, on file). The chemical structures of salmeterol and salbutamol are shown in figure 1.

The aim of our study was to compare the peak bronchodilator response and duration of action of three doses of inhaled salmeterol with those of salbutamol in adults with asthma, and to measure the effects of these drugs on blood pressure, heart rate, and skeletal muscle tremor.

Methods

We studied eight adult patients, seven male and one female, with a documented history of non-atopic asthma (table 1). Each patient had previously shown an increase in FEV₁ of 20% or more 15 minutes after inhaling salbutamol 200 μg. On four separate study days the patients received either salmeterol 50, 100, or 200 μg or salbutamol 200 μg according to a randomised, double blind, placebo controlled, crossover design.

Patients arrived at the laboratory at 7.30 am, after a light breakfast. Inhaled β_2 adrenoceptor stimulants

were withheld for 12 hours before the study, oral β_2 adrenoceptor stimulants for 24 hours, and slow release theophylline for 36 hours. Patients taking inhaled corticosteroids continued this treatment at a constant dose, throughout the study. The patients rested in a semirecumbent posture for 50–70 minutes, after which the following measurements were made: (1) Heart rate, determined from continuous electrocardiographic recordings. (2) Blood pressure, determined by a sphygmomanometer. (3) Skeletal muscle tremor, recorded by means of a single plane accelerometer (Grass Instrument Co) connected to a Grass polygraph via a Grass integrator; the accelerometer was fixed to the right hand middle finger and recordings were made over 90 seconds.[9] In addition, subjective tremor was scored by the patients. (4) Forced expiratory volume (FEV₁) measured by a Collin's survey spirometer (two recordings made and the higher value used). (5) Peak expiratory flow rate (PEF) measured by a Wright peak flow meter (two recordings made and the higher value used).

After these basal measurements either salbutamol 200 μg or salmeterol 50, 100, or 200 μg was administered and the above measurements were made 20, 40, 60, and 90 minutes and 2, 3, 4, 5, and 6 hours after the drug had been given. The patients were then allowed to leave the laboratory. At home patients measured PEF

Table 2 $\quad$ *Mean (SEM) FEV₁ and peak flow (PEF) before and 0·3–12 hours after inhalation of single doses of salbutamol and salmeterol in the eight patients*

Time (h)	Salbutamol 200 μg		Salmeterol					
			50 μg		100 μg		200 μg	
	FEV₁	PEF	FEV₁	PEF	FEV₁	PEF	FEV₁	PEF
0	2·2 (0·2)	417 (27)	2·1 (0·2)	398 (27)	2·2 (0·3)	428 (39)	2·1 (0·3)	408 (35)
0·3	2·7 (0·2)	487 (32)	2·5 (0·2)	459 (27)	2·6 (0·2)	481 (36)	2·6 (0·2)	488 (32)
2	2·7 (0·3)	491 (30)	2·7 (0·2)	491 (28)	2·7 (0·3)	499 (28)	2·9 (0·2)	508 (33)
6	2·2 (0·3)	426 (30)	2·6 (0·3)	481 (32)	2·6 (0·3)	479 (35)	2·7 (0·2)	494 (33)
12	—	411 (28)	—	460 (33)*	—	469 (32)*	—	489 (27)**

*p ≤ 0·05 by comparison with salbutamol 200 μg; **p ≤ 0·01 by comparison with salbutamol 200 μg.

Salmeterol, a new long acting inhaled β₂ adrenoceptor agonist:
comparison with salbutamol in adult asthmatic patients. *Ullman A, Svedmyr N*

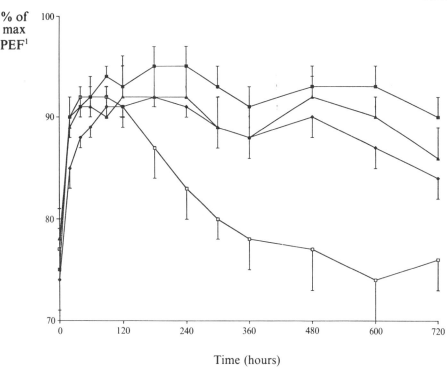

Fig 2   *Peak flow (PEF) after inhalation of salbutamol 200 μg (□) and salmeterol 50 μg (♦),*
100 μg (▲), and 200 μg (■). PEF is expressed as mean (SEM) percentage of the best individual
registration over the four test days.

8, 10, and 12 hours after inhalation of the study drug.

For statistical comparison Friedman's test was used, followed by Wilcoxon's signed rank test when appropriate. The PEF value is expressed as a percentage of the maximum PEF for each patient during the four test days. Tremor is expressed as the ratio between measured and the basal value. Heart rate and blood pressure are expressed in terms of the change from the basal value. Basal values for blood pressure were taken as the mean of recordings carried out 10 and 30 minutes before the study drug was given. The effects of the drugs on blood pressure, heart rate, and tremor were compared by calculating the mean of the individual peak values within six hours of each treatment.

Results

Peak flow Mean basal PEF values were similar on the four study days (table 2). PEF rose after all doses of salmeterol and after salbutamol. The increase in PEF was more prolonged after all the salmeterol doses than after salbutamol (fig 2, table 2). The area under the curve (AUC) for the first two hours after adminis-

tration of the drug was similar and did not differ significantly between the three salmeterol doses and salbutamol, whereas the AUC over 12 hours was significantly greater for all salmeterol doses than for salbutamol ($p \leq 0.01$). The differences in AUC over 12 hours between the three salmeterol doses were fairly small and significant only between the 50 and 200 μg doses ($p \leq 0.01$).

FEV_1 Mean basal values were similar on the four study days (table 2). Both salbutamol and salmeterol produced a rapid increase in FEV_1. The increase over baseline two hours after administration did not differ significantly between any of the different treatments. After salbutamol the FEV_1 had returned to baseline within six hours, whereas a significant increase over baseline remained six hours after inhalation of salmeterol ($p \leq 0.05$; table 2).

Heart rate Mean basal values of heart rate for the four test days were similar. After salbutamol and salmeterol 50 and 100 μg there were small, nonsignificant decreases in heart rate. Salmeterol 200 μg produced an increase in heart rate with the peak effect two hours after inhalation (fig 3). The mean maximum increase over baseline was significantly higher for

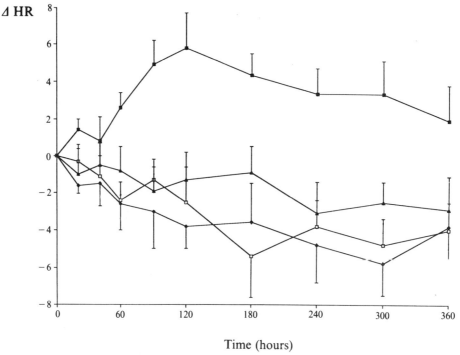

Fig 3 *Changes in mean (SEM) heart rate from baseline (ΔHR) over six hours after inhalation of salbutamol 200 μg (□) and salmeterol 50 μg (♦), 100 μg (▲), and 200 μg (■).*

salmeterol 200 μg (8·2 (SEM 1·8) beats/min) than for salbutamol (1·7 (0·7) beats/min; p ≤ 0·01).

Blood pressure Systolic blood pressure showed only minor and non-significant differences between the different treatments. The maximum fall in diastolic blood pressure was significant only for salmeterol 200 μg (11 (SEM 3) mm Hg; p ≤ 0·05).

Skeletal muscle tremor The ratio between the individual maximum tremor recordings and basal tremor was 1·4 (SEM 0·2) for salbutamol and 1·4 (1) for salmeterol 50 μg, which did not differ significantly. The higher doses of salmeterol produced a greater increase in tremor ratio. It was 1·7 (SEM 0·23) for salmeterol 100 μg (p ≤ 0·05) and 2·2 (0·18) for salmeterol 200 μg (p ≤ 0·01). Subjective tremor, however, was reported by only two patients, after salmeterol 200 μg.

Discussion

These data confirm that in asthmatic patients salmeterol is a potent long acting bronchodilator. All doses of salmeterol produced maximum bronchodilatation similar to that produced by 200 μg salbutamol. There were no significant differences in

the time of onset between the three doses of salmeterol and salbutamol. All three doses of salmeterol had a longer duration of action than salbutamol 200 μg and produced bronchodilatation throughout the 12 hour study period. There was a trend suggesting greater bronchodilatation by 200 μg salmeterol than by the 50 or 100 μg doses. Blood pressure, skeletal muscle tremor, and heart rate did not differ significantly between the 50 or 100 μg dose of salmeterol and 200 μg salbutamol. Salmeterol 200 μg, however, had a more pronounced effect on heart rate, skeletal muscle tremor, and diastolic blood pressure. Our results suggest that salmeterol in doses of 50–100 μg is approximately equipotent to 200 μg of salbutamol, in terms of peak bronchodilator effect. These doses did not differ in their effects on the cardiovascular system or skeletal muscle tremor, but all doses of salmeterol produced bronchodilatation that lasted almost three times as long as that of salbutamol.

The pharmacological mechanism or mechanisms of the long duration of salmeterol are not clear. The plasma half life of the drug approximates to that of salbutamol (Glaxo, on file) providing further evidence that the duration of action of inhaled β₂ agonists is not closely related to their plasma half life. This is not surprising as the bronchodilating effect of inhaled clenbuterol, a β_2 agonist with a plasma half life of about 20 hours, did not differ in duration of action from that of salbutamol, an agonist with a plasma half life of three hours (K Svedmyr, personal communication). Salmeterol was designed by modifying salbutamol to obtain a drug with much greater affinity for its receptors because of increased exoreceptor binding.[10] The consequence of this would be that salmeterol would be localised to and persist in the vicinity of β_2 adrenoceptors. This may be true, but other explanations are possible. For example, it has recently been shown that the airway epithelium constitutes a diffusion barrier through which bronchodilators pass at different speeds (E Widmark and B Waldeck, paper presented to World Conference on Clinical Pharmacology and Therapeutics, 1986). Possibly therefore the airway epithelium acts as a reservoir for bronchodilator drugs.

It has been shown recently that terbutaline, when administered regularly for 14 days, produces a rebound increase in bronchial reactivity to histamine. In addition, the protection against histamine induced bronchoconstriction was found to be lower on day 14 than on day 1.[11] A receptor agonist with such a long lasting effect as salmeterol might produce tachyphylaxis as well as possibly affecting bronchial reactivity. Studies are required therefore to investigate the possibility that tachyphylaxis as well as changes in bronchial responsiveness may result from long term administration of salmeterol.

In conclusion, our results indicate that inhaled salmeterol produces long lasting bronchodilatation in asthmatic patients with no differences in cardiovascular effects or skeletal muscle tremor between salmeterol and equipotent doses of salbutamol. The long duration of action of this drug may be of value in the treatment of asthma, particularly in those patients with nocturnal symptoms.

The study was supported by grants from the Swedish Heart-Lung Foundation and from Glaxo Ltd. We would like to thank Dr Roy Brittain and Dr James Palmer of Glaxo Group Research for their comments.

References

1 Clark TJH. Choice of drug treatment in asthma. *Pharmacol Ther* 1982;**17**:221–8.
2 McFadden ER Jr. Aerosolized bronchodilators and steroids in the treatment of airway obstructions in adults. *Am Rev Respir Dis* 1980;**122**:89–96.
3 Svedmyr N, Löfdahl CG. Physiology and pharmacodynamics of beta-adrenergic agonists. In: Jenne JW, Murphy S, eds. *Drug therapy for asthma*. New York: Dekker, 1987:177–212.
4 Tattersfield AE. Bronchodilator drugs. *Pharmacol Ther* 1982;**17**:299–313.
5 Svedmyr N. Anti-asthma xanthines and adenosine. In: Andersson KE, Persson CGA, eds. *Current clinical practice*. Series No 19. Amsterdam: Excerpta Medica, 1985:135–45.
6 Svedmyr N. Fenoterol: A beta-2-adrenergic agonist for use in asthma. *Pharmacol Ther* 1985;**5**:109–26.
7 Bradshaw J, Brittain RT, Coleman RA, *et al*. The design of salmeterol, a long acting selective β_2-adrenoceptor agonist [abstract]. *Br J Pharmacol* 1987;**92**:590P.
8 Ball DI, Coleman RA, Denyer LH, Nials AT, Sheldrick KE. In vitro characterisation of the β_2-adrenoceptor agonist salmeterol [abstract]. *Br J Pharmacol* 1987;**92**:591P.
9 Thiringer G, Svedmyr N. Evaluation of skeletal muscle tremor due to bronchodilator agents. *Scand J Respir Dis* 1975;**57**:17–24.
10 Brittain RT, Dean CM, Jack D. Sympathomimetic bronchodilator drugs. *Int Encycl Pharmacol Ther* 1981;**104**:613–52.
11 Vathenen AS, Knox AJ, Higgins BG, Britton JR, Tattersfield AE. Rebound increase in bronchial responsiveness after treatment with inhaled terbutaline. *Lancet* 1988;i:554–8.